Developmental Assessment: Theory, Practice and Application to Neurodisability

T0203196

Editor: Hilary M. Hart
Managing Director: Ann-Marie Halligan
Production Manager/Commissioning Editor: Udoka Ohuonu
Project Management: Lumina Datamatics

First published in this edition in 2016 by Mac Keith Press
6 Market Road, London, N7 9PW

British Library Cataloguing-in-Publication data
A catalogue record for this book is available from the British Library

ISBN: 978-1-909962-56-9

Typeset by David Peduzzi

Printed in India by Imprint Digital Ltd.
Mac Keith Press is supported by Scope.

Developmental Assessment: Theory, Practice and Application to Neurodisability

Patricia M Sonksen

Consultant Paediatrician (Emeritus)
Great Ormond Street Hospital for Children
and Honorary Senior Research Associate
at the Institute of Child Health (ICH), London, UK

Mac Keith Press

2016

To the development of children – everywhere

Contents

About the Author

Dr Patricia Sonksen is Consultant Paediatrician (Emeritus) at Great Ormond Street Hospital for Children and Honorary Senior Research Associate at the Institute of Child Health (ICH), London, UK During her 40-year career in paediatric neurology Dr Sonksen's main interest has been in severe visual impairment and for 23 years she directed the Vision Research and Clinical Service Team at the ICH. She has lectured and published widely in the field of neurodevelopment and neurodisability and was principle lecturer and demonstrator for the Developmental Examination Course at the ICH.

Foreword

It is some time since we have had a new look at neurodevelopmental assessment, after those heady years in the 1950s and 1960s where giants of the profession such as Mac Keith, Egan, Griffith and Sheridan recognised the need for clinicians to understand child development and developed standard assessment tools to achieve this. I am now delighted to be able to write a foreword to this book, which will add a refreshed approach for aspiring and established clinicians in the assessment of children's acquisition of skills and abilities. Its contents are particularly important to guide clinicians who are keen to learn how to assess children with sensory difficulties associated with, or independent of, neurodevelopmental problems.

Patricia Sonksen is a leader in the field of neurodevelopmental assessment and, in particular, assessment of children with a visual disability. She is passionate about her subject and is keen to share all the knowledge and practical 'tricks of the trade' she has acquired over the years. Her development of assessment tools, with Joan Reynell, for children affected by visual problems has had an exceptional influence, and with her team she has pioneered the development of newer tools that are currently used nationally and internationally.

Detailed descriptions and wise experience with practical up-to-date advice in this area are overdue and for all clinicians (paediatricians, neurodisability paediatricians, neurologists, therapists, psychologists). For those who want to learn skills in this area, this book has much to offer.

In Chapter 1 we are invited to reflect on what developmental assessments and their division into domains mean. She makes the point that in order to acquire many of the skills (e.g. walking), the infant's cognitive development is involved too. Hence she has gone on in her developmental schedule to assess this in the chapters on social and non-symbolic cognition.

Important chapters follow on the practicalities of how best to assess children, before detailed chapters on assessing vision, hearing, speech, communication and finally motor ability. The arrangement of the chapters reinforces one of the key messages of the book, which is the importance of the other modalities in developmental assessment as opposed to the more traditional focus on gross motor development. Each chapter finishes with a helpful 'Key Points' summary.

In Chapter 12 the author gives the reader pointers on how to formulate the information gathered from the individual domain assessments into a readable report.

Throughout the book, Dr Sonksen uses anecdotal stories drawn from her wide experience in assessing children and her wise observation of typical and atypical development patterns.

This book's historical perspective is important. Clinicians who not only identified the need for developmental assessment but taught us how to approach this in a standardised fashion are too often forgotten or taken for granted with the passing of time. Patricia Sonksen embodies what Newton (and possibly others) is claimed to have said 'If I have seen further, it is by standing on the shoulders of giants'. Patricia Sonksen has enlightened us and helped all those who are learning about and carrying out developmental assessments for children with developmental and visual disability. This book will help today's clinicians to see more clearly how to do this.

Dr Jane Williams
Consultant Paediatrician
Nottingham Children's Hospital
Nottingham, UK

Preface

A sound knowledge base, logical thinking and specialised practical skills are essential in all areas of clinical practice. Developmental practice as described in this book embraces all three. The expertise to unravel the developmental profile of children with multiple impairments is neither innate nor, like 'Rome', acquired in a day. Therefore, the initial focus of this book is on developmental process and progress in typical children from birth to 4½ years and on 'thinking developmentally', i.e. analysing the developmental content of spontaneous behaviours, play, test items and test responses, rather than in 'milestones'. The developmental rationale behind test design and practical suggestions to optimise the flow of assessment are also presented, followed by how this grounding and way of thinking can effectively be applied to the assessment of children with developmental disorders, single and multiple impairments, to the adaptation of test procedures without compromising the target measure and to the design of intervention strategies. The issues are systematically presented in this way for a number of important reasons.

The attainment of the necessary level of clinical skill to assess/manage these impairments and disorders requires active training and supervision by those well versed in the field. Identification of atypical development requires a gestalt (i.e. a detailed perspective) of what is typical; vaguely defined milestones within 'umbrella' avenues of development are no longer fit for purpose. Second, developmental assessment is the cornerstone of diagnosis of developmental disorders and contributes significantly to the diagnosis of neurological impairments (both congenital and acquired), neurodegenerative and neuromuscular diseases, paediatric syndromes and genetic disorders. With the incidence of multiple impairments and developmental disorders rising, the former as a consequence of medical advances leading to improved survival of preterm infants and of those with life-threatening illnesses/injuries, there is a growing requirement for professionals with comprehensive expertise in these areas..

Early diagnosis provides an opportunity to instigate developmental treatment at an age when the brain is more pliant and before secondary delays emerge, and to prevent or reduce the incidence of secondary disabilities.

Assessment findings inform specialist referrals, investigations and intervention strategies and, when carefully explained, help parents understand and manage their child's developmental and neurological difficulties.

Standardised developmental scales are suitable for typically developing children and for those with minor disorders/impairments; however, as a high proportion of children with a severe impairment have a variety of additional impairments, it is difficult to obtain a truly representative normative sample. This problem obviates scales for those with multiple severe impairments (e.g. cerebral palsy). The developmental status of these children can best be explored using the knowledge base and way of thinking developmentally, referred to in the domain chapters and illustrated fully in Chapter 13.

Today many disciplines contribute their expertise to the neurodevelopmental care and assessment of preschool children: community paediatricians, paediatric neurologists, neurodisability and neurodevelopmental consultants, general practitioners, developmental psychologists, health visitors, specialist nurses, physiotherapists, speech and occupational therapists, ophthalmologists, orthoptists, audiologists and audiometricians. The intention is to speak to all these disciplines at every level of training or experience; expand developmental thinking within and between disciplines; rekindle enthusiasm amongst paediatricians to be more proactive in developmental assessment and developmental intervention; and promote an understanding and respect for what each discipline contributes.

The chapters have been structured so that each contains something of potential value to all disciplines. For example, in the domain chapters the domain is introduced with a discussion of developmental process, the neurological substrate and an analysis of the observable characteristics of typical development. The scientific basis and qualitative aspects of history and test delivery at different ages are followed by endpoint criteria and age guidelines. Case vignettes are presented in which the domain findings are viewed in the context of the rest of the profile, and an action plan for the child is developed. Most chapters conclude with a resumé of the most common disorders affecting the domain.

The aim of this book is to impart a sound foundation and a way of thinking developmentally from which to grow professionally and to provide informed and skill-based stepping-stones into the assessment of neurodevelopmental disorder and neurodisability.

Parents derive great joy and delight in watching their baby develop; the joy is mutual and reciprocal. Those of us who share this delight in infant observation and actively seek to harness it to insight into neurodevelopmental processes will find the field of neurodevelopmental assessment intellectually challenging, stimulating, rewarding and fun.

Patricia M Sonksen

September 2015

Acknowledgements

Much of the inspiration in this book reflects the wisdom and enthusiasm for child development of my former teachers, especially Mary Sheridan, Joan Reynell and Dorothy Egan (most particularly and fondly because she was the most wonderful mother and gave me some useful genes). I was fortunate in having two strong mentors, Kenneth Holt and Brian Neville, who believed in me and gave generous support through turbulent times. I never would have ended up in a position to write this book without Glen Smerdon loyally and cheerfully re-retyping sections of my MD thesis.

A powerful succession of enthusiastic and industrious senior registrars, including Alexandria Macrae, Jane Ritchie, Helen Goodyear, Marilyn Black, Mike Pike, Deborah Hodes, Hilary Cass, Rasieka Jayatunga, Robert Surtees, Sarah Aylett, Mary-Claire Waugh, Ewoud Bos and of course Alison Salt and Jenefer Sargent (who both became colleagues and ultimately my successors), kept me on my toes and the Vision Team clinically and academically productive.

Working clinically and on research ventures with specialists from other disciplines is a fantastic learning experience, academically productive and mutually fulfilling. I deeply treasure the opportunities given to me to work with Mary Kitzinger, Helen McConachie and Naomi Dale (psychology); Blanche Stiff (specialist nursing); Molly Moodley (teaching); Nicola Jolleff and Katy Price (speech therapy); Alison Wisbeach; Chris Clarke and Sophie Levitt, (occupational therapy and physiotherapy); Janet Silver, Elizabeth Gould and Ruth Proffitt (optometry and orthoptics), to cite but a few.

In January 1972, Kenneth Holt asked me to organise a week's Developmental Examination Course for doctors. The course has been the trigger for me to revisit typical development and to further refine 'thinking developmentally' biannually for more than 40 years. For the last 2 decades, it couldn't have happened without Claire Lister (course co-ordinator) embracing the challenge of organising a course at ICH *with a difference* – practice and demonstration sessions requiring between 20 and 30 typical babies and preschool children, in a cooperative frame of mind, onsite and in local nurseries!

The book owes its existence to the arm-twisting talents of Hilary Hart and the editing gifts of Udoka Ohuonu, both of Mac Keith Press. Sole authorship is lonely at times and I have been extraordinarily lucky in having Kate Fisher (consultant community paediatrician) ever eager to discuss ideas and to read chapters however busy she may be; her comments are always pertinent and the enthusiasm in her voice and smile unbelievably encouraging and restorative to author morale. Lorna Welsh has given much time to follow her two grandsons around with a camera and to rescue me when modern technology challenges my expertise. I am indeed fortunate to have two talented illustrator in Lorna Welsh and Blanche Stiff, and a family and friends ever supportive of my endeavours.

I warmly thank you all for enhancing my professional growth and hence this book in so many ways. However, my biggest hug is for the children who, together with their parents, have so enriched my life.

Introduction

Medicine is both an art and a science; logical stepwise analysis of symptoms and signs is considered in the context of a gestalt of normality and common sense to arrive at a medical diagnosis. A multitude of physical attributes that change with age are added to the diagnostic equation of paediatric medicine. A myriad of neurodevelopmental parameters that also change with age further escalate the diagnostic challenge neurodevelopmental paediatricians and their multidisciplinary colleagues face. In some categories of developmental disorder (e.g. autistic spectrum disorders or developmental language disorders), physical signs may be absent or minimal and diagnosis is entirely dependent on the developmental profile. In others a combination of developmental and medical findings signpost a specific diagnosis.

The term 'assessment' covers a variety of types and levels of procedures (e.g. screening, preliminary, diagnostic). The design of each procedure reflects its purpose. The original purpose of screening tests was to detect individuals in the population with a specific disease, impairment or disorder (e.g. the Guthrie Test for phenylketonuria); administration had to be quick, simple and cost effective and productivity proven. Screening tests for specific developmental impairments did not live up to these criteria, so currently there is a move towards procedures that screen for groups of disorders. For example the Modified Checklist for Autism in Toddlers, Revised with Follow-Up, was originally designed to screen for autistic spectrum disorders but is showing an excellent potential to pick up a broader spectrum of developmental disorders (Robins et al. 2014). At the other end of the spectrum are fully standardised developmental/psychological scales designed as in-depth assessment tools with a strict protocol of administration that compares the test child's findings with those of a normative population sample. The number and depth in which domains are explored varies with the purpose of the scale. For example, the New Reynell Developmental Language Scales (2011) make an in-depth exploration of several aspects of language development that inform discrepancies within the language spectrum; however, an additional standardised scale is required before the test findings can be considered in the context of non-verbal cognition. In contrast, the Griffiths Mental Developmental Scales – Revised (1996) encompass a broader range of cognitive and motor information in less precisely defined domains and consequently have less diagnostic power. The assessment schedule presented in this book, though carefully structured, is more flexible in its exploration of nine domains (two sensory, four intellectual and three motor). Collectively, the findings represent a preliminary but comprehensive overview of a child's developmental status, confirming whether it is typical and, if not, signposting the likely nature and severity of impairments and content of a plan of action. The items within each domain are a selection that have widely accepted age guidelines or standardised reference ranges. Importantly, the discussion of the developmental issues underlying the test content applies equally well to other test schedules and standardised developmental scales.

Professionals can and do take for granted the behavioural cooperation and comprehension of spoken instructions when assessing the neurodevelopmental systems of older children or adults. These individuals cooperate with repetition of part of the physical, sensory, motor or cognitive/language examination and politely give the assessor time to fill in the test form between items and to refer to the instructions for the next item. The speed of performance of a physical or cognitive-motor task is a valid criterion for success or failure as these age groups will reject internal or external distracting thoughts or events. None of this holds true for very young or disabled children; consequently the demands on the examiner and upon his or her level of skill escalate exponentially.

There is no quick fix to acquiring the requisite levels of examiner skills. The theoretical aspects can be learnt from a book, but their smooth and successful application requires sustained practice and self-critical reflection after every encounter, at every level of practice. The following examples illustrate the value of this approach.

Example 1 The examiner quietly places some bricks on the table in front of a 24-month-old boy and tries to remove the car he is playing with. The boy throws a tantrum and sweeps the bricks and car off the table. Before writing 'child uncooperative' in the notes, the examiner needs to ask herself "why did he behave like that?" and "how could I have introduced the bricks more successfully?"

The boy, appropriately for his age, had maintained his attention on the source of his interest (the car) by rejecting other external stimuli, including the assessor's interference. Had the assessor had a deeper knowledge of the developmental sequence of 'attention control' and its implications for handling young children in an assessment situation, she would have used different tactics to switch task (see Chapter 2 p.30)

Example 2 A 3-year-old girl is presented with a set of miniature toys. She names the objects as they are handed to her and arranges the dolls on the chairs, the cups on the miniature table, pours tea stirring it with a spoon and holds it out to the examiner. Before the toys are put away the examiner should ask himself "have I tested what I set out to test? The answer should be 'No'. Symbolic understanding of miniature representations at a 2½- to 3-year level has been tested, but the test extracted only expressive language at a 1- to 2-year level. Verbal comprehension has not been tested at all. As comprehension and expressive aspects of language are the main aims of the miniature toy test, the examiner should have become an active participant in the child's play, giving some age-appropriate instructions such as 'put doggy under the table' and drawn out expressive speech above the level of single noun labelling. The examiner needs to affirm that the child understands three-component *spoken* commands, not just symbolism in miniature. Inexperienced examiners frequently equate the two.

Possession of a gestalt for typical development from birth through the early years is essential before accepting responsibility for carrying out the assessment of children with impairments or disabilities. Experience needs to cover the assessment of all domains at all age levels complemented by developmentally orientated observation of babies and young children encountered during the course of each day. Piecemeal training (increasingly common since the mid-1980s) leaves senior professionals at a disadvantage when asked for a second opinion on a child outside their comfort zone.

References

Robins DL, Casagrande K, Barton M, Chen C-M, Dumont-Mathieu T, Fein D (2014) Validation of the modified checklist for autism in toddlers, revised with follow-up (M-CHAT-R/F). *Pediatrics* 133: 37–45.

New Reynell Developmental Language Scales (2011) London, UK: GL Assessments.

Griffiths Mental Developmental Scales – Revised: Birth to 2 years (1996). Oxford, UK: Hogrefe Ltd.

Chapter 1

A developmental approach to the examination of preschool children: thinking developmentally

Infant behaviours and the tests used to assess development all embody their own developmental content. The following story borrowed from AA Milne (1926) reflects a behaviour that could equally well be a developmental test. 'It was Eeyore's birthday. Pooh decided to give him a pot of honey but regrettably felt a little peckish on the way to the party, and subsequently, after he had checked that it all tasted as good as the first mouthful, he arrived with an empty jar! Piglet's present was a balloon but he tripped on the way bursting the balloon. After initial disappointment Eeyore was seen gloomily but contentedly putting the remains of the balloon in and out of the empty jar.'

> Q In terms of human development which level, of which sequence and in which domain was Eeyore exhibiting and what developmental age would this represent?
> *Two-component level – structural relationships – non-symbolic cognition – 11 to 12 months.*

The manipulative and visual components are at much lower levels than the cognitive, so in a test situation non-spoken cognition is the primary target.

Development of the neurological substrate

The infant brain at term has a full complement of neurons, and its morphology mirrors that of the adult with respect to structure. Basic neuronal links between sensory, higher (cognition, language, memory, attention, behaviour etc.) and motor topographic areas of the brain are present but require elaboration and refinement for development to progress – the two go hand in hand. Neurones are small and immature but ready at all levels to be 'buzzing' in response to the host of novel sensations and experiences that follow birth. Initially, neurons of the sensory pathways and their corresponding cortical areas respond by growth in size and increase in dendritic spines and in synapse formation within and between their own, other sensory, higher and motor domains, leading chain-wise to the establishment of sophisticated, well-integrated and functional networks and coding templates. After the initial exuberant growth of links between areas of the brain, pruning to adult levels occurs. This process is described as neuronal connectivity or networking, and developmental progress, in all areas, is dependent on its functional integrity and capacity; the process is influenced by both pre- and postnatal genetic factors and experiences. Timetabling of networking in different domains is far from fully established, but evidence suggests that it is to some extent biologically programmed, in some areas spanning many years and in others particularly active during the early months.

Connectivity is not confined to cortical areas but is also forged with sub-cortical nuclei, the basal ganglia and the cerebellum. The importance of the cerebellum in the development and smooth execution of movement has long been recognised; its role in the subconscious execution of higher cognitive, emotional and attentional functions is becoming increasingly so (Koziol et al. 2014). At behavioural level babies are observed initially to actively attend to and visually monitor every new movement sequence; with practice the movement is given less and less attention and becomes increasingly automatic, rapid and stereotyped. At neurological level the cerebellum appears to learn to recognise the context in which a particular pattern of movement is required and to decode signals from the premotor cortex that trigger the total motor response earlier and earlier. A body of evidence from primate and patient research and fMRI studies is accumulating in support of these ideas. Thus, two-way disturbances of cortical–cerebellar connectivity may play a role in the genesis of attention-deficit hyperactivity, specific language, autistic spectrum and developmental coordination disorders.

Developmental domains traditionally used for assessment; how well do they serve us?

The purpose of dividing early development into domains that embody their own developmental sequences should be to clarify the thinking and facilitate the task of the assessor – testing, interpreting, diagnosing and formulating a plan of action. Developmental domains and our way of using them in the assessment of babies and preschool children are fashioned on thinking current in the middle of the twentieth century. Skills are grouped into 'umbrella' domains such as social adaptation and play, hearing and language/speech, vision and fine movements/eye–hand co-ordination and locomotion. The importance of the special senses in triggering the networking process was emphasised earlier. Although vision facilitates the development of hand movements, it also tutors and promotes most other aspects of development – social communication, cognition, language, locomotion etc. So why was vision tied to hand skills when it contributes as much if not more to so many other areas? Why in the past was locomotion selected out for status as the only motor domain, when manipulation and speech production – the two that best demonstrate advances in intellectual processing – were engulfed into 'umbrella' domains (eye–hand co-ordination and hearing and speech/language)? Why deprive the development of fine hand skills (manipulation) status as a motor domain when it too possessed clear-cut sequences in the development of reach, grasp, fine finger control and release? The question is equally applicable to the development of the motor aspects of speech. Thus the special senses, particularly hearing and vision, and fine motor systems (manipulation and speech apparatus) like the intellectual and behavioural domains follow their own developmental sequences, which deserve recognition, testing and recording space in their own right.

Neither the protocols nor recording sheets of most test schedules encourage the assessor to observe, record or analyse beyond the given pass/fail criterion. By emphasizing the peripheral points in the domain title, e.g. eye–hand co-ordination, a trainee assessor is

- left to guess which domain (eye or hand) is the primary focus/main objective of tests in the scale and may assume that both the special sense (vision) and the motor area (manipulation) mentioned are tested at age level when that is not the case. Presentation of a Smartie (M&M; 1.25cm discoid sweet) on a table top is a typical eye–hand task for a 9-month-old; the 'eye' component – fixation of a Smartie – is a 5- to 6-month-old visual behaviour (near detection vision): the 'hand' component – index finger approach and closure of the thumb to the side of the index finger – is a 9-month level of manipulation. So, at 9 months, the main objective is manipulation, not near detection vision.

- not encouraged to give any thought to the cognitive processes that underpin and fire the emergence of hand skills; during the first year the size of the object that arouses cognitive interest in looking, and subsequently in manual exploration gradually decreases, so the size of the object that arouses interest carries important cognitive information that needs to be noted.

Ⓠ If the primary test objective is 'eye' (near detection vision) what size of spherical sweet should the assessor have chosen for a 9-month-old and how would this affect the cognitive and manipulative components?
The appropriate size would be a 1.2mm spherical cake decoration known as a hundred and thousand in the United Kingdom. The level of the manipulative component would

be raised above the competence of most 9-month-olds, so the test is no longer suitable for looking at the emergence of the pincer grasp; however, visual fixation and visual interest in such a small object are visually and cognitively definitive at 9 months.

So changing the size of the object completely alters the areas of the test that are definitive.

Q If the baby were 6 months old what would the main objective/s be of presenting a Smartie/M&M?
At 6 months all three domains – 'eye', 'cognition' and 'hand' – can be definitively explored. A Smartie is an appropriate size for all three – near detection vision, visual interest and manipulation.

Q For which domain would the goal posts need moving?
The manipulative endpoint needs to be adjusted to a 5- to 6-month level, i.e. a raking attempt to pick up the Smartie. The other two would be the same – fixation and visual interest.

No clinician would diagnose the nature of a circulatory problem without considering the functional integrity of the heart. The brain (central processor) is the heart of development. The heights of intellectual development attained by humans is the main feature that sets *Homo sapiens* apart from the rest of the animal kingdom, so surely the cognitive implications of visuomotor tasks warrant active consideration in the mind of the observer of a human baby. The real excitement of seeing a 16-week-old swipe at a hanging toy on her baby gym is the confirmation that her cognitive interest in the toy has been aroused and that she has taken a conceptual leap into realisation that she has arms and hands at her command. This is emphasised because when participants attending a developmental course are asked which domains they are testing for items on eye–hand scales, they usually respond 'hand skills' and/or 'vision' or even 'colour vision'.

All skills involve the three main categories of developmental domain – sensory, intellectual/higher-level processing and motor – often more than one of each category. Thus test items have the potential to yield information about a baby's development in all three categories, and in so doing, expand the assessor's construct of a baby's development laterally across domains as well as linearly within the main/target domain. The ability to engage with and process the breadth of this information 'online' throughout an assessment is professionally rewarding, informative and enabling and could become a goal for every professional and a major feature of training.

Thus the domains highlighted in the scheme of developmental examination in this book are in the three categories mentioned earlier. Of the sensory domains, vision and hearing are selected as they impact more than smell, touch and taste on early 'intellectual' development. The intellectual domains highlighted are social cognition/communica-

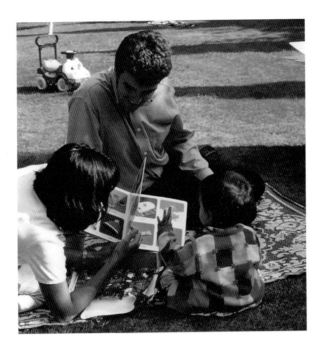

Figure 1.1 Parents are natural facilitators of development.

tion (SoC), non-symbolic cognition (NSC), non-spoken symbolic cognition (NSpSC), spoken symbolic cognition (SpSC)[1] and phonology (Ph).[2] The motor domains are manipulation, locomotion and articulation. The development of each domain and methods of assessment are described in individual chapters – Chapters 3 to 11 inclusive. Subsequently domain assessments are gathered into a comprehensive whole in Chapter 12; the gathering process is illustrated in six tables in that chapter.

Photographs that depict children in everyday rather than assessment situations are chosen in order to

- emphasize the importance of a warm embrace of family and a secure environment to development (Fig 1.1),

- capture facial expressions and interactions that reflect the intellect at work – 'wheels

---

1   NSC is sometimes referred to as non-verbal cognition or performance abilities; NSpSC refers to the understanding of non-verbal symbols such as pictures and miniature toys, and SpSC refers to the understanding of language – verbal comprehension and expressive language

2   For practical reasons phonology is presented in the chapter on speech sound production rather than language.

going round', interest, confusion, triumph, achievement, drive,

- stress the importance of observation (structured or informal) in the developmental assessment of young children,

- hone the reader's ability to interpret and logically think through the developmental content of the scene depicted,

- build the qualitative aspects of the reader's gestalt of normality.

The developmental content of tests

The next paragraphs illustrate how a three-category domain approach expands an assessor's insight into the developmental content of the tests he uses and of the responses he observes. The skill of 'reaching for a toy' and design of a test for it are thought through.

The target domain is motor (manipulation). The main sensory, cognitive (intellectual) and motor components are as follows:

Sensory

- Sufficient vision to see the target and their own hands

- Visual, kinaesthetic and proprioceptive (feedback) from eye musculature to direct gaze and fixate on the target

- Kinaesthetic and proprioceptive feedback mechanisms from core, arm and hand musculature – control of arm movements

Intellectual/higher processing

- Cognitive interest in the target aroused by its visual percept

- Processing coordinates of the position of the target relative to self (parietal processing)

- Concept of arms and hands as prehensile organs that the owner can direct

Motor

- Eye and head movements to focus and fixate target

- Locomotor: head and trunk control and shoulder stability

- Arm and hand movements enacting a reach.

Thus when a baby reaches for a toy the level of integration and functional maturity of the

Table 1.1 Stages in development of reach

Positioning of baby	Quality of arm movement	Average age range (wks)
Supine	'Grasp with the eyes' +/- tensing of arms (small excited movements)	12 to 15
Supine	Incoordinate swiping movement	16 to 19
Supine	More coordinate and more direct movement	20 to 23
Sitting supported on parent's lap	'Grasp with the eyes' +/- general tensing of arms	16 to 19
Sitting supported on parent's lap	Incoordinate swiping/dabbing movement	20 to 23
Sitting supported on parent's lap	More coordinate and more direct reach	24 and >

+/-   with or without

networks and coding templates within and between all of the above are being observed. When designing a test for reaching, the following also need to be taken into account:

Quality of the endpoint criteria

Reaching for a visual target emerges around 12 weeks as bilateral dabbing/swiping movements by supine babies. By 27 weeks the movements are smoother, more coordinated and direct with one hand leading[3] in babies sitting well supported on the parent's lap. This is too wide a time frame and too much variability in quality of movement for 'reaches for a toy' to be age defining under 6 months. How can it be rendered more so? Two variables – positioning of baby and quality of arm movement – could be broken down to define narrower age brackets (see Table 1.1).

Q Why does positioning make such a difference between 17 and 23 weeks?
A supine baby does not have to give attention or motor effort to maintaining posture and is free to concentrate on organising arm and hand movement; a baby-sitting well supported on the parent's lap still needs to give attention to postural control and maintenance of shoulder stability under 24 weeks.

---

3   The rate at which the bilateral movement subsides and the arms act independently varies; but a leading hand should be apparent by 6 months.

Grasp with the eyes, rather than arm movements, is described in two stages in Table 1.1 (see also Figs 1.2 and 1.3).

Q What is the developmental explanation for 'Grasp with the eyes' in each place?
For the supine 12- to 15-week-old 'grasp with the eyes' signifies cognitive interest but not yet realisation of the functional potential of his hands. The sitting 16- to 19-week-old actually has the latter concept because he makes a swiping movement in supine; however, he is unable to demonstrate his conceptual understanding in sitting as so much of his motor effort is given to postural control of his head/trunk and shoulder stability.

The influence of the contributory domains (cognition and gross motor) is evident in Table 1.1. Row 1 emphasises that cognitive realisation of the functional potential of the upper limbs underpins the development of reach. Rows 4 and 5 illustrate the constraint on reaching imposed by the gross motor domain on the quality of movement. Rows 2, 3 and 6 define three age levels between 16 and 27 weeks that could be used as endpoint criteria in the assessment of upper limb development.

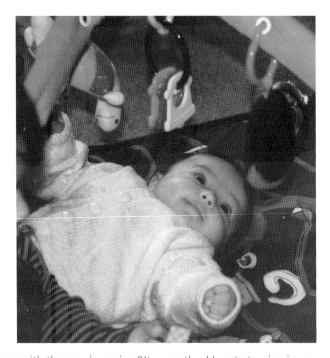

Figure 1.2 Grasp with the eyes in supine 2½ -month-old; note tension in arms and hands.

It is important to ensure that the developmental level of the supporting domains (vision and cognition) is well within the abilities of the age group and not at the ceiling or above; if set too high they will interfere with the interpretation of failure – this was illustrated in the discussion of the hundred and thousand and the Smartie/M&M (mentioned earlier). For the assessment of reach a test item and a mode of presentation that spans the time frame are needed. Assuming the test item is a ball, we need to consider:

- Size – the ball needs to be of a size that arouses cognitive interest in looking and in manual exploration, rather than the smallest that babies can see at the age defined by the test. To be sure that a very young baby is seeing, parents and professionals alike rely on the look of intense interest that accompanies direct gaze and fixation, i.e. upon a functioning visual-cognitive link. In fact the visual acuity of a newborn term baby is sufficient to see a ball of smaller than 1 cm, but such a small target is

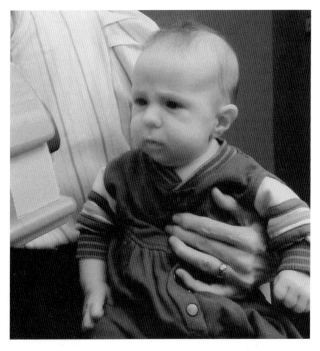

Figure 1.3 Grasp with the eyes of 4½-month-old in supported sitting; arms and hands are similar to those of baby in Figure 1.2. In supine this baby makes a visually directed swipe.

unlikely to arouse cognitive interest until 5 to 6 months. However a 6.25cm ball should arouse visual interest by 6 weeks, so for exploring the development of reach between 16 and 27 weeks a target of that size or larger would be appropriate.

- Mode of presentation – as reaching is dependent on arousing cognitive interest the visual allure of the target is important. A ball of uniform colour dangling limply does not have anything like the visual allure of either a multi-coloured one or one with holes in (to produce light effects) spinning 'on the spot'. Interest can be aroused in a ball on a tabletop by spinning the ball gently. For a sitting baby a squeaky toy of similar dimensions could be substituted as reach, not vision, is being tested.

- Distance from the baby – mobility of babies in this age bracket is limited so the ball is best presented 'within baby arms' reach', i.e. between 30 and 40cm.

- Position in the visual field – the visual field is full at birth but most babies alert and direct their gaze more promptly to a lure introduced within 45 degrees of centre rather than in the extremes of the peripheral field. Spatial processing of visual targets should certainly be adequate by 16 weeks.

- Control of eye movements advances rapidly over the first few weeks, reflecting rapid networking and functionality across the cortical cerebellar circuits that process the visual, spatial and motor aspects of eye movement. Eye movement control should therefore be more than adequate by 16 weeks.

Test procedure/instructions, primary observation and pass/fail criteria evolve directly from the earlier considerations. For each of the three age levels between 16 and 27 weeks test instructions will be the same except for positioning of the baby and mode of presentation of the ball. For a baby of 24 or more weeks:

Test instructions

The baby sits supported on the parent's lap up to a table. Attract his attention to a multi-coloured woolly ball or toy (12.5cm) positioned in his central visual field at a distance between 30 and 40cm.

Primary observation: Reaching movements and the level and quality of the arm movement.

Primary pass/fail criterion: Reaches for the ball with a moderately well-co-ordinated swipe/dab.

Primary record

Reached for ball *Yes No*

If *Yes*, then the developmental level of the arm movement

Incoordinate swipe or dab; Moderately well-coordinated swipe

Interpretation

If *Yes* and *Moderately well-coordinated* have been circled the baby has achieved the main objective of the test (motor domain – manipulation) at age level. This is the moment to think, 'Was everything appropriate in the supporting domains – vision and cognition?' Match what is observed to what would be expected; in this child – fixation and age-appropriate eye movements of normal quality; cognitive interest in looking (6-week level) and 'hands are for reaching' (12- to 17-week level): age-appropriate and normal quality sitting posture.

If *Yes* and *Incoordinate swipe or dab* or *No* is circled the main objective has not been achieved. Repeating the presentation this time with the foci of observation on the cognitive, visual (vision and eye movements) and postural components is likely to highlight potential areas of concern and indicate which, if any, areas should be examined particularly carefully. The following three scenarios are illustrative:

- Scenario 1: Suppose a sitting 22-week-old baby does not reach for the ball. When presented a second time she is noted to fixate the ball with interest; her eye movements and postural control appear age appropriate and without any overt pathological features such as squint, abnormal posturing and low tone. 'Does she understand the potential of her upper limbs for reaching?' should be flashing in the assessor's head.

  (Q) Is there cognitive delay or simply manipulative delay; how could the assessor tell?
  Repeat with dangling ball and baby supine. If she does not attempt to reach or swipe in this position she does not possess the underpinning concept so the manipulative delay is likely to be part and parcel of cognitive delay.

- Scenario 2: A supine 19-week-old baby makes no reaching movement. On second presentation the assessor notes brief visual awareness and interest in the ball and nystagmus; general tone in trunk and limbs appears normal and symmetrical.

  (Q) Which domains are showing delay?
  All three domains – visual, cognitive and manipulative.

  (Q) Which domain would need to be examined with particular care?
  Vision and the visual system.

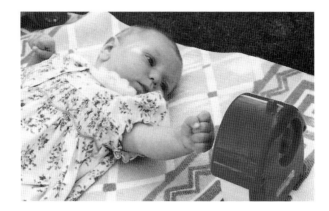

Figure 1.4 While it appears that the baby is reaching for a toy she almost certainly is not. A toy has been placed on the side of the 'fencing' arm of a supine baby already under the influence of the atonic neck reflex. The lifting of her left arm most likely reflects generalised excitement on seeing the toy.

Scenario 3: Figure 1.4 shows a supine 11-week-old.

An appreciation of the developmental content of tests also encourages active engagement of assessors in construction of a diagnostic perspective throughout their assessment in the same way as a clinician does when performing a physical examination. In turn the diagnostic pointers, together with the findings, evolve into an action plan and developmental guidance.

Assessors are advised initially to focus their attention on the target domain and gradually expand it to the supporting domains (secondary observations / bonuses). Readers wishing to hone their developmental thinking may find it useful to reflect upon the developmental content of tests and skills from different domains.

Thinking in profiles

At the end of a preliminary assessment the assessor has a basic construct of the child's functioning within sensory, intellectual and motor domains, in other words a basic profile of the child's development. Analysing the intellectual profile and subsequently considering it in the context of functioning in the sensory and motor domains facilitates diagnosis and formulation of an action plan and developmental guidance. The intellectual profile of seven children, all aged 3.0 years, is presented in histogram format in Figure 1.5.

A line drawn horizontally across the figure through the 3-year-old index on the vertical axis represents the chronological age of each child. First look for discrepancies of a third

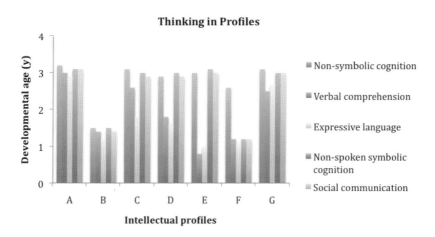

Figure 1.5 Thinking in profiles: 7 children aged 3.0 years

or more in age levels achieved between domains as these provide the strongest diagnostic pointers. There are no discrepancies of this magnitude for child A, B or G; in child A age levels are all clustered around his chronological age – intellectually he is functioning normally; however in child B they are all clustered at approximately half her chronological age – she is globally delayed most likely because of learning disability; child G will be discussed later. Children C, D, E and F present with discrepancies of more than a third between some domains. The best domain to use as a reference/yardstick is NSC. Both expressive language and verbal comprehension are less than two thirds that of NSC in child D and child E, though only expressive language is in child C; with NSpSC and SoC also at chronological age level the most likely problems are specific language delay in child D and specific expressive language delay in child C. Both aspects of language are very severely delayed in child E compared to all other domains; this could represent a severe developmental language delay/disorder. However, in this child an additional small discrepancy provides a subtle clue to a more likely diagnosis; expressive language is slightly (just 2 or 3 months) higher than verbal comprehension; this should start a red light flashing 'HEARING' in an assessor's head. Child F differs from the others in that SoC and NSpSC are also delayed in comparison to NSC, suggesting that the language delay is part of a more widespread disorder of communication – an autistic spectrum disorder (ASD). Note that in child F expressive language is slightly lower than verbal comprehension, like that more typical of children with specific language delays or those with global developmental delay (see children B and D). Returning to child G, his language development is a little delayed, but the language profile suggests that the cause may be a mild/moderate hearing loss, rather than a primary language disorder.

Q Which of the profiles could be the consequence of serious visual or hearing impairments?

Profile B could be the consequence of severe visual impairment though primary severe learning difficulties would be the most common reason. Profiles D and especially E could result from severe degrees of hearing impairment.

Q Which of the profiles could be the consequence of minor visual or hearing impairments?

Profile G is most likely to be the consequence of minor hearing impairment. The other profiles are unlikely to be the consequence of minor degrees of either hearing or visual impairment; however, their presence cannot be ruled out.

Q Apart from profile F which one is most likely to be that of a child with an ASD?

Profile B, as it is the only one with significant delay in both NSpSC and SoC.

There is no fixed relationship between NSC and the other domains in ASD.

Diagnosis, action planning and developmental advice

The diagnostic clues in the intellectual profile are then considered in the context of the primary history (see Chapter 2) and the test findings in the two sensory and three motor domains to arrive at a provisional diagnosis. Further exploration of the primary and secondary medical and developmental histories and some medical examination may be indicated to inform an action plan and/or developmental guidance. For example the intellectual profile of child G suggests a slight delay in language development possibly because of hearing impairment. His parents had not expressed any concerns about his development.

Q What would the assessor want to do before finalising his action plan or giving developmental advice?

Check hearing carefully and examine ears for signs of otitis media with effusion (OME), wax etc., before deciding whether and to whom to refer. Explore the history of URTIs, discharging ear, family history for hearing loss or grommets in childhood and social/cultural and language background. Suppose G has a streaming cold, the assessor could decide to review G in 2 weeks to recheck his hearing and drums before referring him on to ENT/audiology. If positive for chronic OME, the assessor might advise the parents to speak in a louder voice while referral to audiology is enacted. This would hardly be appropriate advice if G does not have any hearing loss. If G's hearing is normal the assessor would be more inclined to give the parent advice on promoting his language development, though if social circumstances are also deprived or English is not the first language of the family, perhaps advising attendance at a nursery, with some one-to-one time with an adult dedicated to language built into his daily program. The ramifications are considerable.

Adaptation of test tasks when disability is suspected or present
Insight into the developmental content of test tasks again gives assessors the confidence to adapt them to a child's disability without degrading the main/target objective of the test. To achieve this requires more advanced developmental thinking and is discussed more fully in Chapter 13. As tasters:

• A 3-year-old severely deaf child requires a test of visual acuity. Obviously, she won't understand spoken instructions 'to match the assessor's letter to one on her key card'. Pantomiming the matching task or assessor and mother demonstrating it can convey the instruction without altering the measure of acuity.

• A 3-year-old child with visual impairment requires free field audiometry. She is not able to see well enough to stack rings on a stick or put bricks in a box. Cognitively she has simple cause and effect.

Q What aspect of the test needs modification?
The response task.

Q Will modification interfere with the test of hearing acuity?
No.

Q Suggest a suitable modification
Give her a soft squeaker; initially the assessor helps her squeak it each time he makes a loud pure tone. Once she starts responding reliably he commences the actual test.

• A 2½-year-old with cerebral palsy and no useful hand movement requires a test of verbal comprehension. At this age he is expected to assimilate a two-component command like 'put dolly on the chair'.

Q How might the assessor modify the test procedure without altering the level of verbal comprehension tested?
Space the items widely and encourage him to eye-point first to single items, e.g. 'Look at/where is the spoon'. Once he is responding reliably raise the command to the age-appropriate level 'Show me the doll and the chair' and observe whether he eye-points to each in turn. The assessor has modified the response task but not the level of the verbal command; the latter still requires the child to assimilate a two-component command.

The principles for adapting tests for children with disability include the following:

- Consideration of the developmental content of the test task in each of the three categories of domain – sensory, intellectual and motor.

- Highlighting which domain is the main objective (the target of the test) and which two are subsidiary. The main one must not be altered; the two subsidiary ones can be adapted to the difficulties/impairments of the individual child.

Allocation of skills to the most appropriate domain
Thinking through the developmental content of skills and test tasks also ensures that in schedules they are allocated to the most appropriate domain. For example, there are a host of cognitive skills hidden in the traditional domains of eye–hand co-ordination, hearing and language and gross motor development. To delineate these and place them into the domain headed non-symbolic cognition (Chapter 6) hones the developmental thinking of professionals and gives more credence to concerns about mental delay, or its absence, during the first 18 months. Sound localisation is a good example.

Sound localisation (locating the direction, relative to self, of a sound source) is traditionally placed in the hearing and language/speech domain; however, its contribution to language development is extremely tenuous. In the author's view the sound localisation sequence represents the development of permanence for sound-making objects/people (sound sources) and thus belongs in the NSC domain. Mary Sheridan first described the stages amongst her sequences of hearing behaviours (Sheridan 1968) but did not flag up cognition. The sense that tutors the cognitive aspects of sound localisation is vision, not hearing (Sonksen 1979, 1983).

Key Points

Thinking developmentally in these ways allows the professional:

- To hone the breadth and depth of her developmental thinking.

- To focus her powers of observation more effectively.

- To build and diagnostically assimilate the picture of a baby's development throughout assessment into domains that are more clearly defined.

- To formulate a clearer diagnostic perspective on which to base both a more robust action plan and individualised developmental advice.

- To design tests and test sequences.

- To adapt tests to a child's disability without degrading the main objective of the test.

- To allocate test tasks in the most appropriate domain(s) and thus strengthen the whole testing schedule.

- To grow professionally from novice tester to one with the knowledge base, expertise and flexibility to evaluate the neurodevelopmental status and problems of children with multiple disability.

References

Koziol LF, Budding D, Andreasen N et al. (2014) Consensus paper: The cerebellum's role in movement and cognition. *Cerebellum* 13: 151–177.

Milne AA (1926) In which Eeyore has a birthday and gets two presents. In: Winnie-the-Pooh, Ch 6. London: Methuen and Co Ltd.

Sheridan MD (1968) *Manual of Instruction for STYCAR Tests of Hearing.* Windsor, UK: NFER Publishing Company.

Sonksen PM (1979) Sound and the visually handicapped baby. *Child: Care, Health Dev* 5: 413–420.

Sonksen PM (1983) Vision and early development. In: Wybar R, Taylor D, editors. *Paediatric Ophthalmology: Current Aspects.* New York: Marcel Dekker.

Chapter 2
Practicalities

Developmental assessment is a dialogue between a child and a professional under the direction of the latter. The influence of external factors, such as emotional stress or poor health, on a child's performance is well recognized, as is the responsibility of the assessor to see that the ambience and physical conditions are optimal for the baby/child to reveal his skills and parents to feel relaxed. In contrast, the skill required of an assessor to drop seamlessly into finely tuned levels of communicative interaction, attention control and behaviour management with every age group and developmental stage is underestimated, and benefits from training; for example, at some ages the development of attention control and of independence combine to challenge the assessor to remain in command. Guidelines for ensuring that ambience and physical setup are optimal in different settings are summarized in Table 2.1. Clearly in home and hospital settings it is the assessor's responsibility to minimize the distractions and optimise the setup.

Tension in parents is readily transmitted to their child, so some strategies for establishing rapport and communicating effectively with parents and child are given in Table 2.2.

Another aspect of engagement with babies and preschool children requires insight into the developmental sequence of attention control, its interaction with other behavioural trends and their implications for handling.

Table 2.1   Guidelines for ambience and physical setup in different settings

Setting	Ambience +s	Ambience -s	Furniture +s	Furniture -s
Clinic				
Waiting area	Welcoming décor and receptionist	Bare and bleak décor	Seating and tables – adult & child sized	Office chairs arranged in rows
		Receptionist lost behind computer screen	Toys/books of suitable age range on view	Broken toys; out-of-date books
Clinic room	Carpeted[a], warm colours	Medical equipment festooning the walls and surfaces	AA furniture already set up <5mo: baby changing mat on AHWT 5–18mo: AHWT 90 x 45cm[b] + 2 adult chairs opposite each other[c] 19–54mo: RNT + 3 Nursery chairs[d]	Office desk covered in piles of notes Office desks unsuitable[e] Adult chairs unsuitable[f]
Home				
	Familiar	Too busy and distracting, e.g. siblings, pets, TV	Coffee and kitchen tables[g] Nursery chair if available Floor: stable	Puff: unstable base[h] Chair of unsuitable height Floor: diverts attention to postural control; leaves toddler too mobile
Ward				
	None	Inherently stressful, busy and distracting	Bed table if available	Bed surface – unstable base Floor: unhygienic + above

[a] infection control permitting, carpet creates homely atmosphere and reduces clutter and shadows; facilitates gross motor assessment. [b] NB 45cm is comfortable distance for introduction of toys and to communicate with baby. 90cm breadth is suitable for non-symbolic cognition tests in this age group – e.g. permanence of objects (see Chapter 6). [c] Wooden tops make less clatter than synthetic tops. [d] A chair with arms helps to 'contain' preschool children. Armless nursery chairs for the parent and assessor bring them down to child's level. N.B. Some assessors (including the author) prefer to kneel. [e] Too big – examiner too far away from child for optimal delivery of tests; no leg room for one adult. [f] Adult chair places assessor's head looming over child, which can be intimidating. [g] Provide a stable base, but height, width or shape may not be ideal and introduce distractions. [h] Frustrates child as towers etc. fall over.

AA, age appropriate, AHWT, adult height wooden table, RNT, rectangular nursery table.

Table 2.2   Guidelines for establishing rapport and communicating with parents and child

Action	Do	Don't
Greeting parent(s) and child	Fetch them yourself Greet mother → 'Hello J'[a] → give attention to parents Once J relaxes, say, 'I've some toys in my room – bring Mummy' Proffer finger while walking[b]	Send someone to fetch them[c] Direct conversation to J[d] Take hold of J's hand
Entering the clinic room	Point 'Look, I've a little table and chair; this one for you and this one for Mummy.' Let him lean on mother or sit on her lap until he relaxes	Expect him to lead the way in without a focus of interest Pick him up or tug his hand Insist he sits on his own chair immediately
Communication with parents	Keep mother relaxed 'How does J go upstairs?'[e] Know your test procedures	Reinforce that J is being 'tested' 'Is he able to/can he walk upstairs?'[f] Write notes or read manual
Communication with child	Remember – young children like to please Praise should convey enjoyment of what he has done rather than that he has passed a test Meet failure with a cheerful 'now let's do this.'[g] Give him your attention throughout[h]	Write 'child uncooperative' without asking yourself 'What did I do wrong?' Imply that he is taking a test, e.g. 'That's right' 'No, but can you do this?' Write notes or consult manuals[i]
Language of engagement	Natural conversational flow[j] Use well-intonated age-appropriate language e.g. 'ooooh what's this?'	Stilted or repetitive Over age level language may confuse assessor's interpretation. Superfluous language confuses and loses the child[k]

[a] Smiling, brief acknowledgement of child. [b] You will be surprised how often it is taken – the child is making the choice. [c] 'Come into my parlour said the spider to the fly'. [d] He needs time to see mother relaxed in your company. [e] Invites mother to generate a description outside the context of age appropriateness. [f] Implies he 'might not' and rubs in the assessment aspect of the situation. [g] Intonation and facial expression more important than actual words. [h] He needs to see interest and enjoyment glowing in the assessor's eyes, facial expression and voice. [i] Conveys a negative message and hard-won rapport will be lost. [j] 'Show me the car? ... and the bike? Where's the cup? Great - now the bus'. [k] 'Now I know you are a clever girl, aren't you, ... umm ... I have some little toys and I want you to tell me what they are when I ask you to name them; do you think you can do that? Tell me what this one is called.'

Attention control, other developmental considerations and handling preschool children

Attention control is a child's ability to control the focus of his attention and was first delineated by Reynell (Cooper et al. 1978). It is a normal developmental sequence and not part of the spectrum of attention-deficit-hyperactivity disorder. The paragraphs below describe children's ability to control the focus of their own attention, other pertinent developmental considerations (OPDC) and implications for handling in an assessment situation at different ages. This information is summarised in Table 2.3. Transition from one stage to the next is gradual.

Under 12 months of age, babies have little control over the focus of their attention.

Birth to 2 months

Attention control: Attention is mainly captured by internal stimuli such as feelings of hunger or contentment. Only near and strong external stimuli, for example a loud noise or an adult face appearing within a baby's near field of vision, capture their attention.

OPDCs: Responses to such stimuli are predominately reflex.

Implications: In terms of testing, external stimuli need to be strong and near. Other absorbing sensations, for example dummies, should be removed.

3 to 5 months

Attention control: Attention is gradually taken by less-strong external stimuli at increasing distance, though internal sensations still dominate.

OPDCs: Cortically mediated responses are emerging; however, alerting, processing and motor response times take several seconds. The sphere of visual attention expands faster than that of auditory attention.

Implications: In terms of testing, sufficient time should be allowed for central processing of the sensory input and the motor response. Internally absorbing stimuli (e.g. dummies) should be removed. The advantage of the small sphere of attention is that activities on the other side of the room do not interfere with the assessment; however, they are not advocated.

6 to 12 months

Attention control: Babies are attracted ('attracted' is preferred to 'distracted' as the latter has a hint of disorder) to any new dominant stimulus in their environment.

OPDCs: At this age babies are unable to prevent the switch of their attention. Visual stimuli remain dominant over auditory and the sphere of visual attention also remains larger. Alerting, processing and motor response times are increasingly brisk. Babies are aware but not wary of strangers, sociable and interested in everything.

Implications: Everything is set fair for the assessor; rapport is online, responses are brisk and definitive. Interest in the same task is easily regained so tests can be repeated if there has been an assessor error. Similarly, tasks can be switched by simply introducing the next item while gently removing the previous one.

Q How do older siblings use this stage of attention control to their advantage?
All they need to do to get the baby's toy is to proffer something else and grab the toy.

Q It is possible to succeed with procedures that older children will reject, for example putting a patch on one eye when testing monocular vision. Why?
Babies may whinge as the patch is put on, but if they are immediately offered a squeaker, it will take their attention and the patch is forgotten.

The next 16 months (13 to 28mo) increasingly become a serious challenge for assessors as toddlers acquire control over the focus of their attention at a period when they are also establishing their independence.

13 to 16 months

Attention control: Babies begin to sustain attention once given by actively ignoring new stimuli.

OPDCs: Babies are still sociable but now wary of strangers and increasingly become distressed when an object is removed.

Implications: The assessor needs to allow more time to establish rapport and should not attempt to remove test items until the child is visually engaged with a new one; alternatively, he should wait for the child's interest in the former to be fading before introducing a new item.

Q The distraction test of hearing becomes more difficult. Why?
Once the child's focus of attention is the distracter's toy, he ignores other stimuli.

Q What happens when an older brother tries to snatch the baby's toy?
The baby's attention will no longer switch to the substitute toy but will remain on the original. He will hang on to his toy and start to wail. His mother or father will appear and the older sibling will be in trouble!

Table 2.3 Attention control and handling

Age	Stage	Attention control	Other developmental considerations	Implications for handling / testing
0–2mo	1a	Unable: taken by internal feelings and 'strong' near stimuli	Response: mainly reflex	Stimuli: strong and near
3–5mo	1b	Unable: taken by internal feelings and less strong near stimuli.	Response: active emerging Alerting time: long Processing time: long Sphere of attention: small	Remove internally absorbing objects (e.g. dummy) Stimulus near Allow time to alert, to process and to execute motor responses Advantages – activities further away do not interfere
6–12mo	1c	Unable: taken by any new dominant stimulus (unable to prevent switch)	Alerting time: increasingly short Processing time: increasingly short Motor response: increasingly brisk; higher level for familiar Personality: aware but not wary, eager, sociable; interested in everything new Sphere of attention: small for hearing, wide for vision	Perfect for distraction and observation techniques Remember sphere of attention Beware of 'strange' stimuli Advantages – easy rapport, interest and switch of task Clear responses Repetition and 'unpleasant' features possible
13–16mo	2a	Able: sustains attention once given by ignoring new stimuli	Personality: becoming wary; interested in adult choice; distressed by removal; imitative	Allow time to establish initial rapport Good for imitation Less good for distraction test – apply stimulus during 'fade'; 'two of a kind'; correct stimulus first time; avoid repeated stimuli Change of task: use 'fade'; attract to new material before removing old Advantages: imitative

Table 2.3 continued

17–29mo	2b	Able: focuses attention absolutely and inflexibly	Actively rejects adult interference or direction once attention focused; danger of escalating tantrum Increasingly negative	Distraction unsuitable Instruction: implicit in material or given with material as a friendly command Next instruction follows immediately – don't stop to praise! Change of task: avoid confrontation; use 'fade'; attract to new; 'ignoring' technique; Offer choices; bribes useless
30–41mo	3	Single channelled but more flexible; can be switched by adult (from task to adult and back to task); child needs to give attention fully at each stage	Realises reward and benefit of allowing adult to participate and direct activities Less negative Pride in achievement	Set child's attention on examiner before giving instruction Actively encourage and praise
42–48mo	4	Single channelled, but refocusing more under child's control	Enjoys age-appropriate developmental task and achievement	'Name' sufficient to transfer child's attention to adult Change of task: verbal suggestion sufficient Actively encourage and praise
49–60mo	5	Two channelled in one-to-one or small group	Keen to participate	Can be given instruction while engaged with materials Praise can be less effusive
61–72mo	6	Two channelled in large group	Enjoys being one of a group; conforming	Instruction: as for 4–5y Change of task: no resistance

Attention control: Toddlers focus their attention on a task absolutely and inflexibly by cutting out all other stimuli. Attempts to alter their focus of interest by an adult are rejected. If the adult persists, an escalating tantrum may ensue.

OPDCs: In parallel, toddlers begin to assert their independence by giving a negative response whenever an opportunity presents.

Implications: Task instructions should be either implicit in the test material or given as conversationally voiced directives, for example 'Put dolly on the chair'.

Any attempt to ask whether 'he would like to' or 'does he think he can' or 'will he' is likely to be met with a firm 'NO'.

Q The test task is to build a tower of bricks. What will happen if the examiner places the box or tips out the bricks onto the table saying 'Look I'm going to build a tower,' as she starts to demonstrate the task?
The child will immediately grab some bricks and start doing his own thing with them.

The examiner is more likely to succeed if she keeps the box of bricks well out of his reach while she places one brick on the table saying 'We are going to build a tower'; then puts a second beside it saying, 'Put it on the top'. As he puts the brick on top she immediately offers the next saying 'and this one,' rather than pausing to admire his handiwork.

Q Why should one avoid praising the child in between bricks
At this stage the child is likely to take any relaxation of the assessor's control of his attention, to switch to his own choice of task. It will be an uphill battle to reset his attention on her choice the task.

Avoid confrontation when changing task – wait until his interest is showing signs of fading before attracting him to new material; alternatively, try an ignoring technique – this involves introducing his mother to the new task; if the adults refrain from trying to engage the child's interest, most will soon want to be part of the new activity. A third technique is to offer a choice between two new tasks, for example 'Which game shall we play – the pencils or the puzzle (insert puzzle)?' Giving a choice removes the opportunity to say 'no.'

Q Why don't bribes like 'I'll give you a raisin if you build me a tower' work?
What has the assessor done? Focused the child's attention on the raisin; nothing else will do until he gets it!

Practice Point A raisin becomes an incentive rather than a bribe when it becomes part of the test, for example substituting a raisin for a brick in the task of finding an item inside a pot with a lid.

Practice Point From now on management of the test situation begins to ease for the examiner.

30 to 41 months

Attention control: Although still single channelled, children are becoming less intransigent and their attention can be switched by the examiner, that is from the task to the examiner and back to the task. They need to give full attention at each stage of the transfer.

OPDCs: Children are beginning to realise the benefit, in terms of fun and learning, of allowing an adult to participate and direct their play; they are also becoming less negative and want to share the pride they feel in achievement.

Implications: Suppose the examiner wishes to test Suzy's comprehension of a two-component command with miniature toys. Suzy is pouring tea; as she puts the little cup and pot down, the examiner says, 'Suzy', in a voice that promises something interesting, leans forward and gently rests his hands above Suzy's and/or gently tips her chin up. As she looks up at him, the assessor says, 'Put the baby in the bath'. Thus, the instruction is issued when Suzy's attention is fully on the examiner. If issued when attention is not fully on the assessor he cannot know whether failure is due to lack of understanding, hearing or attention. This stage is hard work, but rewarding, for the examiner. Flow from one instruction to the next is still important, but there should be time for a 'that's lovely'.

42 to 48 months

Attention control: Remains single channelled but refocusing is increasingly under the child's control.

OPDCs: Enjoys age-appropriate developmental tasks and examiner's participation. Shows clear pride in achievement, and endeavour increases in response to praise.

Implications: The child's name said with 'ooh look' intonation is usually sufficient for the child to transfer his attention to the adult.

Change of task: verbal suggestion in an interested voice is usually sufficient.

Active praise now helps sustain the rapport.

49 to 60 months

Attention control: Children now assimilate verbal directions from the examiner without needing to pause or look up or be called by name.

OPDCs: Children are keen to participate and to co-operate.

Implications: The examiner now gives directions as the child finishes the last instruction, without even calling his name.

Practice Point Attention control tends to get 'stuck' at the 17- to 29-month stage in children with sensory (hearing or vision) problems and in those with developmental language delay. Assessors should be alert to these diagnostic possibilities when an older child presents with this level of attention control and to adapt their presentation of test tasks accordingly.

Organisation of the assessment

Timing the start of the assessment

Medical disciplines take a full history before starting the physical examination. This philosophy is sound, but in developmental examination there is a limited window of opportunity: start before the child is relaxed or after they have become bored and fretful and all is lost. Assessors need to use the window of opportunity when the child is most accessible. If the child is fully awake, go for a skeleton history and switch to the examination as soon as the child has relaxed and wants some attention. The remainder of historical information can be postponed to later. A sleeping child poses a different problem. Some toddlers and preschool children become very distressed if woken from a deep sleep. A highly distressed baby or child requires a large amount of parental attention, which interferes with satisfactory history taking and examination – effectively a waste of professional time. Reception staff can be trained in how to pre-empt this problem.

Order and framework

It seems sensible to start with domains of development that do not require the child to speak, and to test domains in as near the same order as possible at every age; in this way neither items nor domains will be left out. Manipulation, non-symbolic cognition (performance), language (expressive language, verbal comprehension, symbolic play), speech production, social communication, hearing, vision (over 2½ years)[1] and gross motor are suggested. Observation of social communication should be ongoing throughout, though making a habit, during the language section, of checking that one has witnessed age-appropriate behaviours, such as 'follows a pointing finger' is a good practice. Gross motor is left to last as it tends to overexcite preschool children. With small children some flexibility within this structured framework is advisable so that advantage can be taken of a child's spontaneous interest or conversation. For example if on seeing a toy bus a child says 'like go Gannie', it would be sensible to use the visit to Grannie to generate spontaneous expressive language. Order of testing is further discussed in Chapter 12.

Choice of starting level and item of equipment

Unless a parent has voiced serious developmental concerns, or the assessor's preliminary observations of the child's behaviour and play raise doubts, starting at age level will be an economical use of time and will immediately catch the interest of the child. Starting well below age level wastes professional and family time and runs the risk of lowering the child's interest in the situation. Choosing material that embraces a wide age range (e.g. bricks) has the advantage that if the child has difficulty with the age-level task, the assessor can switch to an earlier level without making the failure too obvious to the parent or child.

Relative position of child and assessor

There are three different positions in common usage: next to the child, at right angles to the child and directly in front of the child. The first two limit the examiner's ability to control the child's attention and his view of the child's hand, eye and lip movements. The latter facilitates managing the child's level of attention control because she has only to look up to attend to the examiner (rather than look up and turn towards the examiner). The examiner is in a perfect position to observe visual fixation, eye movements, arm and fine finger movements, and lip and tongue movements throughout the examination.

History taking

Although earlier in the chapter a rationale was presented for moving from history taking onto the developmental examination as soon as the child indicates she is ready to interact, this was not intended to imply that the developmental history is not important. A developmental history explores not only a child's developmental journey to date but

---

1   See vision chapter (Chapter 3) for rationale.

also the pertinent aspects of the medical, social, emotional and cultural climate in which it has taken place. It needs to be tuned to the context of the assessment and fine-tuned during the assessment. The primary and secondary history each have their own style and aim. The purpose of primary history is to alert the assessor to the presence or not of parental concerns about development and of potentially significant medical risk factors. The purpose of secondary history is to clarify functional levels within specific avenues of development and causal relationships of problems detected. Drawing a distinction between primary and secondary history taking becomes less and less appropriate the greater the severity of disorder or disability; however, in the context of this book it has value.

Primary history

After explaining simply that she is going to look at Jamie's development, including his vision and hearing, the assessor introduces questioning with one that doesn't have any implication of inferring abnormality. She then follows with globally exploratory questions covering the medical and the developmental background, phrased in a way that encourages mother to quickly recall the whole time frame and the whole perspective of development.

Introductory question: 'Is Jamie your first baby?' or 'Does Jamie have brothers and sisters?' 'How old …?'

Medical background: 'Did everything go smoothly while you were pregnant, during and after delivery?' She puts out a few probing questions if she feels the mother's answer needs clarification: for example 'I was in bed for 3 days in the fourth month.' 'Why was that?' 'Any rash or fever?' Then she checks for potentially serious postnatal events, 'Has Jamie ever been ill enough to worry you or your doctor or health visitor?'

Developmental background: 'Do you have, or have you ever had any concerns about Jamie's development?' 'Has your doctor or health visitor ever expressed any concern about his development?' Again probe further as you feel her answers indicate. Replies, like the following, often camouflage a real concern, for example 'I think he's just lazy but ….' Young children are rarely lazy; if unwell they may be lethargic; 'I know he's not deaf but ….' 'He listens when he wants to …,' 'I know children are all different but ….'

Cultural background: If English is obviously not the mother's first language, ask her 'What language do your family speak at home?'

Social background: Explore social circumstance at a superficial level, for example number of children, presence of partner/supporting relatives, working status, etc.

The above questions are merely a framework on which individual assessors can hang their personal phraseology. The assessor is now alerted to areas that should be given special attention through further history taking and examination; this frequently coincides with the child's readiness to participate. Assessment findings will further indicate which aspects of the medical,[2] developmental and social, emotional and cultural climate warrant further consideration.

Recording the primary history: The different aspects of the primary history are recorded under separate headings as this facilitates logical report writing.

Secondary history

Each of the chapters on specific domains of development has an early section devoted to secondary history in which developmental and medical questions particularly pertinent to that domain are highlighted. The style of secondary questioning needs to be probing and specific unlike that of the primary history.

Developmental questions

Vague questions about development lead to vague answers and to a tendency in the questioner to uncritically assume an age-appropriate level. The answers, even to apparently well-framed questions, may not be as definitive as they at first appear.

The assessor wishes to explore 4-year-old Johnny's language level through parental questioning. She asks, 'What do you think he understands of what you say?' Mother replies, 'Everything' and/or 'He fetches his shoes for me when I ask him to'. Should the assessor assume that Johnny analyses an age-appropriate four-keyword spoken phrase like 'Johnny fetch your shoes'. No, for all she knows, the mother may also be tapping his shoulder (to get his attention) and then pointing to his shoes while speaking, in which case he could be responding to touch and gesture rather than to any of the spoken words – appropriate for a 12- to 15-month-old. Questions need to be as definitive as possible from the outset so that the mother doesn't feel that the examiner is 'nit-picking' or does not believe her when she probes further. For the 4-year-old, the assessor could start by asking the mother, 'Do you think he would understand if you said "Johnny, bring me your shoes" without touching him or pointing/looking (eye-pointing) at his shoes?' If the mother looks doubtful or says 'no', the examiner then asks 'Which of these do you think he would understand "Where's Johnny's shoes?" "Johnny's shoe?" with a "where" gesture, or an intonated "shoe?" with a "where" gesture, or do you usually point as well?' Verbal comprehension was chosen because this is the area that parents and many professionals most often overestimate, not realising how many additional methods of communication are being used at one and the same time.

---

2   While telling the history, parents sometimes mention medical 'signs' as opposed to 'risk' factors that they have noted, e.g. 'Her left eye squints when she's tired' or 'I don't know if it's anything but her eyes sometimes roll up two or three times for no obvious reason'. These should be explored and recorded under medical signs of potential diagnostic significance.

Next the examiner wishes to explore a 21-week-old's development of reach (see Chapter 1 for an in-depth analysis or reaching). She composes an apparently probing question *'When lying on her back under the baby gym does she try to swipe at the hanging toys?'* If the mother's answer is 'yes', chances are that this is a visually directed and cognitively motivated swipe, but it could also be random spontaneous movements of the arms that sometimes contact one of the toys by chance. The answer 'sometimes' further increases the likelihood of the hand–toy contact being chance. The answer 'no' probably represents delay in achieving this skill. All these answers would need a series of even more targeted questions to pinpoint the baby's level of achievement.

Although these two illustrations may sound a bit pedantic, they highlight the pitfalls of assessment through questionnaires and the advantages of informed observation; they also emphasize the importance of being as rigorous in eliciting developmental symptoms as one would be in eliciting physical ones.

Medical risk factors
Most medical risk factors are common to several developmental disorders and categories of disability. As these factors and the developmental and disability problems form part of the foundation paediatric curriculum, only a general list of medical risk categories is presented below. Readers will be alerted to those specific to each developmental domain in the relevant chapter. The list is representative and not exhaustive.

Prenatal

- Events

  - Embryonic dysgenesis (systemic and neural)

  - Alcohol or drug abuse, certain medications

  - Intrauterine infections – rubella, toxoplasmosis, cytomegalovirus, acquired immunodeficiency syndrome, herpes, etc.

  - Pre-eclamptic toxaemia, placental abruption

- Chromosomal abnormalities

  - Down syndrome, Fragile X syndrome

- Genetic syndromes

  - Refsum disease, Hurler syndrome

- Familial (genetic) traits

  - Developmental language disorder, autistic spectrum disorders

  - Strabismus, refractive errors

- Sensorineural deafness, otitis media with effusion

Perinatal

- Events
  - Hypoxia, ischaemia, hyperbilirubinaemia, hypoglycaemia
  - Infection – meningitis, gastroenteritis, middle ear infections
  - Complications of preterm birth (<1500g)
  - Complicated term birth – breach delivery, cord around the neck

Postnatal

- Events
  - Infections – mumps, measles, meningitis
  - Metabolic disorder – homocystinuria, hypothyroidism, phenylketonuria,
  - Epileptic disorder
  - Illness requiring chemotherapy or radiotherapy
  - Hypoxia complicating major surgery
  - Trauma – accidental/non-accidental – severe head injury
  - Toxic – side effects of medicine, for example gentamicin, vigabatrin

Recording assessment findings

Accurate recording of assessment findings is paramount but difficult when multitasking and while gaining experience in procedure and delivery; asking a colleague to record during this phase is helpful; later pausing to record between each domain may suffice (see also Chapter 12).

Interpretation of findings

Normative data sets are fundamental to meaningful interpretation of test findings. However, the scientific strength of norms in the field of child development is very variable and too often based on non-representative samples of inadequate size. Sometimes tests and test schedules developed in one culture are applied, both clinically and in research, to child populations from cultures that are totally different to that of the host standardisation sample. It takes only a few moments of 'developmental thought' to realise the pitfalls of such a practice. Developmental tests are not immunisations. Western professionals should be sharing their insight into the neurodevelopmental processes within and between domains, stages of development, test design and standardisation and supporting choice of materials and language that are developmentally and culturally appropriate. Although the tests in this book have not been standardised as a package, the normative guidelines are well founded on Western populations.

Normative Guidelines

In the domain chapters, normative guidelines are given at the end of each test description. The guidelines are referred to as 'reference ranges' when the test is fully standardised and as 'age guidelines' when the norms are extrapolated from standardised scales[3] or based upon the published works and experience of respected individuals in the field. The following abbreviations denote sources referred to throughout the book:

Sh, R, E, S – experience of Sheridan, Reynell, Egan, and Sonksen, respectively;

RDLS – Reynell Developmental Language Scales;

ETS – Egan's Test Schedule;

EBPT – Egan Bus Puzzle Test;

GMDS – Griffiths Mental Development Scales;

RZS – normal controls for development of the Reynell–Zinkin Scales for visually impaired children;

SonkLT – Sonksen logMAR Test;

SSAS – Sonksen Silver Acuity System

Source(s) of normative data are referenced in square brackets followed by the age when 50% achieve in italics and when 80% and/or 90% do so in bold type. For example

Age guideline: [GMDS, Sh, E] *24–***28** months

The mean age informs examiners' choice of test and age appropriateness of the child's response, while the 80% and/or 90% achievement levels facilitate identification of the lowest functioning children, that is for some tests the lowest 20% and for others the lowest 10%, respectively. In other words, if the skill is not present by the age in bold type, the assessor's index of concern should be alerted to explore the domain in greater depth and consider the finding(s) in the context of the overall profile in order to create

---

3   In some instances the test procedure varies slightly from that given by the source.

an effective action plan. Domain findings are gathered together into a comprehensive whole in Chapter 12.

The normative data for some reference ranges, for example the Sonksen logMAR Test, are presented in the form of a centile chart, allowing the assessor to plot the child's achievement over time. As the level of skill varies directly with age, the 50th centile tracks the ages at which 50% achieve succeeding levels; the 90th and 10th centiles track the ages at which the best and the worse 10% achieve succeeding levels of acuity.

Terms like 'average', 'above average', 'below average', 'well below average', 'well above average' and 'in the average range' are used rather loosely by professionals to describe a child's development. In this book these terms are applied as follows:

- 'Average' and 'in the average range' refer to those functioning around/closest to the mathematical mean, that is between the 35th and 65th centile for age.

- 'Above average' and 'well above average' refer to those between the 65th and 80th and >80th centile for age, respectively.

- 'Below average' and 'well below average' refer to those between the 20th and 35th and <20th centile for age respectively

Assessment should be a mutually enjoyable activity for both assessor and child. Professionals new to developmental testing are bound to feel anxious about their ability to control children in this age range. It is all too easy to blame the child when the interaction ends in tears or a tantrum. Assessors need to be free to devote a sizeable portion of their attention and energy to ongoing analysis of primary and secondary observations. Test protocols therefore need to be 'on automatic'; that is a successful assessor should never need to refer to the test form or test instructions to affirm what item comes next or how to administer it. The author suggests that assessors give themselves sufficient practice in communicative engagement, handling and test protocol for tension to be replaced by enjoyment before moving on to assessment of children with developmental disorders and disabilities.

Key Points

- Take care not to inadvertently increase parental anxiety.

- Take responsibility for 'setting the scene'.

- Actively observe and engage with the child throughout.

- Establish a structured framework of assessment.

- Become flexible within framework only once sufficiently experienced.

- Practice engaging and handling – especially attention control.

- Get administration of the tests you use 'on automatic'.

- 'Enjoy' assessing the child.

- Be constructively self- and colleague-critical, not child critical.

- Think about how you phrase developmental questions.

- Probe further if parental answers are not definitive.

- Introduce tests at 50% achievement level.

- Set delays, disorders and disabilities in medical and socio-cultural context.

Reference

Cooper J, Moodley M, Reynell J (1978) *Helping Language Development: A Developmental Programme for Children with Early Language Handicaps*. London: Edward Arnold Ltd.

Chapter 3

Vision

Currently, most Western nations use nurses (community nurses, paediatric nurses and health visitors) or orthoptists to screen the preschool population for visual problems. Suspected visual problems in otherwise healthy or disabled children are further assessed by orthoptists and ophthalmologists in district paediatric eye clinics. Consequently, assessment of vision is no longer seen as an essential part of the training of community paediatricians or indeed of neurodevelopmental and neurodisability paediatricians. Be that as it may, in the context of this book – to give readers a deeper understanding of developmental processes and the skills with which to achieve a comprehensive developmental review of babies and young children – assessment of vision is pertinent. Sensory input is the starting gun of all developmental processes, and the impact of vision on development in the first year is all embracing and more evident than that of hearing, so it seems logical to allocate the first domain chapter to vision. Early detection of severe visual impairment (SVI), while the neurological substrate is most pliant, facilitates optimal time-tabling of developmental intervention to promote general and visual development and, thus limit a spiral of cumulative negative developmental consequences (Sonksen 1983a, Cass et al. 1994). Early diagnosis of SVI due to disorders of the lids or globe is also important as some conditions are visually treatable and/or require urgent medical intervention, e.g. cataract, corneal opacity, glaucoma, retinoblastoma, and ptosis. Although minor degrees of visual impairment are compatible with normal early development, it is important to attempt to identify families at risk of refractive errors or strabismus so that preventative measures can be instituted before secondary complications arise (e.g. hyperopia $\Rightarrow$ strabismus $\Rightarrow$ amblyopia; myopia $\Rightarrow$ divergent strabismus), because once established treatment is an uphill task for professionals, children and families.

Epidemiology

In Western countries the incidence of strabismus in young children at any age is 2%–4%; that of minor refractive errors requiring correction or likely to induce amblyopia is similar, although the balance of causes differs with age. The prevalence of moderate to profound degrees of visual impairment (corrected visual acuity in the better eye of 6/18 or worse) in the UK is approximately 1.2 per 1000 live births (Surman et al. 2008). The visual impairment is cerebral in origin in about 25%, and most of these children have additional impairments. Refractive errors, strabismus and mild through severe degrees of visual impairment are much more prevalent in children with positive general risk factors (see Chapter 2, p.36) and in those with cerebral palsy, neurodevelopmental disorders, neurodegenerative diseases and dysmorphic syndromes. Although not the focus of this book, this subgroup should all receive careful visual assessment. Similarly, children identified with SVI or other disorders require specialist neurodevelopmental assessment including hearing assessment, as over 60% have multiple problems. Our understanding of both the spectrum and variety of visual dysfunction presenting in children with cerebral visual impairment (CVI), together with their neuronal correlates, have greatly advanced in the last two decades and importantly have led to the development of rehabilitative strategies (Dutton et al. 2010, Phillip and Dutton 2014).

Neurological substrate

The visual pathways are extremely complex and represent two distinct evolutionary phases of the visual nervous system of mammals; the older system developed to provide sensory control of movements and the more recent, 'sight,' to provide the perceptual impetus for cognitive development and conscious thought (Goodale 2010). In humans the two evolutionary pathways are separate yet closely integrated at all levels of the central nervous system.

Visual information is conveyed beyond the occipital cortex to numerous areas of the brain along two main projections known as the dorsal and ventral streams. The dorsal stream is responsible for the real-time control of movement (action) and projects to the parietal lobe. The ventral stream, in association with cognitive networks, is responsible for recognition (perception) and projects to the inferior temporal lobe (Goodale 2010).

As mentioned in Chapter 1, neuronal connectivity in the supra and subtentorial (cerebellum and basal ganglia) visual nervous system in sighted babies proceeds apace after birth. At retinal level, cones migrate into the central fovea with achievement of adult densities by 15 months. From birth to 4 months, neurons in the way stations along the 'sight' input pathways, such as the lateral geniculate bodies and in the visual cortices, increase in size and sprout dendritic spines that form synapses with those in other higher visual, cognitive, language and motor areas; 'pruning' to adult levels is largely complete by 15 months. Myelination of the input pathways from optic nerve to primary visual cortex follows a similar timescale. The impetus for neuronal networking is a quality of vision sufficient, initially, to arouse cognitive interest in looking (Sonksen et al., 1991). In the presence of adequate vision, cognitive interest thus becomes the catalyst for self-perpetuating cycles of development both within the visual system and beyond. At behavioural level the outcome of this neuronal activity manifests as (1) rapidly increasing macular and peripheral visual acuity and mature control of eye movements long before mature control of systemic or speech musculature, and (2) functionally active links between visual and higher cognitive centres in the early months. Experimental studies in mammals by Blakemore (1991) and Price et al. (1994) confirm that connectivity is proceeding apace in the visual nervous system throughout the early months. Why such a visual explosion? If permitted a teleological argument, the visual system needs to 'get its act together' quickly because it, of all the sensory systems, orchestrates most aspects of early development. Observation of sequences of visual behaviour through the early months provides parameters for the assessment of vision in infancy.

Assessment

Assessment contains elements of history and examination. At all ages the examination has three distinct aspects:

- Assessment of developing vision/visual acuity (clarity of vision)

- Assessment of the development of eye movement control

- Detection of strabismus, eye movement disorders and lid or globe pathology.

The first two are interrelated developmental sequences. The third reviews medical pointers to visual problems, such as strabismus. In children without overt signs of eye or visual pathology the wise assessor carries out the assessments of vision and development of eye movements within the body of the developmental examination, leaving the more intrusive examination for strabismus, plus or minus pathology, until the end in order not to jeopardize the former. Apart from strabismus, pathological physical eye signs are rare in the otherwise 'not at risk for visual impairment' population. The majority of these signs are overt and therefore noticeable the moment one gazes on a child's face and observes their spontaneous visual behaviour; others have to be actively sought (see the pathology section at the end of the chapter).

History

The primary history (see Chapter 2, p. 34) will have clarified whether or not a child is neurodevelopmentally at risk. The following open-ended question targets both developmental and medical (sign) aspects of vision: 'Do you, or have you ever had any concerns about her vision/eyesight or her eyes'? A smiling, 'No, she's very alert and looks at everything' should lead straight on to the medical risk questions specific for the visual system (see the following discussion). However, sometimes the parent's response will set off alarm bells, for example 'My friend's baby looks at her when she's feeding but Amy just gazes at the ceiling' or 'She smiles when I start her musical mobile but doesn't watch it' or 'She startles and cries when I pick her up'. Such responses clearly require further age-appropriate visual behaviour and medical (sign) probing.

Medical (sign) responses such as 'I sometimes think her eyes wobble' or 'Her left eye sometimes turns in/doesn't look in the same direction as the right' or 'Sometimes I think there's a white speck in his left eye' or 'In this photo one of his pupils is red and the other grey; is that OK?'

Q Which pupil should she be worried about and why?
The grey one: coloboma, large and very white optic nerve head or retinoblastoma may be causing the white shadow.

Clearly all require further questions and careful examination.

The parents of a 5-year-old say that twice in the last week he has asked 'which one?' when she's asked him to point to a picture in a book; the parents have not noticed any change in behaviour and his school report is excellent. On testing, acuity in each eye is normal; a small intermittent strabismus is seen in the right eye; there is a family history of strabismus in early childhood.

Q Would you offer to review in 6 weeks' time or refer urgently to a paediatric ophthalmologist? What would be the reasons for your choice?
Diplopia could be due to an intracranial or orbital mass lesion and therefore needs to be seen urgently before acuity drops because once it has it is unlikely to fully recover.

Practice Point Parents tend not to notice mild to moderate reductions in a baby's acuity so any concern mentioned should be taken very seriously as it is likely to signify SVI. On the other hand, parents are often better than non-eye specialists at suspecting strabismus or eye movement problems so again their concerns should not be lightly dismissed – they are better placed to do so as both may be more noticeable when a child is unwell or tired.

Strabismus and refractive errors, particularly myopia and hypermetropia, tend to run in families; congenital visual disorders are frequently genetically determined so medical (risk) questions specific for the visual system should explore

- Family history of strabismus in childhood.

- Family history in childhood and adolescence of need to wear glasses or contact lenses and of refractive errors.[1]

- Family history of eye diseases/visual disorders in childhood (e.g. infantile cataract, glaucoma, retinoblastoma and retinal dystrophy).

Examination

Visual acuity

Visual acuity matures from birth until at least 9 years, most rapidly in the preschool years. The cognitive element of the test task governs the choice of method used at different ages. The cognitive ability governing standard tests for adults is letter recognition that the testee demonstrates by naming. The cognitive ability to match letters emerges between 30 and 36 months of age, so 33 months creates a natural point at which to advocate the use of the adult standard. Methods for younger children naturally subdivide into those of less than 19 months and those of 19 to 33 months.

Birth to 18 months

The objective test system for measuring visual acuity in babies and toddlers depends upon their preference to look at a pattern rather than a blank (Fantz 1962). Originally the Teller Acuity Card test was developed to investigate the development of acuity in babies and has since been adapted for clinical use (Teller et al. 1986). In the UK, the Keeler Acuity Card Test serves a similar purpose (Keeler 1988). These systems are widely used in specialist eye or neurodevelopmental/disability units; the following description provides essential information only.

Grating Acuity: Each Keeler card (Fig 3.1) has two circular inserts, each 10cm in diameter; one contains a grating of standard spatial frequency and the other a blank of identical luminance.

---

1   Note whether mother, father or a sibling is wearing glasses (contact lenses aren't so easily visible so they need a specific question). Also ask the age of first prescription and the reason — short sight, long sight, astigmatism or 'lazy eye'.

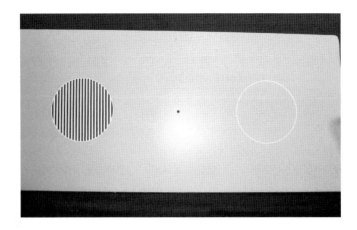

Figure 3.1 A card from the Keeler Acuity Card Test: Babies preferentially gaze at the patterned insert.

The test distance is 38cm and the unit of measurement cycles/degree (c/deg) at 38cm. From 1 to 13 months grating acuity increases from 0.72c/deg (equivalent to Snellen 6/250, 20/800) to 12.5c/deg (equivalent to 6/14, 20/50). As a rule of thumb, acuity in c/deg at 38cm is roughly equal to age in months, up to 12 months of age. Combining data from different national studies suggests that grating acuity has matured to a Snellen equivalent of 6/6, 20/20 (logMAR 0.0) by 3 years of age. Unfortunately, failure of grating cards to identify some children with significant amblyopia remains a concern.

Detection vision
For babies and toddlers, schedules of Observable Visual Behaviours have traditionally presented the most practical way of looking at visual development (Sheridan 1968, Atkinson et al 2002). Unfortunately, many schedules test and record assessment of acuity and control of eye movements under a single term: 'Fixes and Follows', thus blurring the distinction between them. In this chapter they feature in different sections in order to emphasize that they represent two different aspects of development, although in practice it is natural to assess following, convergence and accommodation once fixation has been observed. Secondly, in many developmental schedules the endpoint is 'picks up or pokes' the detection target. Thus the assessor's attention is directed to a manipulative endpoint rather than the visual one of fixation. The Near Detection Vision (NDV) scale monitors the development of fixation for increasingly small objects through the first 9 months (Sonksen 1993).[2]

---

2   Over years of clinical and research work with severely visually impaired (SVI) babies and young children the NDV scale has been adapted to suit the assessment needs of the SVI – the NDV-VI (Sonksen 1983a, Sonksen and Dale 2002).

Scale of Near Detection Vision

The scale is a reflection of increasing visual acuity rather than a measure of visual acuity. The reason is twofold. First the detection of a single target does not fulfil the conditions of the Snellen principle which require visual resolution of the integral components of a visual target e.g. of the component strokes of a letter. However, both usually utilize the macular pathway. Detection requires less acuity than discrimination of a letter of similar overall size – at least five times less. The width of the stroke of a Snellen letter is 1/5th its overall size. The stroke of a size 6 Snellen letter is 1.2mm wide, i.e. the same as the diameter of a cake decoration (known as 'hundred and thousand') – yet adults are often amazed that they can detect a hundred and thousand from a distance of 6m and assume that a child who can visually locate a hundred and thousand from 30cm must have sufficient acuity to read small print – some have and others have not. Second, a baby's cognitive interest has to be aroused by objects the size of the detection target for him to look at or fixate it. The scale therefore reflects the development of visual cognitive interest in increasingly small objects, i.e. the smallest size of object is not necessarily the smallest that babies can see/detect at a given age but the smallest that captures their interest sufficiently to initiate looking/fixation.

Protocol

As for other behavioural scales, adherence to both item specifications and protocol for presentation of the lure is essential to the credence and consistency of findings. The test is carried out with both eyes open, starting with a target one or two sizes larger than the definitive one for age.

Item specifications

In the UK, the lures of the NDV range from diffuse light to a 1.2mm hundred and thousand. Except for the first two items the physical specifications of test lures in terms of size, shape, colour, background and presentation distance are standard. These specifications are presented in Table 3.1. The table top-lures (Fig 3.2) are all yellow or white to ensure standard contrast to the green baize background and spherical[3], because the image impinging on the retina from a sugar strand of similar cross-section or a piece of cotton of smaller cross-section, would both effect a larger image on the retina, i.e. equivalent to their respective lengths.

Procedure, endpoints and age guidelines

Procedure, endpoints and age guidelines for each test item are described in this section.

---

3   Except for the 2.25cm cube/brick as the risk of inhalation of a round bead of this size is greater.

Table 3.1   Specifications of near detection vision lures

Visual lure	Size (cm)	Shape	Colour	Presentation distance (cm)
Diffuse light				
Assessor's face				30
Woolly ball	12.5	Spherical	Yellow and black	30
Plastic ball	6.25	Spherical	Yellow	30
Wooden cube	2.25	Cube	Yellow	30
Smartie	1.25	Spherical	Yellow	30
Saccharin	0.5	Spherical	White	30
Hundred and thousand	0.12	Spherical	White or yellow	30

The endpoint is always visual fixation at full test distance (30cm) – except for the diffuse light source. Fixation implies direct pupil to target gaze. Any reduction in quality of gaze (e.g. searching, peering, roving eye movements, nystagmus, eccentric gaze) is suspicious of a significant degree of visual impairment. The age by which each target should be fixated is given at the end of each section and in Table 3.2. The behaviours are of course present in many babies well before the age given.

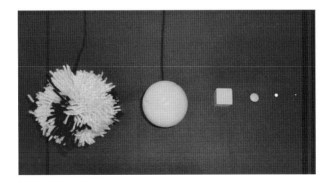

Figure 3.2 Table-top items from the NDV scale.

Table 3.2   Near Detection Scale: Age guidelines

Behaviour	2wks	8wks	14wks	22wks	26wks	30wks	36wks	42wks
Turns to diffuse light	+	+	+	+	+	+	+	+
Fix face	+	+	+	+	+	+	+	+
Fix 12.5cm dangling ball	±	+	+	+	+	+	+	+
Fix 6.25cm dangling ball		±	+	+	+	+	+	+
Fix 6.25cm stationary ball			±	+	+	+	+	+
Fix 2.25cm cube				±	+	+	+	+
Fix 1.25cm Smartie (M&M)					±	+	+	+
Fix 5.5mm saccharin						±	+	+
Fix 1.25mm 100/1000							±	+

Fix, Fixates; ± behaviour present in some babies; + age guideline by which behaviour should be present, i.e. concerned if not present.

Source of diffuse light

A window with Venetian blind, an X-ray viewing box and on a dull day, daylight through a window make suitable sources. The assessor (back to the light source) lays the baby supine along his arms supporting the head in one hand, then turns slowly through 90° and then back through 180°.

Q Why does the assessor turn slowly?
   To avoid stimulating the vestibular system.

Endpoint: head and eye turning towards the light source to both sides

Age guideline: should be present from birth. Asymmetry especially in speed of response
   warrants a closer examination of the eye nearest the source of the diffuse light on
   the slower side.

Adult face

Holding the baby similarly, though now with her head about 30° above the horizontal and with her face about 30cm from his own, the assessor moves his head minimally and makes smiling, silent social overtures.

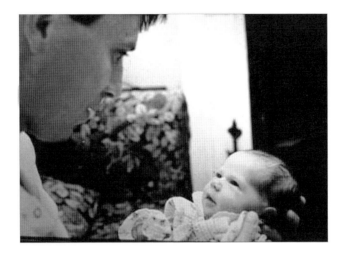

Figure 3.3 Newborn baby fixating an adult face; note the intensity and directness of gaze of both participants.

Q Why should the social overtures be silent?
To avoid stimulating the auditory system.

Endpoint: fixation on assessor's face – Figure 3.3

Age guideline: frequently present at **birth**; should be by **2 weeks**

12.5cm woolly pom-pom/6.25cm plastic ball attached to a thin black shoelace

Place babies of less than 14 weeks supine on a changing or play mat, at table height or floor level. Older babies with effortless head control can sit supported on their parent's lap. The assessor should stand (or kneel) at a supine baby's head end or in front of the sitting baby. Start the ball 'spinning on the spot'[4] 30cm from the baby's eyes.

Practice Point Most assessors require practice to make a dangling ball 'spin on the spot'.

---

4   'Spinning on the spot' increases the visual attractiveness without changing the effective size of the lure; in contrast a swinging or pendulum motion considerably increases the size of the image impinging on the retina

Endpoint: fixation on the ball

Age guideline: 12.5cm – should be by **8** weeks

6.25cm – should be by **14** weeks

6.25cm ball, 2.25cm cube, 1.25cm sweet Smartie (M&M), 0.55cm saccharin tablet 1.2mm hundred and thousand

The parent supports the baby in sitting on her lap at a table covered with dark green baize. The assessor sits opposite and presents a single item at a time.[5] The first prerequisite of placement is that the baby is aware that the assessor has something interesting in his hand, so he holds up the lure saying 'ooohh look'. As soon as the baby's interest is engaged he sweeps his hand across the table surface from his left to his right (right-handed assessors), releasing the lure somewhere en passant – distance from baby's eyes about 30cm – all the while watching the baby's eyes for fixation. The speed of hand movement is fast enough to hold the baby's interest but not so fast that the released target is instantly outside his peripheral field of vision. An alternative placement technique, if interest is not sustained for the two smallest items, is to drop it from the baby's eye level onto the cloth and look for fixation once the saccharine tablet or hundred and thousand is stationary. Releasing the lure where the assessor's hand touches the table is not satisfactory because the child may only need to see something as large as a hand to look at the spot.

Endpoint: fixation of age-appropriate target

Age guidelines:

- 6.25cm ball – should be by **22** weeks
- 2.25cm cube – should be by **26** weeks
- 1.25cm M&M/Smartie – should be by **30** weeks
- 0.55cm saccharin – should be by **36** weeks
- 0.12cm hundred and thousand – should be by **42** weeks

Interpretation: Achievement of the age-appropriate endpoint suggests normal visual behaviour for age. It does not exclude mild or moderate impairment of acuity. Failure to achieve the age-appropriate target may be due to impaired vision, delayed cognitive development or an eye movement disorder.

---

5   Touching items effect a larger image on the retina; multiple items increase difficulty for tester to judge which, if any, individual item the child is fixating.

Practice Point If monocular testing is indicated this is best left until other aspects of the developmental assessment have been achieved because patching causes distress in this age group and rapport may be lost. However, 6- to 11-month-olds tolerate patching better than 18- to 36-month-olds .

Q Why do 6- to 11-month-olds tolerate patching better than 18- to 36-month-olds?
Because their attention control is more malleable.

Q How may acceptance of patching be increased in the younger age group?
By introducing a novel stimulus, e.g. a squeaky duck, immediately the patch is secured; the attention of the younger group is taken by the toy and the patch forgotten. Not so by the older age group.

18 to 33 months

The Cardiff Acuity Card Test (Woodhouse et al. 1992) is a well-researched tool that appeals to and provides standard measures for this age group; the response task accommodates preferential looking, pointing and naming. Unfortunately, the test is too expensive for screening and like Grating Acuity Cards has been shown to underestimate the presence of significant and potentially amblyogenic refractive errors (Sharma et al. 2003, Howard and Firth 2006).

From early in the second year children communicate their recognition of realistic coloured pictures through gesture or vocalizations (e.g. car through a steering gesture, 'brmm – brmm' noise, 'tar' or 'car'). Coloured pictures, like the everyday scene, are made up of subtle changes in colour and hue, whereas optotype charts present clear-cut black shapes against a background of more than 90% contrast. Figure 3.4 illustrates how at the same level of defocusing the Snellen letter (H) is easier to identify than the item depicted in the coloured picture (a half peeled orange) many times its overall size, and hence the potential of coloured pictures to screen for problems of acuity.

The Sonksen Picture Test (SPT) was developed as a screening test and evaluated (Sonksen and Macrae 1987, Hodes et al. 1994). The authors noted that children with 3/4.5 for single optotypes had difficulty with one or more Grade 3 pictures. Vervloed et al. (2001) subsequently showed that visual acuity was more important than contrast sensitivity for recognition of the pictures. The SPT was never produced commercially, but the research showed the potential of the method to identify children with problems of acuity.[6]

---

6   The SPT pictures can be sourced from Ladybird books remaining in circulation; the source of individual pictures is documented in the 1987 and 1994 publications.

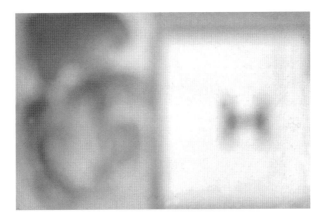

Figure 3.4 Although in monochrome the Snellen H is much easier to identify than the half-peeled orange many times its size.

Thus, definitive measures of acuity are not available to professionals working in the community with this age group.

2 years 9 months and over

Developmental considerations
The youngest age group that can comply with a standard optotype[7] test of acuity is 33 to 39 months. At this age the test is at the ceiling of their ability, in terms of the cognitive demand of the response task (matching letters), interest of materials, ability to give and sustain attention at 3m and acceptance of occlusion. In other words, it is a lot to ask of this age group and a higher rate of success is achieved if time is taken to ensure they understand the response task (matching) and what is required at each stage of testing. By 42 months these constraints have largely resolved with the exception of resistance to occlusion. Optotype tests are therefore suitable for routine testing of children of 42 months and over and although the test takes longer under this age, it is time well spent, if parents or assessor are concerned about vision – over 89% can achieve a binocular linear measure (Salt et al. 1995, 2007). Increasingly, children over 48 months prefer to name the letters and as long as the names they give to individual letters are consistent they are allowable (e.g. 'kiss' or 'cross' for the X or phonetic sounding rather than alphabetical name).

---

7   Optotypes = black letters or pictograms drawn to standard specifications on a white background – contrast 95% .

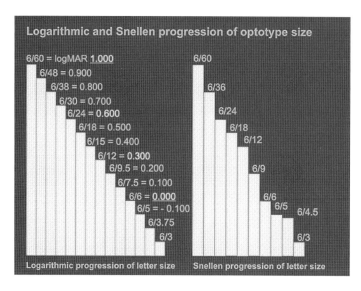

Figure 3.5 Snellen and logMAR scaling.

Standards for optotype test displays

The two most widely known standards for optotype test displays are the Snellen and the logMAR (Snellen 1862, Bailey and Lovie 1976). The log of the minimal angle of resolution (logMAR) scale has superseded the Snellen scale as the International Standard (The Consilium of Ophthalmologists 1988). Any variations from standard specifications introduce errors into measurement and reduce the comparability between results obtained using different tests for follow up of individual patients, in group studies and multi-centre research. The advantages of logMAR over Snellen scaling are a regular progression of letter size, an equal number of letters at each level and a system of scoring that includes every letter correctly identified, leading to increased sensitivity and repeatability of measurement. Of particular relevance is the increased number of levels at the better acuity end of the range, that serve to accommodate the rapid changes in acuity from 2½ to 5 years. Figure 3.5 illustrates these points of difference between Snellen and logMAR scaling.

The basis of logMAR scores

Two examples of the way in which logMAR measures of acuity are derived and relate to Snellen scaling are given below.

Example 1
- The angle subtended on the retina by a size 6 (20) Snellen letter viewed from 6m (20ft) is 1 minute of arc

- The log of 1 is 0,

- So logMAR acuity of 0.000 is equivalent to Snellen acuity of 6/6 (20/20), 3/3 (10/10)

Example 2

- The angle subtended by a size 60 Snellen letter viewed from 6m/20ft is 10 minutes of arc

- The log of 10 is 1

- So logMAR acuity of 1.000 is equivalent to Snellen acuity of 6/60 (20/200), 3/30 (10/100)

Thus, numerically smaller logMAR scores indicate better acuity than larger ones. Acuities better than logMAR 0.000 (6/6, 20/20) are prefixed by a negative sign, so acuity of logMAR –0.050 is not as good as logMAR –0.125.

There are several excellent logMAR tests available for children – Lea logMAR Symbol Tests (Good-lite Ltd), Kay logMAR Crowded Book Set (Kay Pictures Ltd), and Keeler logMAR Test (Keeler Ltd, Windsor, UK) based on the Glasgow Acuity Cards (McGraw and Winn 1993) and Sonksen logMAR Test (SonkLT) (Sonksen 2006, Wade et al. 2006, Salt et al. 2007, Sonksen et al. 2008). Of these the Sonksen logMAR test, described in the next section, is the only test to date with norms derived from a data set that represents the general population with respect to acuity.

The Sonksen logMAR Test

The test displays are drawn in strict accord with the logMAR standard; a standard, age-related test protocol is provided, together with age norms in the manual. Norms for binocular and monocular distant linear (and single) acuity are in the form of centile charts, similar to growth charts.

Practicalities and administration

Practical recommendations are equally applicable to other logMAR tests.

General: The letters on the SonkLT keycard and in the training booklet are of the same size as this helps the youngest children grasp the concept of matching. The test booklets and charts are designed so that displays are arranged in sequence from largest to smallest. The assessor slips his thumb under the tabs to flip successive booklet displays over to face the child.

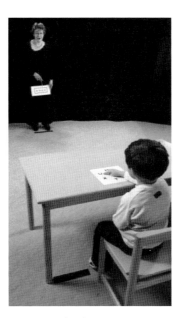

Figure 3.6 Testing linear binocular acuity (3m).

Setting the scene: The acuity test comes towards the end of the developmental session so the child is already sitting at a nursery height table and chair.[8]

Order of testing: In an ideal world both binocular and monocular measures for both distant and near acuity would be obtained. Preschool children quickly tire of a letter-matching task so the most informative measures need to be obtained first. Specialist eye clinics for school-age children traditionally have commenced with monocular testing as the focus of their work is detection and treatment of refractive errors, strabismus and amblyopia; as the work of these professionals has extended to encompass preschool surveillance they naturally continue with this practice. However, in the setting of developmental overview of preschool children the author advocates the following order. (The rationale for this order is given in the section headed Rationale and Evidence base on page 63.)

- Place a marker 3m from the front edge of the child's chair[9] – Fig 3.6

- Train matching using key card and training booklet – Fig 3.7

- Level find using singles test booklet (3m)

---

8 Another advantage of the nursery height table is that a standing assessor has an excellent view of the key card; if allowed to pick up the card most children hold it upright facing themselves, with the assessor unable to see the letter they are pointing to.

9 A piece of non-stretchable cord knotted at 3m and 40cm (near test) is a useful alternative.

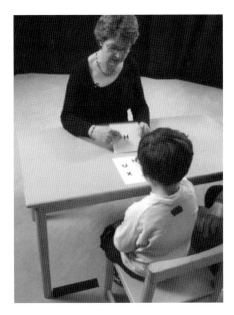

Figure 3.7 Training matching.

- Measure distant acuity with both eyes open (BEO) (binocular) using linear test booklet A – Fig 3.6

- Level find using 'end of line' letters on near chart

- Measure near acuity BEO (binocular) using near chart A – Fig 3.8

- Occlude one eye

- Measure distant then near acuity of non-occluded eye (monocular) using booklet and chart B

- Occlude other eye

- Measure distant then near acuity of non-occluded eye (monocular) using booklet and chart A

Training matching 33–42 months: Place the keycard in front of the child saying 'these are Michael's letters – look, there is one like this and one like ------' pointing to each letter in turn; then pick up the training booklet 'and these are mine.' Point to the first letter saying 'I've got one like this, where's Michael's?' or 'where's the other one?'[10] – Figure 3.7.

---

10   Children understand and use the expression 'other one' from about 24 months, whereas they remain puzzled by 'same' and 'different' until about 42 months.

- If Michael points to the correct letter on the keycard praise him – 'clever boy' and flip over to the next letter 'and where's this one?' It is wise to familiarise children with all six letters before actual testing.

- If he 'fails', place the training booklet upright and directly in front of the same letter on the keycard saying 'look it's this one, here's the other one' pointing backwards and forwards between the two. Failure to understand after the third letter suggests that the task is conceptually too difficult and the test should be abandoned.

Q If the child were (a) 2 years 9 months or (b) 3 years 11 months what would your thoughts/actions be?
(a) Suspect that the child is one of the 20% not yet cognitively ready to match letters and consider less-demanding ways of checking vision. (b) Suspect significant cognitive delay, note it in the cognitive section and ensure other aspects of cognitive development are careful examined.

Level finding: Take the test booklet of single letters to the 3m mark while saying 'Now I'm going to show you some more from over here.' Present the 0.7 letter asking him 'where's yours' then alternate ones until he fails; the smallest size seen is the assessor's guide to the starting level in the linear test booklet (see later in this chapter). It also provides a measure of binocular acuity for single optotypes (see p. 63 regarding limitations of this measure).

Practice Point   If, in this or subsequent sections, the child fails while alternate levels are being shown, vision for the 'missed out level' needs to be ascertained.

Distant measure for linear displays of letters –Test displays should be held vertically at the child's eye level (not at the assessor's chest level) (Fig 3.6).

With a 'I've got some more here' present the display in first linear booklet two sizes larger than the singles level achieved and point[11] to the first letter 'where's this one and this one …' progressing systematically along the line – with small children it pays dividends to be systematic; 'jumping about' only confuses them. Continue to present the next and subsequent lines until three letters in succession are 'failed'. If any of the letters at the starting level are not seen, present preceding larger displays until a full line is seen.

Level finding/near measure for linear displays. With a 'now I've got some teeny-weeny ones,'

---

11   Pointing is discussed in the section headed Rationale and evidence base.

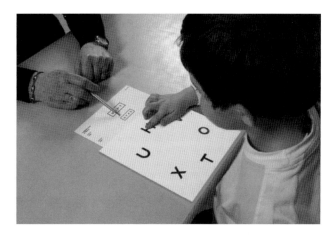

Figure 3.8 Testing linear binocular acuity (near).

place one of the near test charts on the table – side with smaller letters uppermost and facing the child;[12] slide it under the keycard – Figure 3.8. The lower crowding bar of the largest test line should be clear of the key card but the line below should not be visible. Check that the distance of the test display is 40cm from the child's eyes.[13] The mother's hand on the child's shoulder can help to maintain the correct distance. Point to the first letter 'Where's Michael's?' To level find use the first letter of alternate lines as for the distant test until the child fails or leans in to peer. Slide the key card up to display the line two sizes larger and proceed as described for the distant test showing each letter in turn etc.

Occlusion and monocular testing

Most children under 3½ years will have tired of the task before this stage is reached. Although increasingly accepted after this age, no child under 5 years of age is entirely comfortable. Assessors should choose the method that they personally find most successful – a hand, a tissue held in the hand, an eye patch, a square of micropore or occlusion spectacles. The author favours occlusion spectacles as these come in a variety of bright colours and 'choosing the colour' takes the child's mind off occlusion.

Occlude and repeat the distant and near tests first for the right eye and then for the left using the alternative booklet/chart for the right eye and the original for the left; in each instance start two lines above the respective binocular distant/near measure.

---

12   The larger displays are for visually impaired patients.
13   Use a piece of non-stretchable string with knots at 0cm and 40cm.

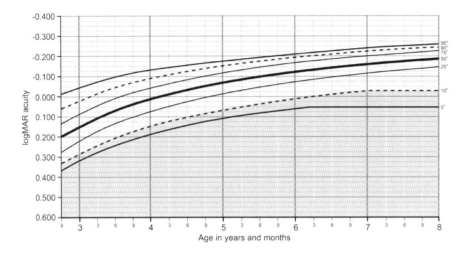

Figure 3.9 Normative curves for binocular acuity (3m).

Scoring and recording

The steps of the logMAR scale are uniform so the size of letters on adjacent lines differs by 0.1 logMAR unit (Fig 3.5). There are four letters to a line so each letter has a value of 0.025 log units. All letters correctly identified contribute to the score. Letters larger than the smallest whole line seen are assumed to be correct.[14] For example:

- All letters on display 0.275 to 0.200 are correct, two on display 0.175 to 0.100 and none on display 0.075 to 0.000 – acuity 0.150

- All letters on display 0.275 to 0.200, three on 0.175 to 0.100 and three on display 0.075 to 0.000 – acuity 0.050

The same principles apply to scoring the near chart. Methods for adjustment of logMAR scores for different test distances are available in the manual (Sonksen 2006).

Age references

Norms for binocular and monocular distant linear acuity are derived from 2,991 children representative of the population of the UK aged between 24 and 104 months (Sonksen et al. 2008) and are in the form of centile charts (similar to growth charts).

---

14   It is not practical with such young children to expect them to go through the whole of each chart.

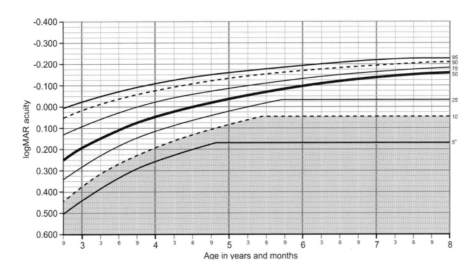

Figure 3.10 Normative curves for monocular acuity (3m).

Children above the 90th centiles have 'exceptionally' good vision with respect to the majority and are not of clinical concern, whereas those below the 10th centile have 'exceptionally' poor vision and are the subset that will contain most of the children in need of specialist eye services.

The norms for binocular and monocular linear distant measures are illustrated in Figures 3.9 and 3.10, respectively.

Visual acuity is shown on the left-hand vertical axis, age along the horizontal axis and designation of the centile curves on the right-hand vertical axis. Visual acuity improves from the bottom to the top of the chart; thus logMAR scores with a negative sign indicate the best levels of visual acuity. The area under the 10th centile is shaded mid-grey to assist clinicians in identifying the 10% of children with the poorest visual acuities for age. The point of intersection of a horizontal line from the logMAR score with a vertical from the age in years pinpoints the position of an individual (or group) score relative to that of children in the general population. For example the binocular linear visual acuity (Fig 3.9) of a child scoring logMAR 0.100 (6/7.5, 20/25) at age

• 2 years 11 months would be better than average (75th centile)

• 3 years 4 months would be average (just below 50th centile)

• 6 years 3 months would be in the 'exceptionally' poor range (below the 5th centile).

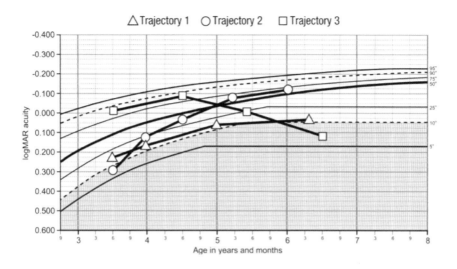

Figure 3.11 Plotting and interpreting changes over time.

Binocular vision tends to be better than monocular vision at all ages and this is likely to reflect binocular summation. Binocular acuity for single letters is significantly better than for linear arrays under 5 years with the difference increasing with decreasing age, being maximal – approximately 0.150 log units (six letters/one and a half lines) for the 50th centile – at 2 years 9 months. This emphasizes the pitfall of equating single optotype measures in the under-fives with their linear counterpart and that the primary purpose of the singles booklet is level finding. However, if a linear measure is not practicable, a binocular singles measure should be interpreted using the binocular singles centile chart. Always aim for a linear measure.

Plotting acuities on the centile charts over time[15] assists the clinician to better evaluate the significance of change in acuity measures. For example in Figure 3.11 acuity measures in child A (triangles) improve at each visit; he is in fact following his own centile, i.e. his vision is making expected developmental progress; were he undergoing ophthalmic treatment the improvement could not confidently be attributed to it, although in the past it probably would have been.

In contrast child B (circles) is crossing centiles upwards at each visit and one can estimate

---

15   Within the limitations of cross-sectional as opposed to longitudinal data.

the treatment response in log units by dropping a vertical from subsequent measures to the projected developmental centile. Child C (squares) initially follows her own centile, but at the third visit her acuity has fallen back to the original level. Although, still in the normal range the clinician is alerted to a fall from just under the 90th to the 25th centile that should raise his index of concern; almost certainly in the past the actual measures would not have done so. Plot actual measurements and be alert to crossing centiles – in either direction.

Rationale and evidence base

Linear measures. Linear rather than single optotype/letter tests are essential because single optotype measures frequently overestimate acuity by one, two or more lines and thus falsely reassure (high false negative rate/low sensitivity); they also tend to miss strabismic amblyopia. Our team's research and experience suggests that a distant linear test is more productive than a near linear test in picking up refractive abnormalities (Jayatunga et al. 1995). In addition the proportion of preschool children accepting a patch and achieving monocular measures is significantly higher once they are fully conversant with the test task and have completed a binocular linear measure; this effect is most marked in those under 42 months (Salt et al. 1995, 2007).

Binocular before monocular testing. Large epidemiological surveys in the seventies and eighties found that acuity was normal in the better eye in only 1–2% of children without strabismus who had two or more lines difference in acuity, suggesting that little reliability is lost by testing children without strabismus binocularly (Alberman et al. 1971, Peckham 1986).[16] More recent studies support this hypothesis (Hodes et al. 1994, Jayatunga et al. 1995). As discussed earlier in the chapter, examination for strabismus is an important aspect of developmental overview and when suspected or identified requires referral to a paediatric eye team in its own right.

Pointing. There is ongoing debate about the effect of using a pointer when testing. Some clinicians feel that 'pointing' helps amblyopic eyes to fixate better and thus decreases the likelihood of detecting amblyopia early; however evidence based studies are lacking. The SonkLT includes a slim line black pointer because the author feels the developmental case for pointing in preschool children is sound. One of the first objectives of teaching a child to read is to impart understanding of the systematic way words are arranged on a page – from left to right and top to bottom (Western societies). To demonstrate this parents and teachers point to each word in turn. Only a few children under 4½ years will have acquired this concept so the main aim of pointing is to ensure that the child is sure which letter the examiner wishes him to match next; it also helps to draw any 'wandering' of his attention back to the task.

---

16   These studies also highlight the importance of identifying and referring children with squints for an expert opinion.

The proportion of preschool children who 'give up' quickly when the linear test cards are presented increases considerably if the assessor does not point. Consequently, a 'non-pointing' assessor is left with no way of knowing whether the measure obtained truly reflects the limit of the child's vision or is an underestimate because he is confused about what he is supposed to do. The pointer is held vertically, directly above or below the target letter and should not impinge on the crowding bar (see Fig 3.6). Encroaching on or over the crowding bar alters the optical properties of the stimulus and introduces errors in measurement.

Despite great advances in testing the special senses in young children, particularly visual acuity, major methodological issues persist.

Eye movements

The development of eye movement control takes place in parallel to the development of acuity. Term babies exhibit a full range of horizontal and vertical eye movements when inspecting their surroundings; these are concomitant most of the time. The range of horizontal or vertical following movements are full if interest in the target can be sustained for long enough – interest is usually brief in the newborn baby. Saccades tend to be jerky and to overshoot the target. Movement of the eyes to fixate a target introduced into a peripheral field of vision (fixation shift) can be elicited in some newborn babies. Frequency of use, concomitance and smoothness of movement gradually improve so that by 4 months of age control of these categories of movement is smooth and proficient. Convergence on near targets is present to a limited degree in some newborn babies and should be strong and symmetrical by 4½ months of age. Power of accommodation is limited at birth with a relatively fixed focal length for the first 6 to 8 weeks of 20 to 30cm.

Examination

First observe and note the developmental aspects of eye movement control in spontaneous looking behaviour, fixation shift behaviour, following behaviour and finally convergence. Each of these behaviours needs to be elicited in turn as they form separate sequences. These observations also form part of the examination to detect strabismus and eye movement disorders – discussed later.

In order to achieve a natural flow in babies under 5 months examination of eye movements is often done as an extension of fixation on the examiner's face in those less than 10 weeks and on the 12.5cm dangling ball in those of 12 weeks and over. When carried out in this order it is important to make sure that the NDV aspect (fixation) is noted before examining eye movements. Each aspect is better looked at separately from 5 months to avoid interrupting the flow of presentation and observation of NDV items on a table-top.

Spontaneous looking behaviour

When a baby is looking around her surroundings observe (1) eye movements (in horizontal, vertical and other plains) and (2) different positions of gaze, noting range, concomitance and symmetry of pupillary light reflexes.

Fixation shift

Ask the parent to cradle her under 5-month baby and to entice him to gaze at her face; assessor then introduces her face (smiling and silently expressive) into the periphery of the baby's field of vision. In an older baby obtain fixation on a toy positioned directly in front of him, then introduce a novel lure (e.g. an 'Oogly' translucent monster figure) on a pen torch at about 55° first to one side and then to the other. Observe the child's eye movements.

Endpoint: a shift of fixation to the examiner's face/the new target.

Age guidelines: 4 weeks; 8 weeks. The movement should be brisk and accurate by 18 weeks

Following behaviour

Babies of 6 weeks or less lie supine along the assessor's arms; those from 6 to about 14 weeks on a changing mattress; those with effortless head control and older children sit on their parent's lap/own chair. The examiner's face is the lure under 10 weeks and a 12.5cm spinning woolly ball thereafter. Once baby fixates the lure observe the range and quality of first horizontal and then vertical following movements. It is often difficult to hold interest in the same lure for long enough to evaluate all directions and aspects of following behaviours. The lure can be changed as often as necessary (e.g. to a glove puppet or a flashing toy) to regain visual interest. Babies and young children tend to turn their heads as well as their eyes and tend to 'freeze' or become distressed if their heads are restrained; so to obtain full horizontal gaze the excursion of the lure frequently needs to be more than 120° from forward.

Endpoint: Full range of following movements in both directions.

Age guidelines: Following a face 4 weeks; 8 weeks – horizontal and vertical following should be full range. Saccades may be jerky with overshoot and only briefly sustained; by 18 weeks they should be smooth in both directions.

Table 3.3 Testing vision and visual behaviour

Test	Average age (wks)	Age for AC (wks)	Timespan
[a]Turn to diffuse light	1	2	
[a]Fix face	2	4	
Fixation shift	4	8	
Following face ⇔⇑	4	8	
[a]Fix 12.5cm dangling	4	8	
Following 12.5cm ⇔⇑	6	12	AEAT
[a]Fix 6.25cm dangling	6	14	
Converge 12.5cm	12	18	AEAT
	(mo)	(mo)	
[a]Fix 6.25cm (stationary)	4	5	
[a]Fix 2.25cm cube	5	6	
[a][b]Fix 1.25cm (Smartie)	5½	7	
[a][b]Fix 5.5mm (saccharin)	7	8	
[a]Fix 1.25mm H/T	8½	9½	AEAT until 33mo
Sonksen logMAR Test	28	33	AEAT – use centile charts for norms

[a] Near Detection Vision (NDV); [b] items used to introduce NDV between 8 and 33 months. AC, assessor should be concerned if not present; AEAT, appropriate as every age thereafter.

⇔⇑ horizontally and vertically.

Convergence

Positioning as for following movements. Obtain fixation on a novel lure located between a third and half a metre directly in front of the baby/child and slowly bring it to 10cm from the bridge of the nose. Observe the degree and symmetry of convergence.

Endpoint: convergence movements and their symmetry[17] and sustainability.

---

17   Remember to check the symmetry of the epicanthic folds when evaluating asymmetry of convergence.

Age guidelines:

- 8 weeks – a small degree of convergence should be present though is likely to be asymmetrical and only brief

- 18 weeks – should be full and symmetrical though may still be better sustained by one eye longer than the other

- 24 weeks – should be equally well sustained by each eye

Table 3.3 summarises assessment of vision and eye movements with age guidelines and, for some items, time span of usefulness.

Detection of strabismus, eye movement disorders and lid and globe pathology

Strabismus

Examination for strabismus is an essential part of developmental overview because there is a dynamic relationship between strabismus, refractive errors, amblyopia, binocularity, stereo-acuity and visual acuity; problems are all more common in children with developmental delays, disorders and disabilities. Strabismus, therefore, can reflect past, pre- or postnatal neurodevelopmental events and others can herald the onset of serious orbital or neurological pathology. Strabismus is a strong marker of unequal acuity: 21% of children with strabismus or a history of strabismus have more than one line difference in Snellen acuity whereas the incidence in those without is only 1–2%. The evaluation and treatment of strabismus in children is complex and is rightly the specialty of orthoptists and paediatric eye teams.

Manifest strabismuses are cosmetically unattractive. Recent studies have shown that the psychosocial and educational implications are wider ranging and more significant than previously perceived. Some medical and visual associations of squint are listed in Table 3.4.

Examination

The assessor will have already had opportunity to observe the child's eyes, spontaneous eye movements and light reflexes at distance. The formal examination of following movements in the developmental section will have provided ample opportunity to note any limitations of the range of eye movements, asymmetries of the light reflexes, manifest strabismuses or abnormal head postures. Review these observations and re-examine as necessary.

Table 3.4 Some medical and visual associations of strabismus

Normal	Abnormal
During the first 3 months the visual axes of many babies are occasionally and briefly not fully aligned; this is normal but should become very infrequent after 3 months and disappear by 6 months.	Constant strabismus at any age is abnormal.
When tired, some children's eyes turn slightly upwards and outwards. If symmetrical this may represent the early stage of drifting off to sleep (Bell's phenomenon) rather than a bilateral divergent strabismus of significance.	Babies who remain hypermetropic or anisometropic after 9 months of age are at particular risk of strabismus, amblyopia and failure to develop binocular vision/defective stereo-acuity.
Alternating convergent strabismus is of little visual significance and does not prevent the development of binocularity.	Divergent strabismus is more likely to be associated with severe visual impairment and/or other neurological abnormalities than convergent strabismus.
Pseudo-strabismus due to wide epicanthic folds are of no medical or visual significance.	A unilateral convergent strabismus is commonly associated with amblyopia.

Q In the context of strabismus why was observation of full horizontal gaze stressed in the previous section?
Unless full abduction is obtained VIth nerve palsy may be missed.

Two further tests are available to the physician – Hirschberg's Test and the Cover/Uncover Test.

Light reflexes (Hirschberg Test)

Light reflexes using a pen torch at near should be formally examined in different positions of gaze. The light source should be at the same distance from the child as the observer. Large deviations will be obvious: small or latent deviations may be missed by this technique as may those that are only apparent when the child is tired or those with an accommodative component.

The Cover and the Uncover Tests

Manifest strabismus can be confirmed with the Cover Test: The child fixates a target held by the examiner. The examiner covers one eye whilst observing the other eye. If the uncovered eye shifts to take up fixation it is the one with strabismus. The test is repeated, this time covering the other eye.

A latent strabismus can be demonstrated with the Uncover Test:

The child fixates a target held by the examiner. The examiner covers one eye. With the child still fixating the target with the uncovered eye, the examiner closely observes the covered eye as he removes the cover; if that eye moves to take up fixation it has a latent strabismus. The test is repeated for the other eye.

The two aspects of the Cover/Uncover Test are done in sequence. Adults and older children obligingly maintain fixation on the target so that the examiner can focus on her observations. However, with babies and preschool children their attention is diverted to the cover every time it approaches or moves; some toddlers are disconcerted as the examiner's hand approaches their face. It is therefore a waste of time to get the child fixating the target and then introduce the cover, as he will immediately look at the cover and try to grab it or push it away. Performing the test in the following stages is likely to be more successful:

- Proffer the cover and let the child handle it if they wish

- Say 'I'm going to hold it up here' and gently move it to his forehead level above one eye, stabilising its position in relation to his forehead with the little finger

- Introduce the target with 'oooh look' and as he fixates it, lower the cover over the eye;[18] continue as indicated above.

The target is in direct competition for the child's visual attention with the cover/examiner's hand, so it needs to have features that can be varied by the examiner, for example an 'Oogly' on a pen torch can be switched on and off as the examiner pretends to blow it 'on' and 'off'; a glove puppet can talk and wave to the child. The examiner therefore needs to control the target in one hand and the cover in the other whilst directing most of his attention to small movements of the child's eyes. This requires slick control and timing and therefore practice. A few sessions with an orthoptist pays dividends.

Disorders of eye movement and pathology of the lids and globe

In the absence of acuity or developmental eye movement problems or strabismus, other eye or visual system pathology is unlikely in children without general medical risk factors or signs in several areas. Pathology of the lids (ptosis, blepharophimosis) or the globe (microphthalmia, anophthalmia, corneal clouding, white pupil, reflections from the pupil, one or both eyes/irises growing faster than expected) or abnormal eye movements (head thrusts, nystagmus, roving eye movements) are all hall marks of visual disorder

---

18   It is better to introduce the cover from above because the superior orbital ridge limits the child's awareness of the cover whereas the temporal field is unsheltered and movement of the cover is immediately noticed.

and should have been noted during initial observations. Several of these need priority referral to paediatric ophthalmology as assessment and treatment may be available and/ or needed urgently – ptosis (amblyopia), white or grey reflections in the pupil (retino-blastoma), rapid eye growth plus or minus photophobia/tearing (glaucoma), corneal clouding, and white pupil (cataract). The latter may not always have been noticed by the parents or observed by the examiner so doctors examining the visual system of a baby/young child for the first time should always examine the fundus and the intactness of the red reflex. This, like other intrusive medical examinations, is best undertaken after the developmental examination is complete as there is a risk of losing rapport. Abnormal eye movements suggest a neurological component. Congenital disorders of the globe, retina or optic nerves are frequently associated with central lesions that contribute to a child's visual and neurodevelopmental problems; the reverse is also common, e.g. the incidence of strabismus and significant refractive errors is high in children with CVI. Thus significant degrees of visual impairment are usually multi-factorial or 'mixed' in origin.

The following exercises may serve to put the visual examination into perspective. Answers to these exercises are provided on pages 71–72.

Exercise 1: A typical-looking 10-month-old baby girl. Setting: a developmental check

1.1 How would you examine 'acuity'? Which item would you start with? What end point would you look for? Which item would you expect her to see?

1.2 How would you look at development of eye movements? What lure would you use? What would you look for? Apart from the following movement what else might help you judge if the movements are concomitant? What might you miss if you stop before getting full abduction? What other eye movement would you want to induce? At this age would you expect it to be strong and symmetrical?

1.3 Would you look for strabismus at this point in the assessment? When you look at strabismus how will you start if the visual exam so far has been normal?

1.4 How long would you expect the visual exam to have taken?

Exercise 2: A normal-looking 35-month-old boy. Setting: a developmental check.

2.1 What test would you use to assess acuity? How would you start? What are the chances of him being able to match letters? Would you expect him to complete a binocular linear distant measure? If he succeeded, would you try a binocular linear near or monocular linear distant next and why?

2.2 Would you look at the development of eye movements and strabismus in the same or a different way to the 10-month-old?

2.3 If his binocular linear acuity was on the 25th centile, his eye movements were normal and there were no signs of strabismus or obvious eye pathology but he refused occlusion, would you refer him on to a paediatric eye clinic?

2.4 How long would you expect the visual exam to have taken?

Key Points

- Master sense for early development.

- Motor control of eyes matures more rapidly than any other motor system.

- Take parental concern about visual behaviour seriously.

- Endpoint for NDV is fixation (not poking at or pick up).

- Failure to fixate age appropriate NDV target may signify significant degree of VI.

- International standard for optotype tests of acuity – logMAR scaling.

- Sonksen logMAR test

  - Population norms available as centile charts,

  - Time spent training matching pays dividends,

  - Binocular linear test before occlusion pays dividends,

  - Do not equate single with linear measures,

  - Strive for linear measures,

  - Centile charts identify 10% with poorest acuities for age,

  - Be alert to measures crossing centiles over time,

- Examination for squint essential.

- All children with manifest squints should be referred.

- Risk of missing amblyopia by using a binocular linear acuity test is low in those without strabismus.

Answers to Exercises

Exercise 1

1.1 NDV; Smartie; Fixation from 30cm; 1.2mm white 'hundred and thousand' cake decoration

1:2 Initiate following; Dangling spinning ball, 'Oogly' on a pen torch, glove puppet, i.e. something with built-in animation to hold visual attention; *Full* range of concomitant horizontal and vertical eye movements; Light reflections; VIth nerve palsy; Convergence; Yes

1:3 No, wiser to wait until other developmental aspects are completed; Formal look at light reflexes using a pen torch in different positions of gaze; Cover/Uncover Test

1:4 2 to 2½ minutes

Exercise 2

2:1 A recognised paediatric logMAR test, e.g. The Sonksen logMAR test ; By training matching; Good 94% of 30- to 36-month-olds can do so; Good 80% can do so in this age group; Binocular near as up to 40% of this age group reject occlusion

2:2 Essentially the same way only the 35-month-old is likely to understand simple directions like 'look at my 'Oogly''; 'is the light on?'

2:3 No, the chances of a non-strabismic child having a significant monocular error is very small (1–2%)

2: 4 About 6 minutes; the median time to complete a binocular measure in this age group is just over 3 minutes – at least half of which is the time spent training matching.

References

Alberman ED, Butler NR, Sheridan MD (1971) Visual acuity of a national sample (1958 cohort) at 7 years. *Dev Med Child Neurol* 13: 9–14.

Atkinson J, Anker S, Rae S, Hughes C, Braddick O (2002) A test battery of child development for examining functional vision (ABCDEFV). *Strabismus* 10: 249–269.

Bailey IL, Lovie JE (1976) New design principles for visual acuity letter charts. *Am J Opt Physiol Optics* 53: 740–745.

Blakemore C (1991) Sensitive and vulnerable periods in the development of the visual system. *Ciba Foundation Symposia* 156: 129–147.

Cass H, Sonksen PM, McConachie HR (1994) Developmental setback in severe visual impairment. *Arch Dis Child* 70: 192–196.

Consilium Ophthalmologicum Universale (1988) Visual Functions Committee: Visual acuity measurement standard. *Ital J Ophthalmol* 11: 15.

Dutton GN, Cockburn D, McDaid G, Macdonald E (2010) Practical approaches for the management of visual problems due to cerebral visual impairment. In: Dutton GN, Bax M editors *Visual Impairments in Children Due to Damage of the Brain.* Clinics in Developmental Medicine No 186. London Mac Keith Press, Chapter 14; 217–226.

Fantz RL (1962) Pattern vision in newborn infants. *Science* 140: 296–297.

Goodale MA (2010) The functional organisation of the central visual pathways. In: Dutton GN, Bax M, editors. *Visual Impairments in Children Due to Damage of the Brain.* Clinics in Developmental Medicine No 186. London Mac Keith Press, Chapter 1; 5–19.

Hodes DT, Sonksen PM, McKee M (1994) Evaluation of the Sonksen Picture Test for detection of minor visual problems in the surveillance of preschool children *Dev Med Child Neurol* 36: 16–25.

Howard C, Firth A (2006) Is the Cardiff Acuity test effective in detecting refractive errors in children? *Optom Vis Sci* 10: 578–582.

Jayatunga R, Sonksen PM, Bhide A, Wade A (1995) Measures of acuity in primary school children; their ability to detect minor errors of vision *Dev Med Child Neurol* 37: 515–527.

Keeler Acuity Card Test (1988) Windsor, Berkshire, UK: Keeler Ltd.

McGraw PV, Winn B. (1993) Glasgow Acuity Cards: A new test for the measurement of letter acuity in children *Ophthalmol Physiol Opt* 13: 400–403.

Peckham C (1986) Vision in childhood. *Brit Med Bull* 42: 150–154.

Phillip SS, Dutton GN (2014) Identifying and characterising cerebral visual impairment in children: A review. *Clin Exp Optom* 97: 196–208.

Price DJ, Ferrer JM, Blakemore C, Kato N (1994) Postnatal development and plasticity of cortico-cortical projections from area 17 to area 18 in the cats visual cortex. *J Neurosci* 14: 2747–2762.

Salt AT, Sonksen PM, Wade A, Jayatunga R (1995) The maturation of linear acuity and compliance with the Sonksen–Silver Acuity System in young children *Dev Med Child Neurol* 37: 505–514.

Salt AP, Wade AM, Proffitt RV, Heavens SJ, Sonksen PM (2007) The Sonksen logMAR Test of visual acuity. I. Testability and reliability. *JAAPOS* 6: 589–596. Epub 2007 Jul 27.

Sharma P, Bairagi D, Sachdeva MM, Kaur K, Khokhar S, Saxena R (2003) Comparative evaluation of Teller and Cardiff Acuity cads in two-year-olds. *Indian J Ophthalmol* 51: 341–345.

Sheridan MD (1968) *The Fixed Ball Test. Manual of Instruction for STYCAR Tests of Vision.* Windsor, Berkshire, UK: NFER Publishing Company Ltd.

Snellen H (1862) Letterproeven tot repaling der guzigtascherpto. Van der Weijer, Utrecht, cited in Bennett AG (1965) Ophthalmic test types. *Brit J Physiol Opt* 22: 238–271.

Sonksen PM (1983a) Vision and early development. In: Wybar R, Taylor D, editors. *Paediatric Ophthalmology: Current Aspects.* New York: Marcel Dekker.

Sonksen PM (1983b) The assessment of 'Vision for Development' in severely visually handicapped babies. *Acta Opthalmologica* Supplement 157: 82–91.

Sonksen PM (1993) The assessment of vision in the preschool child. *Arch Dis Child* 68: 513–516.

Sonksen PM (2006) The Sonksen logMAR Test of Visual Acuity for children and adults from 2 ½ years. Instruction Manual. Novomed, UK

Sonksen PM, Dale N (2002) Visual impairment in infancy: Impact on neurodevelopmental and neurobiological processes. *Dev Med Child Neurol* 44: 782–791.

Sonksen logMAR Test. Medstore Medical, Portmarnock, County Dublin, Ireland.

Sonksen PM, Macrae AJ (1987) Vision for coloured pictures at different acuities: The Sonksen Picture Guide to visual function *Dev Med Child Neurol* 29: 337–347.

Sonksen PM, Petrie A, Drew KJ (1991) Promotion of visual development in severely visually impaired babies: Evaluation of a developmentally based programme. *Dev Med Child Neurol* 33: 320–335.

Sonksen PM, Wade AM, Proffitt RV, Heavens SJ, Salt AP (2008) The Sonksen logMAR Test of visual acuity. II. Age norms 2 years 9 months to 8 years. *JAAPOS* 1: 18–22.

Surman G, Newdick H, King A, Gallaher M, Kurinczuk JJ, Annual Report (2008) *Four Counties Database of Cerebral Palsy, Vision Loss and Hearing Loss in Children.* Oxford: National Perinatal Epidemiology Unit.

Teller DY, McDonald MA, Preston K, Sebris SL, Dobson D (1986) Assessment of visual acuity in infants and children: The acuity card procedure. *Dev Med Child Neurol* 28: 779–789.

Vervloed PJ, Ormel EA, Schiphorst SAM (2001) Measuring everyday visual discrimination in visually impaired children with the Sonksen Picture Guide to visual function. *Child: Care, Health and Dev* 27: 365–376.

Wade AM, Salt AP, Proffitt RV, Heavens SJ, Sonksen PM (2004) Likelihood-based modelling of age-related normal ranges for ordinal measurements: changes in visual acuity through early childhood. *Stat Med.* 23: 3623-3640

Woodhouse JM, Adoh TO, Oduwaiye KA et al. (1992) New acuity test for toddlers. *Ophthal Physiol Opt* 12: 249–251.

Chapter 4

Hearing

In the last decade, most nations in the developed world have introduced automated screening programmes for the identification of congenital hearing loss in newborn babies. In the UK a thoroughly researched programme – The Newborn Hearing Screening Programme – has been in place since 2006. The Automated Otoacoustic Emission (AOAE) test is complemented in babies in whom the findings are not definitive, by repeat AOAE plus or minus the Automated Auditory Brainstem Response (AABR) test (Kemp 1978, Davis et al. 1997, Wessex Universal Neonatal Hearing Screening Trial Group 1998, Bamford et al. 2005). Evaluation studies indicate that the programme is more effective in picking up children with moderately severe to profound congenital hearing loss than when community paediatricians and health visitors carry out hearing tests dependent on behavioural responses between birth and school entry. The programme is therefore an important advance but does not provide a secondary net to catch false negatives and 'not testeds', nor address identification of babies with mild/moderate losses or preschool children with developmentally significant acquired sensory or conductive losses. There is an increasing body of evidence suggesting that at least 8.5% of those who pass the neonatal screening test are found to be hearing impaired before the age of 10 years, with an average delay in diagnosis and treatment of 4.5 years: almost half of these children have profound hearing impairment (Dedhia et al. 2013). In addition to the Newborn-Hearing Screening Programme, UK parents are given a checklist of sounds which babies are expected to react to 'Reactions to Sounds', and another of sounds they are expected to make, 'Making sounds checklist', during the first 12 and 24 months, respectively. They are advised to contact their doctor or health visitor if they are concerned about their baby's hearing for referral on to the audiology clinic designated for children in their district. These checklists shift the onus for voicing concern from professional to parent and their effectiveness is yet to be fully established. Nevertheless, the bonus is that those identified benefit from early access to aids or cochlear implantation in respect of speech and language development.

One side effect of the introduction of the Newborn Hearing Screening Programme is a diminishing pool of paediatric professionals (doctors and nurses) with expertise in the assessment of hearing in the preschool age group. Indeed training of young community paediatricians and health visitors in the development of hearing behaviours and behaviourally based test techniques is in danger in the UK, despite clear guidelines specified in the RCPCH curriculum for training in Community Paediatrics … 'be able to *assess,* investigate and diagnose a broad range of developmental, visual and hearing disorders… An informed view, as opposed to an exact measure, on hearing status is an essential part of preliminary developmental examination. For example consider the preliminary examination of a 2½-year-old, whose parents are worried about her language. The professional's role is first to confirm or refute the presence of a language problem and secondly to determine which of the three core areas subserving language – sensory (hearing), cognitive (specific language or global cognition) or motor – is responsible. Without the expertise to assess the child's hearing status – normal or in the mild, moderate, severe impairment range – the preliminary examination is incomplete. Moreover the examiner is not in a position to transmit an opinion on the likely nature of the problem or to formulate a provisional investigative and treatment plan to the parents or in his referral letter to audiology – this is an unsatisfactory start to the parent–professional and interprofessional relationship. Responsibility for initiating and overseeing care lies in the campus of the developmental/community paediatrician.

Epidemiology

Recent studies suggest that Neonatal Hearing Screening Programmes are identifying approximately 1.06 neonates per 1000 live births with permanent bilateral hearing loss greater than 40dB; by 9 years the prevalence has risen by between 50% and 90% (Fortnum et al. 2001, Russ et al. 2003). Suggested reasons for the shortfall are children who slip the neonatal net, screened but not detected, impairments acquired postnatally, of late onset or progressive; the two latter probably account for the majority. The incidence of this level of hearing loss is even higher in subpopulations of children with other single or multiple disabilities, e.g. 7% of Children on the Victorian Cerebral Palsy Register (Reid et al. 2011). Otitis media with effusion (OME) refers to the presence of fluid in the middle ear without signs or symptoms of acute ear infection. OME is particularly common in the preschool years, with 50% experiencing it during their first year and 90% doing so by 5 years with a point prevalence of 15–40%. Most episodes resolve spontaneously within 3 months although 30%–40% have recurrent episodes and in up to 10% the condition becomes chronic. The effusion leads to conductive hearing loss of mild to moderate degree (<20 to 55dBHL), which in frequently recurring and chronic patients often impacts on attention control, behaviour, listening and language. Thus the pool of children developing hearing problems after the neonatal period is several times larger than that of those born with one; these children need closely linked audiological and paediatric services. Clinical practice guidelines for OME were updated by the American Academy of Paediatrics (2004).

Descriptive terminology

In clinical practice the thresholds at 500, 1000, 2000 and 4000Hz are averaged and the finding used to describe the degree of hearing loss is as follows – mild 20–39dBHL;[1] moderate 40–69dBHL; severe 70–89dBHL, profound 90 or more dBHL Hearing losses are described as *conductive* if the pathology lies in the external or middle ear, *sensorineural* (SNHL) if it lies in the inner ear or auditory pathways and *mixed* if it lies in both. Electrophysiological research is delineating a subgroup of SNHL, known as auditory neuropathy disorder/ dys-synchrony spectrum (ANDS) in which speech and language outcome is poorer than would be expected from hearing thresholds; in these children the outer hair cells of the cochlea appear to function well and the problem is hypothesised to lie in the inner hair cells or the synapses between them and the VIII nerve or in nuclei of the nerve and that disordered or desynchronized transmission may lead to disordered language development at cortical level (Starr et al. 1996, Sharma et al. 2011).

Neurological substrate

Sounds are conveyed by the auditory nerve from the cochlea to the contralateral primary auditory cortex and planum temporale for initial acoustic and acoustic-phonological processing (Friederici 2011). The arrangement of cells along the basilar membrane of the cochlea and in the primary auditory cortex of the superior temporal lobe is tonotopic, i.e. organised by frequency. The speed of conduction from the cochlea and speed of initial acoustic and acoustic-phonological processing increase rapidly between birth and 15 to 24 months. The messages are transferred on for further processing to the rudimentary temporo-frontal language network. To be effective the systems need to become high speed, selective and integrated with attentional, cognitive, language, memory and motor areas and with those from the other senses. This highly complex connectivity process continues throughout childhood into adolescence, and although research is rapidly advancing understanding of the genetic and neurological basis of syndromic and non-syndromic sensorineural disorders of hearing, there is much left to be unravelled.

---

1   dBHL – decibels of hearing loss

Role of hearing in early development

Hearing like vision is a major input sense for many aspects of development, subserving communication, language, speech, musical skills, sound recognition and sound location, which in turn foster attentional, cognitive and emotional development and self-confidence. Language development is better in babies with bilateral hearing loss greater than 40dB who are diagnosed and given intervention before rather than after 6 months of age (Yoshinaga-Itano et al. 1998). The impact of hearing impairment, although major, is not as obvious to parents or professionals as that of visual impairment during the first year, as the influence of hearing on manipulative, gross motor, non-symbolic cognition, non-spoken symbolic and social communicative development is relatively small and its influence on spoken language development, although accumulating from birth at neurological level, is effectively hidden at behavioural level until 10 to 15 months when it typically crystallises out as comprehension of key words. Hearing loss has to be in the severe range before difficulties with recognition of everyday sounds and location of sound becomes apparent, because most sound-making toys and everyday environmental sounds – dog barking, door shutting, vacuum cleaner, phone ringing – are loud (>60dB). Although a parent's gentle vocalisations may not be audible to a baby with a moderate loss, the development of 'two-way proto-conversations' is not noticeably disrupted; at neurological level the baby accesses and processes all the other communicative facets (facial expression, mouth movements, eye expression, warm embrace) of her communication and as vocalisation is an inherent part of the baby's responsive network the response includes vocalisation. Differences in vowel and consonant–vowel vocalisations between normally hearing babies and babies with hearing impairment, even at 8 or 10 months, are usually too subtle to be detected by parents or professionals. If hearing loss is severe, situational phrases such as 'row, row, row the boat?' appear to be understood because the baby assimilates the carer's contextual clues, e.g. rocking movements and facial expression. If hearing loss is mild to moderate the rhythm and intonation of the vowel sounds becomes sufficiently familiar to provide understanding: at any level of voicing vowel sounds are louder than consonants by up to 30dB. For all these reasons it seems common sense not just to flag up hearing as an important consideration of preliminary paediatric examination but to actively explore it.

Assessment

History

The primary developmental and medical histories will flag up whether the parents have or have ever had any concerns about hearing, and whether there are any risk factors for neurodevelopmental problems or deafness in childhood in the family. One should not assume the referrer has adequately covered these; the following case history reveals one such lapse.

The question in 3-year-old Susan's referral letter was 'Susan has global learning difficulties but is she also autistic?' My umbrella primary medical question for pregnancy 'Were you well throughout pregnancy – no fevers, rashes, illnesses, hospitalisations, medicines … etc?' received the response 'I had German measles at about 10 weeks ….' There had been no mention of this event in the referral letter. Susan's only problem was severe sensorineural hearing loss resulting from her mother's rubella infection.

Secondary developmental history

First 24 months. A history of typical two-way vocalisations and spontaneous babble and of comprehension or even use of situational phrases does not exclude hearing loss; one of delay in their emergence is more likely to be part of global delay and one of disordered sound content (with or without oromotor signs) of neuromotor disorder. Similarly, a history of startling to very loud noises, such as doors slamming, does not inform about 'hearing for speech'; indeed it does not even exclude severe or profound hearing loss as such sounds generate vibration in the physical surroundings. Looking up when called is typically well established by the second half of the first year; however, a positive response does not necessarily rule out mild to moderate loss as children learn their names as they hear them and parents and carers subconsciously raise their voices to levels that induce a response. Thus, in the context of detecting a hearing loss or establishing that hearing is normal a history of early vocalisations is fraught with interpretive hazards. However, listening to and thinking about a child's vocalisations during the assessment can bring rewards.[2]

Over 24 months. A history of delay in both aspects of spoken language development should always flag up 'Hearing?' as well as specific language disorder, global learning or communication difficulties. One of delay in expressive language but normal comprehension is more likely to be due to a specific expressive language delay/disorder than a problem with hearing; comprehension is usually more delayed than expressive language in the presence of hearing losses from mild to profound degree, though the magnitude of the discrepancy is usually only 2 to 4 months (see Chapter 1, Thinking in Profiles). The examiner's index of concern for hearing impairment should rise to parental comments like 'I know he's not deaf but….' and to replies such as 'when he wants to' or 'sometimes' to questions like 'does he fetch his car/ball when you ask?' For one age group these replies might reflect normality.

---

2   A 2-year-old boy, referred as possibly globally delayed, was being assessed. He was composed and cooperative, looking at the speaker and smiling communicatively; as he relaxed he started to vocalise in strings of mainly vowel sounds. However, the sounds he made were guttural and the intonation was German. It transpired that his nanny was German and his parents were frequently abroad. His language was delayed by a combination of moderate high-frequency hearing loss and mixed language background.

> Q Normality of which aspect of development for which age group?
> *From 18 to 30 months these replies might reflect age-appropriate levels of attention control and behavioural independence – see Chapter 2.*

> Q How would your thinking differ if the child were above this age range?
> *A sensory impairment is likely; one of hearing is the most common reason for a child to fail to move on to the next stage of attention control and of behavioural development – see Chapter 2.*

It is important to keep in mind that parental and professional concerns about behaviour may have a hearing problem underpinning them. For example

- Johnny, a 23-month-old referred for global developmental or language delay. When replying to probes about language his mother suddenly said quite vehemently '… and he's so rude doctor.' Surprised, I asked 'In what way is he rude?' 'Yesterday evening while I was talking to my Mum on the phone, he stood there and put his hand over his ear and went like this…' she made exaggerated mouth and smiling facial grimaces. 'When I shouted and waved my arms angrily he just laughed and danced around'

> Q What could be the reason for Johnny's responses?
> *Not as rudeness because this age group aren't intentionally rude. My immediate thought was 'perhaps he is deaf'.*

Johnny was severely deaf. Initially he was showing age-appropriate symbolic/domestic play; as he couldn't hear his mother talking it would be natural for him to voicelessly mouth and copy her facial expressions. Her shouts of anger even if just audible would lack any cadences of anger and her waving arms would excite him to join in what seemed to him a fun situation. An explanation was all that was needed to restore harmony between mother and son.

> Nicholas, a 6-year-old, was referred for behavioural problems and inattention at school possibly secondary to problems in the home. His mother genuinely seemed puzzled as to why she had been referred because she found Nicholas responsive and well behaved at home; she felt his language development had been normal and she had never been concerned about hearing. The school reported that Nicholas daydreamed in class and when asked a question would give a cheeky answer unrelated to the question, which made all the other children laugh and disrupted the class. During cognitive and language testing he interacted normally with me and performed age appropriately. As puzzled as she, I went over the history in my mind. The only thing I had noticed was that his mother had a very loud voice, so I paused the assessment to ask if there was anyone in the home with a hearing

problem. 'Yes my husband has had poor hearing and been unable to work for the last 7 years'. He was at home all day and she had become accustomed to raising her voice. Nicholas had a 35 to 40dB loss because of very chronic OME. He could hear at home and in the quiet assessment room but not in the noisy background of a classroom; when he realised that everyone was waiting for him to answer the teacher he said the first thing that came into his head. The 'clown' of the class and his family were redeemed and successfully treated, but the story might have been different if exploration of hearing status hadn't been part of my professional repertoire.

Examination

The aim of audiological clinicians is to arrive at as exact thresholds as possible, across the frequency range of speech (250 to 8000Hz), whereas that of paediatric professionals is to establish a realistic and informed estimate of hearing status, i.e. whether hearing is in the normal range or impaired and if the latter to what degree – mild, moderate, severe or profound; also whether there is a significant discrepancy between high and low frequencies.

Objective tests. Objective hearing tests require no response from the child and are the province of the audiological services, requiring expensive equipment, specialist time and expertise and sometimes sedation. The excellent programmes for screening the neonatal population (AOAEs +/− ABRs) were discussed in the first paragraph. Otoacoustic emissions and brainstem evoked responses, together with tympanometry and steady-state responses are valuable diagnostic tools throughout the preschool period but should be reserved for children with recognised hearing problems and the few whose responses to behavioural testing are not clear, e.g. are confounded by movement disorder, epileptic status, profound learning difficulty and cortical inattention.

Behavioural tests. Behavioural tests are used by both audiological and paediatric clinicians. They require a response from the child so interpretation contains an element of subjectivity. It is the essence of good test design to identify and consider the developmental factors from all developmental domains that underpin the test method. When a method covers a broad age band the effect of individual factors change as each matures. Assessors need to adjust delivery accordingly, and once experienced also accommodate the impairments of children with multiple disabilities. Therefore the description of each test method incorporates a discussion of developmental factors, how they change over time and how to adjust test delivery in the light of them.

Essentially four cognitive competencies are used in testing preschool children:

• Alerting to sound

• Location of out of sight sound sources

- Selection of pictorial or three dimensional representations of spoken noun labels

- Responding in a prearranged way to an auditory signal

In other words, general behavioural, distraction, speech discrimination and conditioned response tests, respectively.

General behavioural test

In order for attention to be captured, newborn and under 18-week babies need to be awake and content and stimuli near and dominant. During this period the clinician can use loud sounds of short duration to trigger reflex responses such as startling or turning of the eyes and head towards the source. Emerging listening behaviours can also be utilised. From about 6 weeks 'stilling' in response to sounds that continue for more than 15 seconds (musical mobile, the parent singing or the washing machine) emerges. From about 12 weeks, smiling, excited movements or vocalisations to unseen familiar sounds of mild-moderate intensity (parental voice, own musical toy) appear and reflect an early cognitive ability: recognition of a familiar sound. Actually, quieter levels of sound are responded to throughout this period, by stirring from light sleep: so *don't waste a sleeping baby!* Rouse the baby to light sleep by gently rubbing her sternum; as she begins to sink back make as quiet a sound as possible, using your voice, a soft squeaker or by stroking the bristles of a baby hairbrush gently, close to one ear;[3] watch for re-arousal and repeat for the other ear as she starts to sink back again.

The distraction test

This method could be referred to as the 'attraction test' because the assessor's task is to *attract* a baby/toddler's attention to a minimal sound stimulus delivered at a moment when his attention to anything else is minimal, rather than to *distract* him from something that is currently absorbing his interest. The two most critical skills required are the ability to (1) capture then fade a baby's attention and (2) judge the moment of maximum fade and deliver the test stimulus at that precise moment, i.e. before the baby switches his attention to something new.

Traditionally, the distraction test requires two professionals – a distracter and a sound maker who work together as a team. The distracter is responsible for capturing and fading the baby's attention and sound maker for judging the moment of maximum fade so the test stimulus is perfectly timed. Much of the literature suggests that the distracter's role is more difficult but judging the moment of maximum fade from behind is equally so.

---

3   Taking care not to create a tactile stimulus such as a puff of air.

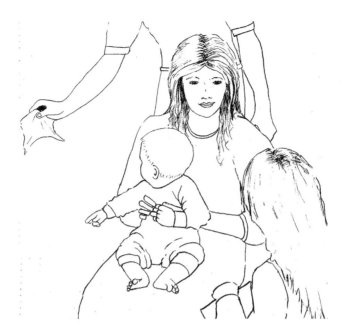

Figure 4.1 Baby responds to novel soft sound as he is not listening to adult's conversation.

During the first 4 months the templates and connectivity underlying the eye and head turning response to locate sounds made out of sight are established and integrated at neurological level. The main domains involved in this networking are hearing, vision, cognition, attention, behaviour and motor (visual and systemic).

Listening behaviours
Sphere of listening attention. The sphere of listening attention is a third to half a metre at birth; by 4 months (the age of introduction of the distraction test) it has reached two-thirds of a metre, and by 6 months 1m

Q The recommended test distance for testing 4- to 6-month-olds is two-thirds of a metre. Why is this?
To avoid interpretative confusion between hearing loss and normal levels of development of sphere of attention.

Selective listening. Newborn babies selectively listen to sounds as they become meaningful, e.g. parent's voices, splash of milk in their bottle, musical mobile over their cot.

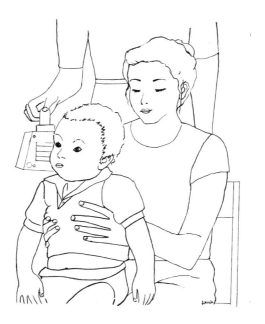

Figure 4.2 Thirteen-month-old puzzled by unfamiliar quality of sound and reverts to earlier level of response – stilling rather than brisk head turn.

Initially these sounds are experienced in a multisensory context. Once meaningful, babies select the sound from other ambient sounds and attend to it even when it is out of sight, evinced first by stilling and later by smiling and excited movements and finally by active looking/turning towards the source. The ability to selectively listen gives us the capacity both to select and attend to voices and sounds of interest that are softer than the ambient noise level and to establish hearing status in rooms that are not sound proofed! The 8-month-old in Figure 4.1 has turned to the test sound even though his mother and the specialist nurse are deep in conversation; their conversation (level of voicing 25 to 55dB) is not meaningful to him so he is not listening and is 'ready' to respond to softer, and to him more interesting sounds. Testing hearing in such circumstances is not recommended.

Familiarity. The level of response is higher throughout the first 18 months to sounds that are familiar, so it is important that test sounds have an everyday quality and are not totally outside the baby's experience. Strange qualities of sound may cause babies to respond at levels typical of a younger age. The baby in Figure 4.2 is 13 months; he stills and looks confused to the (to him) 'strange' sound emanating from the pure tone audiometer with no attempt to locate it; however, he briskly located the test rattle in all horizontal planes and above and behind his head. This showed he was neither developmentally delayed nor hearing impaired.

In recent times babies are exposed to more 'bleeping' sounds in the home such as televisions, mobile phones, digital cookers, washing machines, and laptops, and once they have understood simple cause and effect these sounds become interesting rather than strange. However, exposure does not always lead to arousal of interest; babies hospitalised for long periods are exposed to the constant 'bleeping' of hospital monitors that they perceive as meaningless background noise and therefore ignore. Unlike the 13-month-old in Figure 4.2, they may not even still to pure tones used to test their hearing.

Practice Point In the setting of a distraction test of hearing be alert to both the possibility of over or under familiarity of an individual baby to the test sounds. Warble tones have a less 'strange' quality and arouse greater interest in babies and toddlers than pure tones and hand-held audiometers are commercially available.

Ambient noise. Ambient noise levels in a carpeted paediatric clinic room will be 55 or more decibels. On the whole neither adults nor babies selectively listen to background environmental noise; therefore, unless ambient levels are intrusively loud or of an unusual character, meaningful and novel sounds of a *lower* decibel level are selected out by babies of 6 months and over.

Practice Points

(1) The position of the test sound in a distraction test (see below) is equidistant from the parent's, the sound maker's and the baby's ears, so 'if the sound maker and the parent can hear and select out the test sound so should the baby'.

(2) One reason that the statistical productivity of distraction test screening proved unsatisfactory was that assessors too freely explained a baby's failure away on ambient noise, i.e. the baby was given the benefit of doubt rather than being recalled for re-testing.

Vision/cognition
The visual domain plays a major tutoring role in establishing the cognitive foundation of the response. Babies can hear quiet sounds from birth. They look towards quiet sounds emanating from sources within their field of vision such as their mother's voice while she coos smilingly to them, i.e. when the sound is part of a global sensory experience that includes visual information. However, sounds made outside the field of vision need to be loud (50 to 75dB) to trigger a reflex turn of eyes and head to the side of the sound resulting in visual fixation of the source (Figs 4.3a and 4.3b).

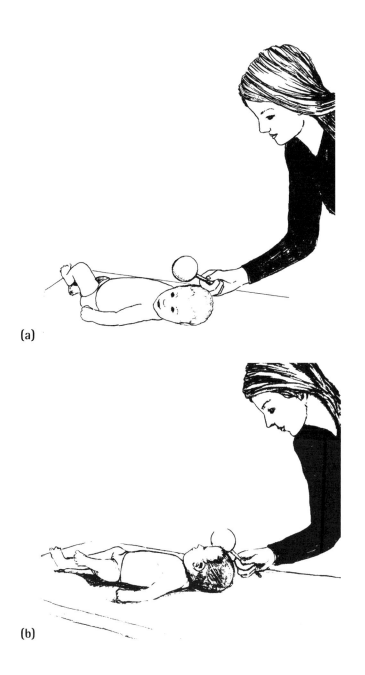

(a)

(b)

Figure 4.3a and 4.3b Reflex eye and head-turning response to loud sound, made out of sight to either side, at 6 weeks.

Practice Point From 3 to 4 months many babies still or look animated to mother's gentle vocalisations made out of sight, demonstrating that they hear and recognise her voice and that it is the reflex that requires a louder sound.

At neurological level the visual components from both types of experience inform the following cognitive templates:

• The permanence of sound-making objects, i.e. that sounds come from substantive sources

• The location of the sound source relative to self – where it is

• The nature of the sound source – what it is

By 16 to 18 weeks a basic cortically mediated circuit is in place for babies to actively turn to loud and soft sounds. However, two factors impact on test delivery: (1) processing time is slow at 4 months; it rapidly increases over the next 2 months; (2) 4-month-olds can only locate sounds when the source is at ear level. Over the next 6 months they perfect location of sound to each side above and below ear level. The tutoring role of vision is again clear. Initially, babies still and listen to sounds made in these positions; between 7 and 9 months, their eyes and head turn horizontally to the side of the sound and catching sight of the source in their peripheral vision they then shift their gaze up or down to it; the response is in two clear stages – two-stage response. By 10 months the movement of head and eyes is direct to target – one-stage response (see Fig 4.4).

Practice Point From 4 to 6 months babies need time to alert and assimilate the auditory input and to organise their motor response. Allow 2 seconds for each stage (2 seconds for alerting + 4 seconds of silence for processing and motor organisation) before moving the sound source. Moving the sound source to the other side quickly results not in turning but a bemused expression on the baby's face. As transmission and processing speed up responses become brisker. They should be brisk by 6½ to 7 months.

As location in different horizontal planes develops over many months the wise assessor takes care to always position the sound source at ear level irrespective of the child's age. This is because when a 10-month-old fails to turn to a test sound made above ear level the assessor doesn't know whether the failure is due to poor hearing or delayed cognition.

Although we use sound locating ability to test hearing it is a visually dependent cognitive skill with its own developmental sequence.

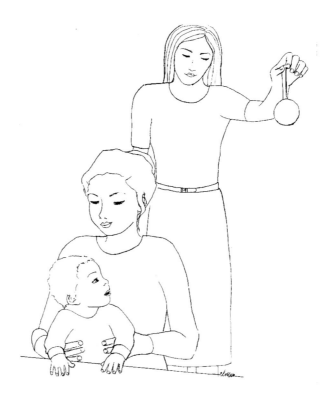

Figure 4.4 Sound location one-stage response – 10-month-old looks straight up to the rattle.

Practice Point Babies with light perception or less vision show the eye and head-turning reflex in the first trimester but fail to develop the active cortically mediated response in the second.

From 11 to 12 months onwards other aspects of cognition develop that increasingly render distraction testing less productive: (1) second and third presentations of test sounds are no longer novel as babies now conceptualise the whole object from its sound and can decide whether or not to ignore it; (2) they quickly become cognisant of the presence of the sound maker behind them and start looking for her.

Practice Point When either of these scenarios occurs during testing the paediatric assessor has the advantage of being able to break off the hearing test to explore another domain and then return to hearing, thus recreating an element of novelty and surprise.

Motor development
The eye and head turning response is also dependent on the developmental level and functional integrity of the visual and systemic motor systems. In typically developing children a full range of controlled eye movements is available well before 4 months of age and most babies sit stably with minimal trunk support on parent's lap by this age.

A wise assessor looks informally at eye movements, head control and trunk control during the early part of the developmental assessment and takes care to ensure that the parent gives sufficient support to counter any delay in either of the latter. This will minimize the possibility of failure to turn being due to delay in postural stability rather than failure to hear, i.e. clarifying interpretation.

Thus by 4 months the sensory – cognitive – motor connectivity is sufficient to support an active cortically mediated response to sounds made out of sight, at ear level.

Attention control and behaviour
This section puts development of attention control and behaviour into the context of testing hearing (a re-read of the appropriate section of Chapter 2 and Table 2.3 is suggested). Lack of any active control over the focus of attention during the second half of the first year leaves babies prey to every new stimulus: theoretically, perfect for distraction testing because any errors in technique, e.g. sound too loud/incorrectly timed can be resolved by repeating. However, with the emergence of control of their chosen focus of attention by actively ignoring or rejecting new stimuli from 12 months the distraction technique rapidly runs out of steam and the professional test duo increasingly fail to get a second chance.

Practice Point To a toddler the distracter's toy/lure is much more interesting than the minimal sound from a high-frequency rattle (HFR); once focused on the toy the toddler continues to attend to it by actively ignoring other stimuli including the test sound. Behaviourally she wants the toy and becomes increasingly frustrated when denied. An escalating tantrum may develop with the hearing test ending unsatisfactorily.

Distractions

Distractions in the test room of any sort are counterproductive, yet most guidelines fail to stress that visual events are more disruptive than auditory ones. This is because visual events attract and hold the attention of babies more than auditory ones. The sphere of visual attention is also wider than that of auditory attention; by 4 months the former is out to room size while the latter is still confined to a metre. Thus visual events across a room are much more likely to interfere with a hearing test than auditory ones, for example, a colleague silently opening the door and creeping across the room mouthing 'excuse me', to fetch something is much more disruptive than children talking and laughing in the corridor. Even an observer crossing their legs or turning a page of their notes will immediately steal a baby's attention. Colleagues, family and observers should be made aware of this.

Distraction lures. Distracters are rightly advised to use visual lures (e.g. glove puppet or toys that move or flash 'on the spot')[4] in order to ensure that gaze remains forward and steady. Initial presentation has high intensity in order to capture attention. However, some guidelines suggest that the distracter looks down or adopts an impassive expression and/or puts the distraction lure into their lap or behind their back. Looking down prevents the distracter from seeing the baby's response and like an impassive expression sends negative messages that puzzle some babies and cause them to withdraw. Putting the lure behind the distracter's back may excite older babies to look to each side in expectation of its reappearance, i.e. producing the opposite of fade and altering the parameters of the visual field.

Any hint of an enquiring expression or a glimmer in the distracter's eyes will alert the baby to look for something. The distracter looking towards the test source or up at sound maker may cause the baby to follow her gaze.

Practice Point Distraction lures should be presented at the baby's eye level to ensure he is looking straight ahead when the test sound is delivered – keeping all the parameters 'squared' up facilitates the distracter's and the sound maker's judgement of visual fields and test sound positioning.

In contrast, auditory test stimuli are initially presented at minimal decibel level and are of relatively brief duration, thus placing the auditory aspect at a considerable disadvan-

---

4   For example, standing animals that can be made to collapse, spinning discs, finger puppets, 'Oogly' on a pen torch etc. A 12.5cm colourful woolly ball held 3cm below eye level and thrown up *no more than 6cm* two or three times, also works well, because eye excursion is minimal in the vertical and zero in the horizontal plane; and the distracter fades attention by holding on to the caught ball after a prearranged number of throws.

tage in terms of attracting attention. Obviously some developmental thinking needs to be applied to the situation.

Practice Point The most effective way to reduce this 'disadvantage' is for the distracter to use the same sound as the test stimulus. For example an HFR is visually not as attractive as a glove puppet, but when shaken at moderate intensity is sufficiently attractive to capture attention and then, by ceasing the sound and shaking motion, to fade it; a perfect state for recapturing attention with the same sound introduced (1) at the moment of maximum fade but before attention is taken by anything else; (2) at test intensity; and (3) out of sight to one or other side.

This technique can be managed in two ways; either the distracter manages capture and fade and the sound maker re-attraction or the sound maker manages all three. Figures 4.5a, b and c show the sound maker managing capture, fade and re-attraction in a baby 'who wants' everything he sees. Six weeks earlier the sound maker would not have needed to give him the rattle but simply have stilled it to induce fade – a great technique when both members of the duo are not available. When the distracter is present the method can also be used to test hearing for low frequency sound (humming) and speech sounds; for example the distracter hums the toddler's favourite tune and as she pauses the sound maker continues it.

Properties of sound

Intensity

As we have seen, loud sounds to one side trigger a reflex response in the first trimester that tutors sound localising ability. In contrast the lifelong startle reaction to sudden very loud sounds does not contribute to this learning process.

Practice Point As mentioned earlier this reflex can be used clinically to exclude severe and profound hearing loss during the first 4 months. Test sounds should be of minimal intensity from 4 months.

Duration

In the first 6 months sounds of less than 2 seconds duration may not gain a baby's attention.

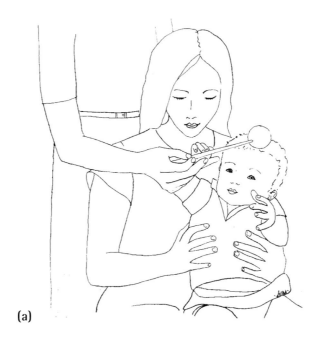

(a)

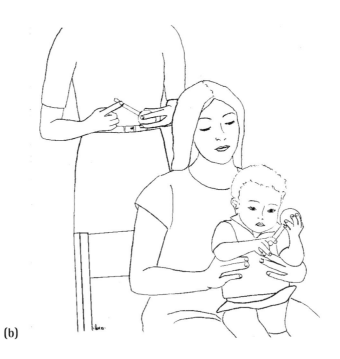

(b)

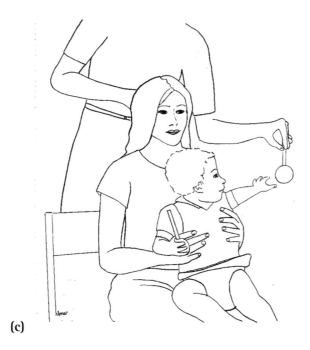

(c)

Figure 4.5a, b, and c Two of a kind technique (baby at level of attention control when he 'wants' every new stimulus) – reaching eagerly for rattle → interest fading → alerts immediately to same sound made to other side.

Practice Point Test sounds should therefore be of at least 2 seconds duration during the first 6 months and at least 1 second thereafter.

Test sounds

As we have seen it is important that test sounds have an everyday quality, endure for at least 1 second (2 seconds between 4 and 6 months) and feature voiced/speech sounds; the latter because hearing for a full range of speech sounds is so critical to development of the language template during the first 15 months.

Warble tones
Technical equipment such as warble tone generators provide a choice of five frequency bands with switches that control intensity and duration; the intensity switch is calibrated so that the reading reflects the level of sound reaching the ear when operated at standard test distance.

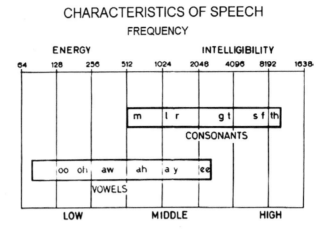

Figure 4.6 Characteristics of speech sounds.

Specialised rattles
Toy rattles should *never* be used as they produce white noise with some elements at very high intensity even when shaken gently and thus provide no information on frequency and only exclude very severe degrees of deafness. HFRs are available; when shaken minimally/maximally at standard test distance sound reaches the ear at 15 to 20db and 60 to 70dB, respectively. Assessors should familiarise themselves with the manufacturers specifications and instructions etc. The sound maker controls the duration of the test sound.

Speech sounds
The frequency range of human speech is approximately 128 to 8000Hz. Vowel sounds fall into the low and lower-middle and consonants into the middle and high-frequency bands. Speech phonemes at the same level of voicing vary in both intensity and duration; the intensity by up to 30dB and the duration from milliseconds for the high-frequency consonants, e.g. 'p', to as long as a speaker can sustain expiration for some vowels, e.g. 'aaah'. When the word 'thaw' is spoken the 'th' will not only be 30dB quieter than the 'aw' at all levels of voicing but of much briefer duration. Figure 4.6 shows the relative intensities of speech phonemes and illustrates why the low-frequency vowel sounds provide the carrying power and the consonants the intelligibility of speech while highlighting the plight of an individual with a high-frequency loss struggling to make sense of a series of vowel sounds.

Practice Point High-frequency phonemes such as 't', 'f', 'th' are very brief and therefore need to be repeated several times in quick succession. It is hard however, to speak these phonemes without adding 'er' after the consonant (e.g. 'ter', 'ter',

'ter' or 'fer', 'fer', 'fer)'; 'er' is low to mid frequency, louder than the high-frequency component and smothers the attempt to test the latter. The high-frequency components are more effectively isolated if prefixed by a voiceless 'i' e.g. '(i)t', '(i)t', '(i)t' or '(i)f', '(i)f', '(i)f.

Particular caution needs to be taken with the high-frequency phoneme 's' as, unlike the others it can be extended to 'sssss…'. (forced SSSS), which tends to be both louder and cover a wider range of frequencies than prefixing 's' with a voiceless 'i' – '(i)s', '(i)s', '(i)s'.

As mentioned earlier, duration is not a problem for low-frequency phonemes such as 'oooh', 'aaah' and 'aw'; humming with the lips shut is an alternative way of producing low frequencies. However, when produced quietly and steadily both have a slightly strange droning quality with the result that babies are more likely to revert to stilling and listening than actively turn. Unfortunately, adding interesting intonation to either method – a 'what's this' or 'jolly' intonation to 'oooh', or humming the baby's favourite tune is difficult without see-sawing the decibel level.

The 'two of a kind' technique increases the success rate of both methods: the distracter attracts attention with a conversationally voiced, interestingly intonated 'oooh' or hum; the distracter stops and the sound maker continues at test intensity. .

Practice Point Production of voiced sounds at minimal test intensity is a skill acquired and retained through practice and periodic checks of the intensity reaching the ear with a sound-level meter.[5]

Peripheral fields

When looking straight ahead the limit of the temporal fields is about 90 degrees right and left. The limit may be more like 120 degrees in children with proptosis, craniofacial dysostosis, widely spaced eyes or divergent strabismus; it also varies with the direction of gaze.

Practice Point The sound maker should check that his hands when in sound-making position (see below) do not impinge or cast shadows that impinge on the temporal field. The distracter attracts the baby's attention forwards and observes for

---

5   Sound-level meters are expensive, so practice 'in the bath': periodically check and moderate the intensity of your test sound repertoire at the district audiological centre.

directness of gaze and any voluntary or involuntary eye movements while the sound maker wiggles his fingers silently to each side in turn at the point where test sounds will be made.

The distraction test requires the assessor and parent/child duos and furniture to be re-arranged – sufficient reason to test hearing after table activities are complete. Orientate the parent's chair 'squarely'[6] in the room leaving sufficient space (at least 1½m) behind it for sound maker to operate. Place the distracter's chair a metre in front facing the parent and child's chair. The sound maker stands a quarter of a metre directly behind the parent's chair in a 'I am a uterus' (IAAU) pose[7] – upright with minimal anteflexion at the hips and with the arms abducted and minimally flexed at elbow and wrist; this places the hands in an ideal position for delivery of test sounds and allows the sound maker to remain stationary throughout.

Q What are the disadvantages of standing to one or other side?
Movement introduces additional stimuli that draw a baby's attention to the sound maker's space, e.g. footsteps, rustling clothes, wafts of perfume and shadows. Positioned behind and to one side a sound maker's head is more likely to impinge into the child's peripheral field as she needs to bend forwards to deliver speech sounds at ear level. Sound makers with back problems are better to remain directly behind the parent's chair, turn through 90° and bend forward.

Many toddlers of 18 months and over require a distraction test as their understanding of noun labels is too tenuous for use of a language-based one.

Q Would you leave him seated on a nursery chair and ask the distracter also to sit on one or ask the parent/child and distracter to sit on adult chairs – and why?
Full-size chairs are preferable because it is physically difficult for the sound maker to position the sound source at the child's ear level without impinging part of herself into his visual field when nursery furniture is used.

In order not to re-enforce the presence of the sound maker it is best if (1) the distracter continues to look at the parent/baby and speaks her interpretation in a conversational

---

6   So the chair seat is parallel to the walls of the room – this facilitates symmetrical delivery.

7   To demonstrate the relative position of female organs in the body our Professor of Anatomy adopted this pose.

voice ('yes', 'no', 'not sure/not convinced', 'possibly seen rather than heard', etc; (2) the sound maker conveys her thoughts through gesture or facial expression – thumbs up/down, oscillating hand, enquiring expression, etc.

Delivery
Delivery is summarised in Table 4.1 in two columns to emphasize the duet played by the distracter and the sound maker.

Continuation

Babies who respond at age-appropriate level to test sounds at minimal level
The duet continues with the distracter varying the lure and the sound maker varying the test sounds and the side tested (R or L) as each judge appropriate. Distracter's lures are changed as soon as their effectiveness begins to wane (effectiveness tends to wane faster with increasing age). The side of test sounds is randomised, as even 8-month-olds rapidly cognise and anticipate regular alternation. Similarly, in 'older' babies, test sounds are more likely to remain a dominant attraction if varied. A break in testing is sometimes advisable (mentioned above).

Babies who respond at less than age-appropriate level (e.g. a 10-month-old who clearly stills and listens to the test sound but does not turn)
With the benefit of findings in other domains the duo can adapt delivery and response expectation accordingly, for example if cognitively the baby functions at a 5-month level they increase the duration of the test sound, and the time allowance for processing and accept and expect the response level to be 'stilling and listening', 'alerting and smiling' or slow eye and head turning; in fact it would have been wiser of the duo to start the test with this expectation if they had already established the baby's cognitive level.

Babies who do not respond to the test sounds at minimal level
The three most likely explanations and ways to proceed are as follows:

- The baby couldn't hear the test sound. The sound maker slowly increases the intensity until the baby responds, or fails to respond at maximal intensity. The sound maker notes or subjectively estimates the decibel level at which a response occurs or the maximum intensity.[8]

- The delivery was suboptimal in some way, e.g. suboptimal management of baby's attention or of positioning and duration or intensity of the test sound. With experience, a test duo recognise and assimilate such errors as they happen and modify delivery accordingly without loss of flow.

---

8   Notes it if the stimulus is a warble tone hand held audiometer. It is sensible to practice estimating the range of decibel levels produced by other test sounds (HFR, voice, hum) regularly using a sound level meter positioned at standard test distance.

Table 4.1   Duet nature of delivery of the distraction test

The distracter	The sound maker
Explains the procedure, do's and don'ts to mother and asks her to do the following: To support baby with her hands sitting 'squarely' on her lap, about 4in. forward of her body To ignore the SM and test sounds e.g. not to • lean round to see if baby has heard the test sound, • turn and look at TS herself, • turn baby towards TS.	Unobtrusively moves behind the mother's chair with sound making equipment – HFR, +/– warble tone, own voice[a]
Picks up a visual distraction lure	**Positions self in 'IAAU' position**
Attracts baby's attention directly forwards at baby's eye level	
Fades attention	Checks that TS and shadows will be outside visual field
Re-attracts baby's attention directly forward	Picks up TS1
	Abducts the arm holding TS1
Then fades it ...	At moment of maximal fade but before spontaneous switch, introduces TS1 at minimal dB level
Continues to look at baby with the same natural expression. Why[b]	
Observes and notes level of response	**Observes and notes**
• None • Stilling and listening (<18 weeks) • Alerting and/or smiling (<18 weeks) • Slow eye and/or head turning (16 to 30 weeks) • Brisk eye and/or head turning[c] (>27 weeks)	Any movements of the head or trunk towards the side of TS1[c]
Communicate or continue	**Communicate or continue**

[a] Assessor usually takes a bell rattle, a squeaker and a clicker as sources of moderate to very loud white noise in case the baby/child does not respond to the TS and to explore the level of sound localisation once hearing status has been established. [b] So she can observe his response and not alert him to search for something. [c] If the 'older' baby is more interested in the distraction lure than the TS, the movements may be limited to a partial flick of the eyes or twitch of the head.

SM, soundmaker; TS, test sound; IAAU, "I am a uterus posture"; HFR, high-frequency rattle.

(Q) What will the distracter and the sound maker do if the test sound was made when (1) an 8-month-old was looking and playing with his toes, (2) a toddler was focused intently on and reaching towards the distracter's lure; and (3) the test sound was well above ear level?
(i) Repeat making sure test sound is made at the moment of fade and before the baby switches his attention to something else (ii) repeat using a less motivating distraction lure, or two of a kind technique (iii) repeat with the test sound at ear level.

- The baby's cognitive level is below a 20-week level. In this circumstance the duo can try to induce a behavioural response to the sound maker's voice at quiet conversational level 'hello Jamie, where am I?'

(Q) What would you do next if you saw no response and why?
Ask the mother or father to take your place and talk to him in a similar way 'Jamie, Mummy's here'; because at any cognitive level a response is more likely to occur to a familiar than unfamiliar source. Ask the parent to raise their voice to moderate levels.

(Q) If still no response how would you proceed?
Try to induce a startle response or eye and head turning reflex with a source of loud noise – e.g. clicker, drum, plastic rattle.

(Q) If a positive response is obtained to the clicker but not to a raised parental voice what would you conclude about the baby's hearing?
Both voice and clickers cover a wide frequency range so assessor cannot conclude anything about frequency, only that Jamie hears loud broadband sounds and probably not moderate-level sounds.

Practice Point   Never ask parents to 'shout' as they would find this distressing.

The earlier sections emphasize the developmental complexity of the distraction test which, once digested should give assessors the confidence to become flexible within its structured framework, i.e. to modify delivery 'en route' to a child's developmental profile, whilst strictly adhering to auditory requisites and thus arrive at a valid opinion of hearing status. Examples of delivery adaptations for children with single/multiple disabilities are discussed in Chapter 13.

Language-based tests

Language-based hearing tests (LBHTs) are governed by a child's level of verbal comprehension for noun labels. Vocabulary is usually sufficient by 21 months, though some babies as young as 15 months can be tested. LBHTs are more discriminatory in terms of hearing for speech than the distraction test and have greater capacity to highlight discrepancies between high- and low-frequency phonemes. LBHTs require only one assessor who manages the child's attention and test word delivery in a companionable interchange. Altogether, more suited to the developmental ambience of 1-, 2- and 3-year-olds than the distraction technique and therefore should be introduced as soon as noun label vocabulary is adequate. The dependence of language comprehension on hearing, however, negates the effectiveness of LBHTs in children with moderately severe hearing losses: the child fails the test but the assessor then has to delineate whether hearing or language (or both) is the culprit. In this age group language delay may be specific to the language domain or part and parcel of global developmental delay or autistic spectrum disorder. Hence when planning to use a LBHT assessors should first satisfy themselves that verbal comprehension is adequate through language history, active observation of communicative behaviour and language tests (see Chapter 8). A child's spontaneous vocabulary and level of expressive speech usually[9] reflects at least equivalent levels of comprehension.

Developmental considerations

The developmental domains involved are hearing (sufficient to discriminate the phonemes), vision (sufficient to see the material clearly), language (verbal comprehension) and manipulative (motor competence to point or pick up item). Normally all are on line by 15 months; some, for example, vocabulary, continue to increase and provide the assessor with an even more phonetically discriminatory choice of items. Similarly, the number of items from which children can select increases – from three at 13 to 18 months to five at 19 to 30 months to seven at 30 to 42 months – again giving the assessor increasing flexibility in exploration of hearing status. However, as with the distraction test, the greatest challenge for the examiner remains management of attention; the challenge is greatest between 18 and 30 months and lessens with increasing age as each level of attention control is realised. Minimally voiced (10 to 40dB) test words lack attraction or authority and do nothing to counter the assessor's already difficult job of keeping the child focused on the task.

Setting

Children of 21 months and over continue to sit at their nursery table and chair. Young-

---

9   Except in rare cases, e.g. 'party speech' or distant echolalia

er toddlers with sufficient comprehension continue to sit on the parent's lap up to an adult height table.

Characteristics of test words

When designing a hearing test the test words should

- be well within the language capacity and experience of the age group;

- each contain the same number of syllables;

- contain good phonetic discriminations between high, middle and low frequencies.

Language capacity
Names of parts of the body tend to feature prominently in the first word vocabulary. In English we are fortunate that most of the earliest also have one syllable and contain excellent phonetic discriminations. It proves harder to find suitable words amongst 'first word lists' of everyday objects. It is preferable to use parts of the body under the age of 30 months (see Table 4.2).

Number of syllables
A child with a moderate high-frequency loss may hear mainly vowel sounds (e.g. hearing 'aeroplane' as eer-oh-ai, which would stand out when grouped amongst single-syllable words such as 'car', 'bus', 'dog', 'cat', 'fish').

Phonetic discriminations
Pairs or sets of words with good consonant discriminations should have similar sounding vowels or diphthongs (gliding vowel); those with good vowel discriminations should have similar sounding consonants. Two extensively researched tests – the McCormick Toy Test (MCTT) and the English as an Additional Language Toy Test (EALTT or E2L) are in widespread use in the UK in screening 3- and 4-year-olds; the latter is an adaption of the former for children of Asian parents for whom English is not the first language (McCormick 1977, Bellman and Marcuson 1991, Bellman et al. 1996, Harries and Williamson 2000). Both are based on seven pairs of words[10] with each pair containing the same vowel or diphthong but different consonants – thus the discriminations are all of middle and high frequencies (see Table 4.3). Words used in the author's Doll and Picture tests are listed in Table 4.2, these include one or more pairs where the difference lies in the vowel or diphthong while the consonants are the same in order to explore the lower frequencies as well (see underlined vowel sounds in Table 4.2).

Ideally, a test designed in England should be valid throughout the English-speaking

---

10   Two of the pairs are common to both tests – plate/plane and shoe/spoon.

Table 4.2   Sets of words used by the author in relation to hearing loss assessment: early vocabulary for body parts, and everyday objects

Hearing level	Body parts	Pictures of everyday objects
High frequency	Teeth Feet Knee	Bus Bath Fish Dish Tree Key Three
Medium and low frequency	Eyes Nose Toes Ear Hair Hand	Ball Bell Bowl Dog Doll Duck Cup Chair Bear Horse House

world. Not so for hearing tests! Vowels and diphthongs of both assessors and testees vary enormously between member countries (national dialects), regions of the same country (regional dialects), ethnic and social class groups. A normally hearing 24-month-old in Northumberland may not recognise the words 'bus' or 'bath' as pronounced by an assessor from London, simply because his family and friends call them a 'booss' and a 'baathe'. An assessor who adopts the local pronunciation would completely shift the weight of the discrimination from high to low frequency. Overall, assessors with vowels that differ from those of the designer are better to try to acquire the latter and to introduce the test as described below in *Procedure/Practicalities*.

Q Many trainees from other countries propose to translate established hearing tests into their own language. Why should this be avoided?
The phonetic content and frequency discriminations will be totally different; the number of syllables per word is likely to vary and for cultural reasons first words may be very different.

Materials

Children respond by picking up a toy representation of the word in the MCIT and E2L or pointing to parts of a large realistic baby doll (Fig 4.7) or to a selection of A5 size realistic coloured pictures of everyday objects.

Q Why use a large doll?
To be certain that 15- to 24-month-olds recognise that the doll is representative of a baby and to facilitate clear pointing.

Table 4.3 Pairs of words in the McCormick[a] and E2L[b] Toy Tests

McCormick Toy Test	EAL Toy Test
Tree Key	Brush Bus
Shoe Spoon	Sweet Key
Cow House	Car Star
Plane Plate	Bed Egg
Horse Fork	Duck Cup
Duck Cup	Plane Plate
Man Lamb	Spoon Shoe

[a]McCormick (1977); [b]Bellman et al. (1996).

Q Why use pictures rather than toys?

Because pictures initially capture attention just as well as toys, but are less self-diverting and less playable with than toys in children in this phase of attention control. Pictures therefore facilitate the assessor's management of attention control.

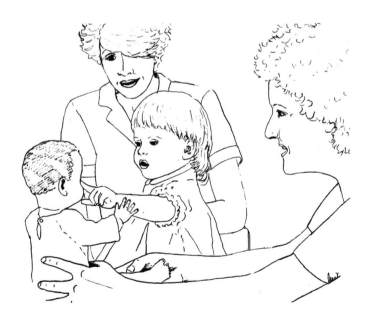

Figure 4.7 Minimal voicing: 2-year-old pointing to doll's 'nose'. Note the position of examiner relative to child's ear and shared mutual enjoyment of adults and child in the task.

Procedure and practicalities

Procedures for the MCTT and E2LTT are available in their respective test manuals. The principles outlined below relate to the Doll and Picture Tests but are generally applicable to other tests.

Position. The assessor kneels to one side of the child, with her mouth about two-thirds of a metre from the ipsilateral ear at ear level – upright kneeling for toddlers sitting on parent's lap and sitting on heels for older preschool children at a nursery table.

Note that this is the only time that sitting beside the child is advocated. The advantages of this position are that

- rapport is facilitated as the child only needs to relate to one person who is comfortably near;

- many children under 3 years are upset if the assessor's lips are covered; the position reduces the need for this as 'the child's looks forwards at the doll;

- young children are stressed by having an ear occluded, however,

  - Whenever the assessor is minimally voicing, sounds reaching the contralateral ear are too quiet to discriminate. In other words the assessor can be confident of testing the ipsilateral ear.

  - Whenever the assessor needs to increase voicing level, occlusion can be achieved by sliding her hand up so that her thumb rests over the ipsilateral occiput while her third finger gently presses the tragus to close the contralateral external auditory meatus. The amount of pressure needed is minimal because the assessor's hand can move naturally with the child's head movements – Figure 4.8.

Delivery. Unless it is already clear from earlier interaction or language tests that vocabulary is adequate, check with the parent.

- Use minimal voicing to speak test words. The words are voiced (not whispered) – with the loudest vowels peaking at 40dB. In whispering the voice box is not used, the sounds are sibilant and carry further than most people realise (only your neighbour will hear if you minimally voice 'I'm bored, let's go for a cup of coffee' though half the room will if you whisper!). Minimal voicing takes practice and needs regular 'recalibration' by checking peak decibel levels with a sound-level meter.

- The words in phonetic pairs/sets should not be delivered sequentially but separated by phonetically dissimilar ones.

- The clearest sign that a child may not have heard is turning to look at the

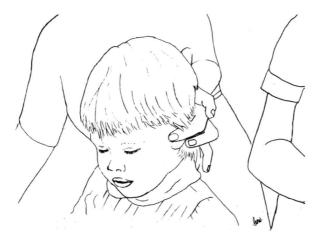

Figure 4.8 Occlusion: Examiner gently presses tragus to occlude the external auditory canal.

assessor enquiringly, although this may also happen if the word is outside his vocabulary.

- To prevent lip reading the assessor tries to direct attention back to the pictures and if this fails passes the fingers of one hand in front of his lips.

- Fiddling with the doll's clothes or gathering all the pictures together is likely to reflect loss of attention.

- Whenever the assessor suspects that a child has not heard, he should repeat the test word at increasingly loud levels of voicing (minimal, conversational, loud and very loud) until the child responds appropriately. The peak decibel level can be checked with a sound-level meter.

- To test the contralateral ear the assessor moves to the other side of the child.

Body Parts. Hold the doll in front of the child and in a moderately loud voice say 'Here's dolly, where's dolly's *hair*?' As the child points use minimal voice to say 'and her *eyes*' As she points '…. and her *feet* …etc.

Q Why should the assessor not acknowledge the child's success?
Because of the level of attention control of 18- to 36-month-olds – having gained attention keep it!

- 'Kiss' is early vocabulary and a good high-frequency word, so the test can be finished with a minimally voiced 'give dolly a kiss'.

Q If she gives the assessor a kiss, would you pass her?
  Of course – it's a hearing not a language test.

Pictures. Select an age-appropriate number of test pictures (mentioned above); in general using the following five: 'bus', 'bath', ' ball', 'dog' and 'doll' as a baseline test.

- As each picture is placed on the table ask 'what's this?' in a *conversational* voice. If his vowels are not 'standard', say 'Yes, I call it a 'bus', shall we call it a 'bus' today?' Most children nod their agreement. Once all are placed double check that he understands your pronunciation in a clear voice.

- Pictures should be placed in a line taking care that members of a phonetic pair/set are not placed next to each other.

- If necessary draw the child's attention forwards by tapping the table and in a *clear* voice say 'Show me/where's the *ball?*'

- As the child points use *minimal* voice to say 'and the *bath*'

- As he points '…. and the doll'

- … etc (repeating 'ball' at some point)

- Make sure phonetic pairs are *not* named in sequence

- Add or substitute pictures as the findings indicate. For example if a child doesn't discriminate 'bus'/'bath' add or substitute another high-frequency pair, e.g. 'tree'/'key'.

Having tested one ear, present *either* the basic test pictures *or* body parts on the picture of the doll, from the other side. The latter is preferable as children in this age group tend to get bored if they are asked to repeat with the same material.

Q You have tested verbal comprehension of a 2-year 11-month-old and his vocabulary is not sufficient for you to use a language-based hearing test. What alternative test methods are available to you?
  The 'distraction test' or free field audiometry.

Q On what would you base your choice?
  On his level of non-symbolic cognition (see below).

Free field pure tone audiometry

Free field pure tone audiometers are expensive and too heavy to be used in a peripatetic way. Nevertheless, specialist paediatricians will find this method useful in establishing hearing status in children with neurodevelopmental disorders and sensory impairments. Frequency ranges from 250 to 4000 or 6000Hz (250, 500, 1000, 2000, 4000, 6000) and intensity from 20 to 80 or 90dB.

Developmental considerations

Free field audiometry requires the testee to respond in a prearranged way to a signal made by the assessor – loosely referred to as 'conditioned'. Strictly, a conditioned response is a reflex response to a stimulus that has become associated with a naturally occurring pleasant or unpleasant event, e.g. Pavlov's dogs. The response required in free field audiometry requires higher level cortical processing in the non-symbolic cognitive domain, in which the testee understands that he should perform a specific action in response to a specific category of sounds generated by the assessor. This level is achieved on average by 30 months and should be present by 36 months. Attention control should not pose a great problem in children of this cognitive level but remember it is more likely to be delayed in those with hearing problems.

Procedure and practicalities

The child sits at the nursery table and chair.

If nothing in the history or exam has led to concern about hearing make a 40 or 60dB sound at 1000Hz out of sight to check that he alerts. If he doesn't, try a louder noise.

Kneel down facing the child with the free field audiometer on the table.

The response task

• Keep the response task as simple as possible.

  • Stacking tasks can be simple or complex – one vertical rod and rings of one size and colour offers little leeway for inventiveness. Whereas, a set of vertical rods of different heights and rings in different colours offers many possibilities to self-distract from the test task of listening for increasingly quiet tones to devising one's own game of arranging the rings by colour and or number.

  • A packet of paper coffee cups make a stable and relatively non-self-distracting stacking task

Delivery

- Place a stack of three cups on the table.

- To ensure that the child understands the relationship between hearing a tone and putting a cup on the top use a combination of simple language and pantomine

  - 'Listen, my box makes noises,'

  - … 'sometimes loud,' 'sometimes small,' 'sometimes squeaky,' 'sometimes deep' – demonstrate tones as you speak varying the loudness and pitch of your voice accordingly.

  - 'When you hear a noise put a cup on the top'

  - Make a tone and put a cup on the top of the stack – 'toot' and 'on the top'

  - Give him a cup 'your turn' Make a tone and observe whether he puts the cup on the top. If he doesn't guide his hand with an 'on it goes'

  - Repeat several times until he starts doing it himself. Children younger than 3 years require more trial runs and greater emphasis on the non-language aspects.

- Basic plan for actual testing

  - Initially a loud middle frequency – 1000Hz at 60 or 80dB

  - Repeat at decreasing decibel levels

  - Randomly vary time interval between successive tones

  - When the child fails to respond, repeat the previous sound at a louder level.

  - Confirm threshold by crossing it several times

  - Repeat for each frequency in the same way

  - Children under 3½ years may not realise that they are expected to respond when a new frequency is introduced; before assuming that the problem is hearing the assessor should assist with a reassuring 'on it goes', i.e. be prepared to retrain to each frequency if necessary, but beware of conditioning a child with hearing impairment to something other than the tone

- During actual testing the assessor needs to be extremely careful not to provide the slightest clue that a tone has been issued whilst keeping the child on task and in communication. Clues come in many guises; the intelligent child with hearing impairment will be alert to the slightest hint of enquiry in the assessor's eyes or facial expression and will watch their hands to try and detect the movement that heralds the making of the test sound; for example, not only should the tone button and fingers be covered by the other hand but the tendons on the dorsum need to be out of the child's view. This requires an actively self-questioning approach during

Table 4.4   Choice of hearing test for typically developing children

Nature of test	Level of sound	Age of Introduction
Behavioural Tests		
• Startling	Loud	From Birth
• Reflex turn	Loud	From 4 weeks
• Rousing from light sleep	Minimal	From 6 weeks
• Stilling to familiar voice	Conversational	From 12 weeks
• Stilling to familiar sounds	Moderate	From 14 weeks
Distraction test	Minimal	From 4½ months
Speech Discrimination Tests		
• Body parts on Mummy	Minimal voicing	From 18 months
• Body parts on large doll	Minimal voicing	From 21months
• Picture or toy tests	Minimal voicing	From 24 months
Free Field Audiometry	Loud down to threshold	From 30 months

testing 'Did I give a clue?' particularly when a child responds in a clinically un-expected way. Susan, a 3-year-old referred as globally delayed, query autistic, was introduced earlier (p. 79). Susan was socially responsive and co-operative; she actively engaged with tests of NSC performing above age level; she became fidgety during language testing but spontaneously arranged and played imaginatively with the miniature toys at an age-appropriate level. I therefore chose to test hearing using free field audiometry. From behind she alerted to a drum banged maximally and to the pure tone of 1000Hz at 90dB but not to a loud squeaker or a rattle. I conditioned her initially to the drum; then extended this to the pure tone at 90dB. Her thresholds for 1000Hz and 500Hz were 90dB and for 250Hz 80dB. She failed to respond to 2000Hz at 90 or 80dB but suddenly did so at 60, then 40 and 20dB. Was I giving her a clue? I observed her carefully and realized that she was respond-ing to the flick of the needle of a sound-level meter that I had left on a table some 1½ metres to her right. She certainly was neither intellectually disabled nor autis-tic!

• As with language-based tests, asking an experienced colleague to observe and com-ment periodically on one's test delivery makes for sound technique.

Guidelines for selecting the most age-appropriate test or starting level and for the age when all but 10% should co-operate are summarised in Table 4.4.

Hearing loss – an important clinical sign?

Hearing losses of mild to moderate degree are most commonly due to OME. If history, paediatric examination and oroscope examination suggest that OME is simple and chronic, then referral to ENT and/or audiology is appropriate. Severe and profound losses usually are sensorineural but may have sensorineural and conductive elements. Hearing loss is a diagnostic feature of many serious paediatric, neurological, syndromic and neurodegenerative disorders so before onwards referral hearing loss needs to be considered in the context of the rest of the developmental and paediatric profile. Without including hearing in their assessment portfolio paediatricians deny themselves diagnostic opportunities that are likely to lead to delays in diagnosis and treatment of the underlying condition.

Key Points

- The pool of children developing a hearing problem after the neonatal period is several times larger than that of those born with one.

- Failure to include estimation of hearing status as part of preliminary developmental examination leads to over referral to audiological services.

- Hearing losses tend to present in a variety of guises – behaviour, language, learning difficulties (e.g. the class clown)

- Query 'hearing' when a child over 2½ years is still entrenched in the 'rejecting adult interference' level of attention control.

- Don't make excuses for a child failing a hearing test. If you and the parent can hear the test sound so should the child.

- If a child is too tired, upset or unwell to test see him again rather than give him the benefit of the doubt.

- To avoid interpretive confusion always utilise the lowest level of a hearing behaviour in test delivery.

- Auditory events are less attractive than visual ones to babies and preschool children.

- Visual occurrences are more ruinous to a hearing test than extraneous noises.

- The distraction technique fast runs out of steam during the first half of the second year due mainly to a normal stage in the development of attention control.

- Groups of test words should contain good frequency discriminations.

- Variation in regional vowel sounds are a major design problem.

- Test words should be minimally voiced, not whispered.

- Never place or deliver phonetic pairs in sequence.

- In free field audiometry, keep response task simple.

- Always use a sound you are *certain* the child can hear when training the conditioned response task.

- Something doesn't fit. Ask yourself 'Did I give a clue?'

- A conditioned response test is an excellent test of cognition for 30- to 36-month-olds.

References

American Academy of Pediatrics (2004) Otitis Media with Effusion. *Pediatrics* 113(5): 1412–1429.

Bamford J, Uus K, Davis A (2005) Screening for hearing loss in childhood: Issues, evidence and current approaches in the UK *J Med Screen* 12: 119.

Bellman S, Marcuson M (1991) A new toy test to investigate the hearing status of young children who have English as a second language: A preliminary report. *Br J Audiol* 25(5) Informa Healthcare.

Bellman S, Mahon M, Triggs E (1996) Evaluation of the E2L Toy Test as a screening procedure in clinical practice. *Br J Audiol* 30 Informa Healthcare.

Davis A, Bamford J, Wilson I, Ramkalawan T, Forshaw M, Wright S (1997) A critical review of the role of neonatal hearing screening in the detection of congenital hearing impairment. *Health Technol Assess* 1(10): 1–176.

Dedhia K, Kitsko D, Sabo D, Chi DH (2013) Children with sensorineural hearing loss after passing the newborn hearing screen. *JAMA Otolaryngol – Head Neck Surg* 17: 1–5. doi: 10.1001/jamaoto.2013.1229. [Epub ahead of print]

Fortnum HM, Quentin Summerfield A, Marshall DH, Davis AC, Bamford JM (2001) Prevalence of permanent childhood hearing impairment in the United Kingdom and implications for neonatal hearing screening: questionnaire based ascertainment study. *BMJ* 323: 526.

Friederici A (2011) The brain basis of language processing: From structure to function. *Physiol Rev* 91: 1357–1392.

Harries J, Williamson T (2000) Community-based validation of the McCormick Toy Test. *Br J Audiol* 34(5): 279–283.

Kemp DT (1978) Stimulated acoustic emissions from within the human auditory system. *J Acoust Soc Am* 64: 1386.

McCormick B (1977) The McCormick Toy Discrimination Test: An aid for screening the hearing of children above a mental age of 2 years. *Public Health, London* 91: 67–73.

Reid SM, Modak MB, Berkowitz RG, Reddihough DS (2011) A population-based study and systematic review of hearing loss in children with cerebral palsy. *Dev Med Child Neurol* 5: 1038–1045.

Russ SA, Poulakis Z, Barker M et al. (2003) Epidemiology of congenital hearing loss in Victoria, Australia. *Int J Audiol* 42:385–390.

Sharma A, Cardon G, Henion K, Roland P (2011) Cortical maturation and behavioural outcomes in children with auditory neuropathy spectrum disorder. *Int J Audiol* 50: 98–106.

Starr A, Picton TW, Siniger Y, Hood LJ, Berlin CI (1996) Auditory neuropathy. *Brain* 119: 741–753.

Wessex Universal Neonatal Hearing Screening Trial Group (1998) Controlled trial of universal neonatal screening for early identification of permanent childhood hearing impairment. *Lancet* 352: 1957.

Yoshinaga-Itano C, Sedey AL, Coulter DK, Mehl AL (1998) Language of early- and later-identified children with hearing loss. *Pediatrics* 102: 1161–1171.

Chapter 5
Social Cognition

Cognition

The Oxford dictionary defines *cognition* as 'the ability to acquire knowledge' and as 'knowledge acquired through perception and information/language,' i.e. primarily through visual and auditory input. The term thus embraces intellect and has symbolic[1] and non-symbolic facets. The understanding and expressive use of spoken, written and sign languages is symbolic whereas understanding of the physical world (objects and environment) and of non-symbolic strategies of communication (social communication/cognition) is non-symbolic. At birth the neo-cortex is relatively underdeveloped compared to the mid- and hindbrain. Networking accelerates at birth in response to a barrage of sensory information and in the normal-term infant the system is soon humming. The primary networks and templates for the intellectual processing of incoming perceptions and information into concepts are constructed and refined; these early concepts are the stepping stones to higher functions such as thinking, reasoning, remembering, problem solving, accessing and empathising with the feelings of others, etc. Processed information is stored in memory and the links between conceptual areas and memory, allow new experiences to be mapped onto old, resulting in sequential development. The sequences of social communication can be accessed from birth or

---

1   A *symbol* represents something else, e.g. the word 'cup' represents the object cup. Some symbols like the spoken or written word 'cup' are entirely arbitrary, i.e. they bear no resemblance to the object, whereas others have some physical resemblance, e.g. a drawing of a cup, a miniature toy cup, the Makaton sign for cup.

shortly afterwards; those of physical world cognition from 2 to 3 months and those of symbolic development not until the final quarter of the first year. Many early developmentalists assumed that connectivity in the symbolic domain is not active until then. On the contrary, the network is busy; auditory information (spoken words) is collated with visual perceptions of situations, activities, objects and people into language concepts that reveal themselves as understanding of the spoken word towards the end of the first year and its use early in the second. It is hardly surprising that the templates for this high level and relatively recent evolutionary achievement take a year to prime. If they were dormant, children with hearing impairment would make a rapid catch up when aided at 12 months. They don't!

These four aspects of intellectual (cognitive) development will be covered in the order in which they can be clinically accessed: social cognition (SoC) in this chapter, non-symbolic cognition (NSC) in Chapter 6, non-spoken symbolic cognition (NSpSC) in Chapter 7 and spoken symbolic cognition (SpSC) in Chapter 8. Phonological development will be covered in Chapter 11 as it is part of speech sound production (SSP) and inextricably intertwined with articulation in the preschool years.

The social (external experiences in the socio-cultural climate) and cognitive aspects of communicative development are closely interconnected and so are dealt with together.

Social cognition

It has long been recognised that newborn babies exhibit instinctive behaviours like crying and screaming when they have colic or are hungry. The primary role of these behaviours is to serve the baby's biological needs rather than socialising. Professionals only acknowledged that newborn babies possess natural sociability and the fundamental importance of this to developmental progress, in the 1970s. This is surprisingly recent, considering that generations of parents (including professional ones) have intuitively cradled and melodically vocalised their joy and welcome to their newborn babies. The babies listen, gaze back into their eyes, open their mouths and make small discrete expressive movements of their fingers and faces; some even vocalise (Fig 5.1). This is a powerful bonding experience for parents and baby – the dawn of a rewarding partnership that will motivate and promote the baby's development. A newborn baby has had some in utero experience of voices, but has never seen her own face or hands or those of her parents, suggesting that the human baby is born with an innate social-communicative network of templates that is functionally responsive to the emotional content of parental communication and which has functional links to the main motor pathways involved in communicative behaviours of the eyes, hands, face and voice. These behaviours can also be elicited in preterm babies born up to 2 months before term (Van-Rees and De Leeuw 1993). The neuropsychological term for responsiveness and emotional understanding

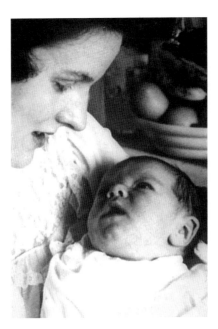

Figure 5.1 The dawn of social communication and of an enduring emotional bond. A mother's first step as facilitator of her baby's development (Archive photograph of author with her daughter).

between two individuals is intersubjectivity. The development of intersubjectivity was thoroughly reviewed by Trevarthen and Aitkin in 2001.

Primary intersubjectivity

At birth a baby shows communicative readiness and often recognizes her mother's face and voice within days, even hours, of birth. The first communicative encounter between mother and neonate quickly blossoms into more elaborate proto-conversations[2] in which both rhythmically regulate their own and each other's contributions; the baby's little grunts become more melodic (rising coos) in tune with mothers'. The rhythms, musicality and intonations that impart the emotional content to a mother's vocalisations are known as 'motherese'. Through these exchanges the baby develops and demonstrates the dawn of self-other (person–person) awareness. Parents naturally smile during these encounters but smiling back is not part of the baby's communicative repertoire until 6 to 8 weeks, i.e. it is a learnt social response as opposed to an innate one. A baby's eyes usually reflect his pleasure and interest as he gazes intently at his parent's

2   Both mother (father) and infant in the communicative state rhythmically look, listen, and express themselves through vocalisations, their facial expressions and their eyes. Thus proto-conversations are conversations without words.

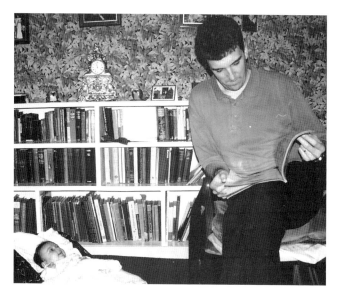

Figure 5.2a "Daddy, I'm here."

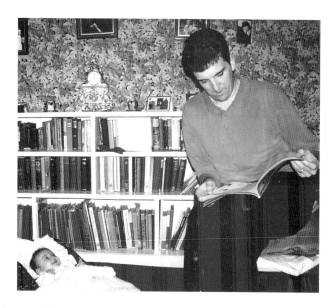

Figure 52.b "Coo-eee, I want some attention."

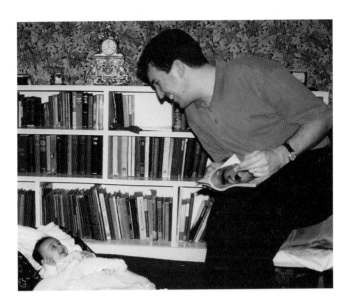

Figure 52.c "At last, now talk to me."

expressive face during early proto-conversations. Although newborn babies sometimes focus on their parent's mouth and may open their own as they do so, they rarely smile when watching the mouth. Eye contact and the visual percept are important factors in learning to smile responsively.

Between 2 and 4 months a baby realises that her voice has communicative power and that she can use it to attract and engage her parents socially. The 10-week-old baby in Figure 5.2a—c gazes intently, smiles, vocalises and excitedly moves her arms until she is successful in commanding the attention of her father.

From 3 months babies listen to the sounds they make and experiment with them ('raspberries', vowel sounds 'ah, 'aroo', 'ergroo'); gradually these vocalisations become more formed and are prefixed by consonants 'ba', 'da', 'ma', 'ga'. The baby makes and listens to a sound – pauses – attempts to repeat it singly ('ah' pause 'ah') and later in strings ('ba-ba-ba' pause 'ba-ba-ba pause, ba-ba-ba-ba'). Parents naturally delight in joining in, at first imitating the baby and between 7 and 8 months intuitively changing the combination after a few rounds ('ba-ba-ba' to 'ma-ma-ma'). Thus they encourage the baby to listen, imitate and turn take; instinctively introducing the person–person communicative element into the baby's solitary practice session.

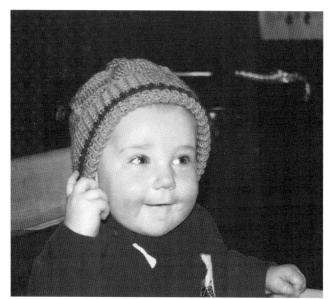

(a)

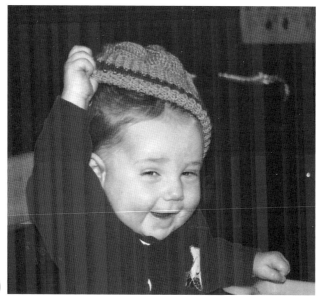

(b)

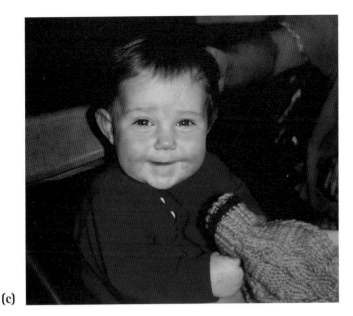

(c)

Figures 5.3a, b and c Dawning sense of fun.

At 8 months parents introduce rhyme games such as 'round and round the garden'; the parent walks two fingers up the child's arm as she sings 'one step, two step' with a tension raising pause before 'tickle you under there'. After two or three exposures he shows the excitement of familiarity but no specific response. In time (9 to 11 months) he signals his anticipation of the tickle by squeezing his arm closer to his chest and a facial expression alive with excited apprehension. Similarly, in 'Row, row, row the boat' understanding by the baby of his social role in the activity is heralded by self-initiated rocking and a spontaneous shriek after 'and don't forget to scream'. These games do more to promote situational phrase understanding in the language domain than inter-subjectivity, although they certainly reinforce the latter.

Babies (including those up to 8 weeks' preterm) are intense observers of facial expressions from birth and start to experiment with the power of facial expression during the early months. In the early weeks babies are disturbed if the facial expression of their parents is unusual, e.g. is blank or doesn't fit with the melody and timing of other aspects of their social engagement. By 4 months wearing a mask may induce a look of alarm and a bout of inconsolable crying. Development of the communicative power of facial expression occurs in parallel with the vocal aspects. Two- to four-month-olds store the motive content of their parent's expressions and begin to express them themselves in the correct context. Between 6 and 9 months some babies indulge in rather exaggerated facial expressions even with strangers. This is sometimes referred to as 'showing off' but more likely is a reflection of the way parents naturally emphasise intonation and facial expression in an effort to convey meaning. Between a year and 18 months babies instinctively look at their mother or fathers' expression to seek information when suddenly confronted with a strange situation or person. Their ability to analyse the facial expression of others is sufficiently well established to instantly tell whether or not the parent 'thinks it is OK'.

A sense of humour and a sense of fun are powerful social attributes that emerge during the first year. Babies use facial expression and laughter to convey their amusement. In the second half of the first year their laughter occurs in response to occurrences rather than to jokes; for example at the sight of mother rushing to retrieve the contents of a packet of frozen peas as they bounce all over the kitchen floor! Mobility is often the trigger that releases a sense of fun; a baby soon learns that his father runs after him when he crawls towards the stairs, so he crawls as fast as he can. When about to be caught the child spins round, his face alive with the fun of the chase to see his father's expression mirroring his own as he says "Got you!" A sense of fun is captured in Figure 5.3a—c.

Secondary intersubjectivity

From 4 months the interest of babies increasingly includes objects and a desire to explore and discover more about them results in rapid advances in manipulation and NSC. Initially, they are totally absorbed by the object (self-object) and it is mother who models shared interest by joining in and directing play with the object/toy; for example she smilingly presents a rattle – the baby grasps it and studies it visually, but doesn't shake it – she either takes it back and shakes it or helps him to shake it, looking back and forth excitedly (visual referencing) between rattle and baby and with vocalisations expressing interest and fun. From 9 months babies actively employ this model to initiate shared interest with another, i.e. they use gaze and vocalisations to obtain their parent's interest and then direct his/her attention to the object of their interest by showing, bringing or looking at it (Fig 5.4 and Fig 5.5). They then jointly attend to the object (person–person–object or secondary intersubjectivity).

Towards the end of the first year babies begin to point to objects they want (request/imperative pointing) (Figures 5.6a and b) and then to objects or events that they wish to share with someone (declarative pointing) (Fig 5.7); in both instances they look to and fro between the caregiver and the object (visual referencing). Figure 5.8 shows a two year old trying to share an event with a 7 month old who is too young to understand pointing.

Q Why, in the context of this chapter is the declarative point the more important of the two?
Because its purpose is to share interest/jointly attend.

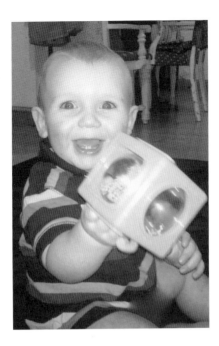

Figure 5.4 Sharing interest in toy – showing.

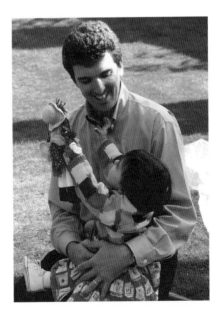

Figure 5.5 Sharing interest and pleasure in a first birthday present.

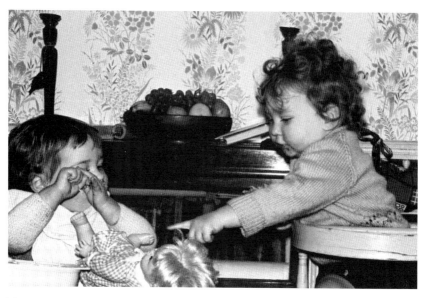

(a)

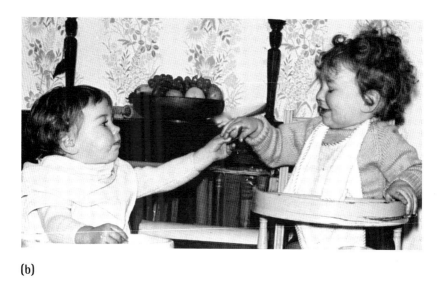

(b)

Figure 5.6a and 5.6b Communication between toddlers: a boy points at something on the girl's tray. The girl follows his pointing finger, 'reads' his communication and picks up the toy and hands it to him. Note his clear satisfaction that he 'got what he wanted'.

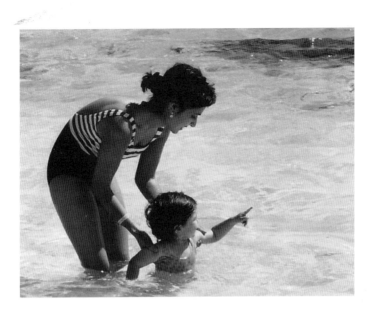

Figure 5.7 Declarative pointing to share an interest (passing fishing boat) with her mother. Pointing was accompanied by eye referencing back and forth between mother and boat.

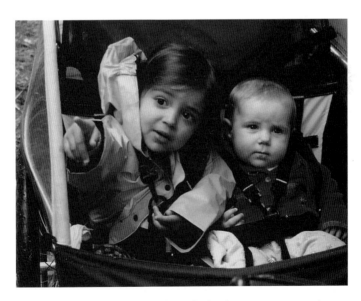

Figure 5.8 A 23-month-old using declarative pointing in an attempt to share an event with a 7-month-old who is too young to 'read' the pointing gesture.

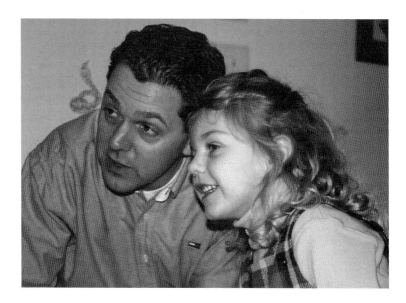

Figure 5.9 Now old enough to share an interest in an event through conversation – no longer any need to point.

Over the next three years, child initiated sharing of interest in events and toys with adults becomes a well-established and increasingly frequent behaviour. As expressive language blossoms the verbal components of these episodes become more elaborate and prominent while the use of pointing and gesture correspondingly reduce (Fig 5.9). In the main sharing of interest and joint attention is reserved for adult caregivers and is only extended to other toddlers when the latter has something the former wants. Unfortunately a toddler's strategy is to grab and run off with the wanted item, leaving the owner in tears and the grabber in trouble! The grabber's thoughts are blinkered on what he 'wants'; the feelings of the owner don't enter his thinking. Sharing interest in toys with peers emerges slowly in the second half of the third year but is not fully established as shared play until the fourth (see Chapter 7).

Towards the end of the first year facial expression shows the dawning of more complex emotions, like guilt when caught doing something they know is not allowed. Once language is available the emotion is also reflected in the tone of the child's voice. A 22-month-old's understanding of the emotional and social aspects of her situation – swallowing a safety pin – may be revealed by a hushed voice when she turns to her mother saying 'all gone', and by her already alarmed expression crumpling into tears. Recognition of emotive states in others emerges more slowly and empathy for the situation of others not until later. A 5 or 6 year old boy might spontaneously interrupt his play to help his great grandmother rise from her chair, but a younger child is very unlikely to do so.

Appreciation of the social effect of what one says is a pragmatic aspect of language that is gradually acquired during preschool and primary school years. At 2½-years of age a toddler exclaiming "Daddy, why that man got 'normous umbella?" as the Bishop appears in full regalia is surprised when father whispers "Ssh darling" rather than answering his interesting question. At this age he still has no conception of the inappropriateness of his words in the context of the social situation. These are the moments that parent's wish they could 'drop through the floor'. Similarly, a concept of 'the little white lie' is rarely present before 6 or 7 years and the social nuances of language should not be expected even at primary school level.

Another aspect of developing pragmatics in the preschool years is to interpret words literally, based on previous experience of their meaning. For example, a 3-year-old whose understanding of the word 'sew' has been his mother mending his clothes, may look baffled when the play leader says 'let's sow these seeds in the garden'.

Non-literal figures of speech are interpreted literally throughout the preschool years and new ones may puzzle 6- and 7-year-olds (e.g. 'It's raining cats and dogs').

Assessment

All or any of the above-mentioned aspects of social understanding and language pragmatics may be delayed or disordered in children with disorders of social communication.

During the first year the development of intersubjectivity (primary and secondary) is the focus of social-communicative assessment; there are no test tools (toys or everyday objects) for primary intersubjectivity, so dedicating time to explore this area is often omitted. Yet these attributes are fundamental to a baby ultimately functioning effectively within the social framework of human societies. History, observations of parent–baby interaction and active examination all have a place.

History

The primary medical history will have alerted the examiner to general medical risk factors for social-communicative disorders.

Specific secondary medical history should enquire into the following:

- Family history of autistic spectrum disorders (ASD), pervasive developmental disorder (PDD) syndromes/disorders that commonly feature autism or autistic features (e.g. fragile X syndrome, Rett syndrome).

- Postnatal depression impacts on a mother's ability to respond to her baby's communicative cues and flattens the emotional content and exaggerated melody of her 'motherese'.

- Preterm birth – apart from the many medical possibilities of damage to the brain in very low birth weight (VLBW) babies, the physical barrier imposed by incubator care disturbs a parent's ability to establish an early emotional bond; in addition the baby's socio-communicative networks are likely to be very immature which will confuse and may depress parents anticipating the responsiveness described earlier.

- Severe visual impairment (SVI) – subtle elements of early social interaction are deviant and tend to confuse and depress parents reducing their motivation to interact and the baby's opportunity to do so in the following ways:

  - SVI reduces a baby's ability to access the emotional content of their parent's social overtures as all but the auditory and tactile components (warmth of being cradled) are denied.

  - When cradled and talked to blind babies tend to still – they don't gaze back – and their facial expression becomes passive (listening intently) rather than communicative.

  - Denied the forewarning that sight gives to a parent's approach a blind baby often stiffens and startles as soon as grasped.

  - Between 2 and 4 months the vocalisations and facial expressions of blind babies usually contain remnants of a newborn baby's response to discomfort/discontent; the rhythm tends to be interrupted; together these are likely to convey a more demanding and less sociable message to the parent than the charming melodic request 'for a chat' of his sighted peer.

  Q Why might the rhythm of a blind baby's vocalisations be interrupted?
  A baby with visual impairment needs to rely on his hearing to tell if the parent is responding/even present (he won't see her gazing smilingly back at him), so he pauses between vocalisations to listen.

  - Modelling of secondary intersubjectivity by a parent is heavily dependent on her baby having sufficient vision to see her gaze referencing, her look of interest and her demonstration of the object/toy. The task of the parent of a blind baby is formidable in comparison.

  Q What might be the reason that two way vocalisations and rhyme song games develop quite strongly in blind babies?
  Because the input sense for both activities is predominately auditory and many of the actions are tactile ('one step two step) or physical – rocking in ('row, row, row the boat').

- Severe hearing impairment eliminates the auditory but not the visual and tactile components of 'motherese'; babies with hearing impairment tend to enjoy socialisation, which suggests that the communicative power of vision (expression in face and eyes) is paramount.

Parents are naturally deeply shocked and saddened, even depressed by news that their baby may have developmental problems. It is therefore important to keep the impact of a depressed mental state on a parent's ability to promote her newborn baby's social-communicative development in mind and to be active in ensuring she gets appropriate guidance and emotional support. In social-communicative disorder: prevention is better and less expensive than cure.

Secondary developmental history

The secondary developmental history explores primary intersubjectivity (plus secondary intersubjectivity), dropping to an earlier level if age level responses are not forthcoming. Questions which engender a description rather than a 'yes'/'no' answer are best. There are multiple facets to communicative overtures so probe for description of each facet as necessary. Choose age-appropriate questions from Table 5.1 and shift up or down as the responses indicate.

Examination

History is second best to informed observation of spontaneous, or assessor-directed, parent–baby interaction or assessor–baby interaction. So follow up parent's descriptions with 'Oh that would be lovely to see, show me'. If the parent seems shy or expected age levels have not been observed already then 'Can I see if she wants to talk/play to me[3]?' The assessor engaging the baby herself at target age level is not only informative, but creates rapport and strengthens the assessor's gestalt of the qualitative and quantitative components of typical reciprocal interaction. In no domain is gestalt more important to an assessor. When assessing social communication in children who are talking, it is also important to separate the social-communicative aspects from the linguistic with each apportioned to its respective domain. Examination protocol, endpoint and age guidelines are detailed in Table 5.1. Many of these age guidelines are not derived from population based normative studies but extrapolated from clinical experience and from the behaviour of typically developing control groups reported in research studies. As usual the age guidelines in Table 5.1 indicate the age when the social-communicative behaviour described is present in typically developing children and the age when the

---

3   A toy is needed for testing secondary intersubjectivity, e.g. present a music box to a 10+-month-old. Having shown her that the music plays when the lid is lifted, stop actively engaging her and observe when and if she actively tries to share her enjoyment of it with you or her parent.

assessor registers concern if it is not. However, also compare the qualitative aspects with the gestalt of typical development. Once well grounded, assessors will find that their index of concern is raised by subtle differences, such as reduction in eye contact or communicativeness of facial expression or the amount of work required to gain and maintain engagement. Table 5.1 is not exhaustive and only explores some aspects in the development of social communication.

As children with an ASD frequently present with a range of atypical behaviours, the presence or absence of some or all of them needs exploration, particularly if the assessor's index of concern is raised by the parent's responses or their observations of the baby to date. Table 5.2 lists a sample of the abnormal behaviours. Suitable questions might be 'Would you say Jamie was a content baby or did he have bouts of intense distress for no apparent reason?' 'Tell me how Johnnie plays with his toy cars', 'Does Susan like going to new places and doing new things?' Recently, the quality of vocalisations made by children of typical development, and those with ASD or developmental delay aged 18 to 24 months has been shown to differ significantly. The vocalisations of babies with ASD or developmental delay, perhaps unsurprisingly, contained a lower proportion of speech sounds than those of typically developing babies. The most striking finding, however, was a much higher proportion of distress vocalisations in the children with ASD than in either of the other two groups. This led the authors to recommend further investigation of distress vocalisations as a potential early indicator of ASD in the second half of the second year (Plumb and Wetherby 2013).

The assessor needs to discuss (1) words and whether these are used spontaneously and appropriately, or only in imitation, and (2) jargon, babbling and non-speech sounds; if the latter to ask for examples and parent's view of their emotional content.

If the examiner's index of concern is raised he should look at the findings in the context of the intellectual and total profile before deciding to refer for administration of a standardised screening procedure, full ASD evaluation or other specialist consultation (see the following discussion).

Disorders of social communication

Recently, the traditional triad of diagnostic criteria for ASDs, reflected in classifications since Kanner's first description (Kanner 1943), has been reduced to 2-factor format in DSM-5 (American Psychological Association 2013), by combining the social and communicative factors into one, with the restricted and repetitive patterns of behaviour, interests and activities comprising the other. Guthrie et al. (2013) tested toddlers with ASD on the Autism Diagnostic Observation Schedule – Toddler Module (ADOS-T) and found it fitted DSM-5 better than any of the previous classifications; their study thus suggests that the pattern of symptoms varies in only minor ways throughout development.

Table 5.1   Assessment of social communicative development: questions and answers

Question	Examination		
	Protocol	Endpoint	Age guidelines
"How does J respond when you cradle and 'talk' to him?"	Cradle and smilingly engage baby socially Fig 5.1	Eye contact, intense regard, listening expression +/- vocalising, mouth opening/finger movements	Birth–**4**wks
"Have you ever seen S upset by an expressionless face?"	[a]Don't ask or test unless other observations concern you. Always explain procedure first.	Baby clearly puzzled or upset	*2–***6**wks
"Does J smile back when you smile at him?"	Cradle and smilingly engage baby socially.	Smiles back with eye contact + sparkling expression in eyes[b]	*6–***9**wks
"Does S ever try to get you to engage with her and if so how?"	Keep an eye open for this behaviour when neither assessor nor parent are engaged with S	Baby vocalises looking at one or both adults in turn trying to 'catch their eye'	*14–***18**wks
"If you try to join in J's vocalisations does he take turns?"	If J vocalises join in. Otherwise engage and vocalise to him - pause for response and repeat x2 or x3	Baby engages visually and vocalises with pauses to allow adult to vocalise	*18-***22**wks
"What rhyme song games do you play with S?" Parent names one. "That's one of my favourites too – how does S join in?"	Ask parent to demonstrate the song routine and observe baby – or do so yourself	Baby engages visually and actively participates in actions.	*44-***48**wks
"What makes S laugh?" "Does S have a sense of fun? Give me an example"	Observe for sense of humour or fun	Needs to indicate a sense of humour (not tickling or rough and tumble)	*39-***52**wks
"Does S point at an object she wants?"	Observe throughout assessment	Imperative pointing	*42-***52**wks
"Does J follow your pointing finger"	During assessment call his name and point at a toy some 2m away	J looks at toy	*44-***56**wks

Table 5.1 continued

"When J is playing with a toy or is interested by a happening, does he ever try to share his interest in it with you or other adults?" "How does he do so?"	Observe whether J actively tries to engender parent's / assessor's interest in a toy or happening by visual referencing and/ or declarative pointing.	Visual referencing and expression inviting adults interest	45–54wks
		+ Declarative pointing and/or vocalisation 'dere'	47–54wks
		+ Meaningful utterance - 'ook'	21–26mo
		+ Simple[c] spoken requests, comments or questions	27–30mo
		+ 'Conversation'[d]	33–39mo
"Does S bring objects or toys to 'show' you?"	Watch for this behaviour	S spontaneously turns holds up or brings an object or toy in which she is interested to 'show' assessor or parent	12–16mo
"Do you think J knows when he's doing something 'forbidden? If so how can you tell?"	(Hard to set up during a preliminary assessment)		14–18mo
"Do you think J 'reads' your facial expressions e.g. that you are upset or sad; that you think a happening is funny? If so how can you tell?"	Watch for either of these naturally occurring during the consultation		12–18mo
			12–18mo
"In a new situation does he look to see if you think it is OK?"	(Hard to set up during a preliminary assessment) unless sibling available		12–18mo
"Does J share his interest in a toy or happening with peers?"	(Hard to set up during a preliminary assessment) unless sibling available		36–48mo
'Does S ever show empathy with the situation of others? If so can you give me an example?"	(Hard to set up during a preliminary assessment)		60–68mo

[a]Risk of upsetting mother and baby; [b]The sparkle is an important sign as it distinguishes the emergence of the social concept from the proverbial 'wind'. [c] oggy dink', 'do ee'; [d]'Who gave you the car?' 'Granny did. Look door opens' +/- with or without

ASD are a heterogeneous group of developmental disorders of multiple interacting aetiologies including genetic influences. The cognitive profile in ASD and its links with genes and behaviour has been recently thoroughly reviewed by Charman et al. (2010). There is increasing evidence from imaging studies in older individuals with ASD that connectivity between the frontal cortex and the cerebellum, caudate and temporal cortex is commonly reduced (Geschwind and Levitt 2007). Based on evidence of brain overgrowth during the first year in babies later developing an ASD, Courchesne et al. (2007) speculate that excessive overgrowth of connections at local level may impede the formation of long-range links with the large-scale templates that underlie social emotional and communicative functions.

Our developmental vision team demonstrated that up to 30% of babies with profound visual impairment (PVI) with congenital disorders of the peripheral visual system and good developmental progress during the first year underwent developmental setback/autistic regression in the second and third year (Cass et al. 1994, Waugh et al. 1998, Dale and Sonksen 2002, Sonksen and Dale 2002). It is not tenable that such a high percentage of babies with PVI were predetermined, genetically or otherwise, to undergo autistic regression; after all, the rate in sighted children is more than 30 times less and in children with hearing impairment between 1 and 2%. An alternative mechanism, operating equally silently/stealthily throughout the first year, which has a similar end result, i.e. underdevelopment and deficient connectivity of social, communicative and emotional circuitry should be looked for. The obvious candidate is visual deprivation; in which case the input in the driving seat for these aspects of connectivity and tem-

Table 5.2   Some atypical behaviours of babies and preschool children with autistic spectrum disorders

Behaviour
Bouts of irritability (first 12mo)
Bouts of intense distress (first 12mo)
High proportion of vocalisations containing non-speech sounds (18–24mo)[a]
High proportion of distress sounds in vocalisations (18–24mo)[a]
Stereotypies, e.g. twirls, flaps hands
Repetitive and often unusual play routines, e.g. spinning wheels of toy car
Restricted interests and activities
Dislike of change to routines and new situations

[a] Plumb and Wetherby (2013).

plate formation is vision, rather than the tactile or auditory components of parental overtures to their newborn baby. Communicative networks are fired the moment baby and parent eyes meet. In visual impairment the baby's atypical body language and facial expression – body and facial stilling without eye contact – degrades all components of feedback to the parents. The baby's apparent lack of interest leads parents to withdraw from an activity that is the cornerstone of social-communicative development further compounding the strain on connectivity. Both sighted babies (later to be diagnosed with ASD) and babies with PVI usually participate in proto-conversations, presumably because the auditory circuitry is sufficient to arouse interest, listening and turn taking. However, many babies in both groups have been noted to be less animated and make less eye contact during communicative interchanges, due presumably in the sighted to the secondary effects of an abnormal brain trajectory and in the babies with PVI to visual deprivation. Despite the very different postulated causative agents and pathways, the male to female sex ratio in both groups is approximately 4:1, which suggests that in boys the social-communicative networks and templates are inherently more vulnerable than in girls.

Year on year the prevalence of children over the age of 2 years diagnosed with an ASD increases, with the latest Centres for Disease Control report of participating states in the USA reporting a rate of 1 in 68 among 8-year-olds (Baird et al. 2006, CDC 2009, 2014). The proportion of children with average and above-average intelligence has risen from a third to a half. However, the ratio of boys to girls remains steady at 4:1 and the prevalence remains higher in children of white, than of either black or Hispanic ethnicity. The reasons for the overall increase in prevalence are multiple and complex and include more effective screening protocols and higher levels of professional and parental awareness and expertise, etc. For example a recent validation study of a two-stage screening tool, the Modified Checklist for Autism in Toddlers, Revised with Follow up (M-CHAT-R/F), has shown that 95% of toddlers attending well baby check-ups, who screened positive after the second stage screen at 24 months were, on detailed assessment, found to have developmental delays and disorders, including 47.5% diagnosed with an ASD (Robins et al. 2009, 2014). As a consequence the children in this cohort with ASDs were diagnosed 2 years earlier than the national average (USA) and as a consequence will have earlier access to appropriate educational support. Similarly, a cohort of 'well' Swedish preschool children who had screened positive for an ASD contained a significant number of children with other developmental disorders (Kantzer et al. 2013). These studies suggest that screening toddlers and preschool children for deficits in social communication has a high specificity for identification of those in need of specialised help for ASD and other developmental disorders.

The earlier studies support the advice in Chapter 1 to 'think in profiles', first within the intellectual profile and then to consider the intellectual profile in the context of sensory and motor findings. In a significant proportion of children failing a screen for social communication the delay in social communication may be part of generalised developmental delay (GDD)[4] rather than an ASD. All children who score poorly for age in tests of expressive language do *not* have a specific disorder of expressive language; in fact the majority will have GDD or an ASD. In other words, one does not make a provisional diagnosis or decide on follow-up or therapy until all areas of the intellectual profile and sensory and motor findings have been explored and considered as a whole.

In times of financial constraint a level 1 screening test like the M-CHAT-R/F with high specificity for many disorders of the intellectual profile including ASD is attractive because it can be more reliably and quickly administered to 18- to 30-month-olds[5] by primary care personnel after relatively brief training at relatively low cost, than tests of symbolic and non-symbolic intellect. However, before this could be advocated it will be imperative to establish the true sensitivity of the test for each disorder in the intellectual domain and to ascertain its ability to identify those disorders without autistic traits.

Key Points

- The earliest access to a baby's intelligence is through social-communicative behaviour so it should be *the major feature* of cognitive assessment in the first 6 months.

- Active parent or examiner engagement with the baby is more valuable than assessment through questions.

- Important aspects:
  - Primary intersubjectivity
  - Secondary intersubjectivity
  - 'Reading' the facial expressions of others and subsequently applying them appropriately
  - Sensing humour and fun in others and the development of a sense of humour and fun
  - Awareness of empathy in 'others', growing into empathy for others

- Examiners suspicious of social, emotional and/or communicative status should:
  - Explore the presence of atypical behaviours found in ASD,

---

4   Currently and more precisely referred to as intellectual developmental disorder (IDD).

5   An age range when the child's level of attention control and negative behaviour require high levels of tester skill and experience.

- Consider findings in context of the rest of the IP before finalising a plan of action.

- Current screening schedules for ASD identify children with a variety of developmental disorders of intellect as well those with ASD; further research is needed to refine these schedules.

References

American Psychiatric Association (2013) *DSM-5 Diagnostic and Statistical Manual of Mental Disorders*, 5th ed. Washington, DC: American Psychiatric Publishing.

Baird G, Simonoff E, Pickles A et al. (2006) Prevalence of disorders of the autism spectrum in a population cohort of children in South Thames: The Special Needs and Autism Project (SNAP). *Lancet* 368: 210–215.

Cass H, Sonksen PM, McConachie HR (1994) Developmental setback in severe visual impairment. *Arch Dis Child* 70: 192–196.

Centers for Disease Control and Prevention (CDC) (2009) Prevalence of autism spectrum disorders – Autism and Developmental Disabilities Monitoring Network, United States, 2006. *MMWR Surveill Summ* 58: 1–20.

Centers for Disease Control and Prevention (CDC) (2014) Prevalence of autism spectrum disorders – Autism and Developmental Disabilities Monitoring Network, United States, 2010. *MMWR Surveill Summ* 63: 1–21.

Charman T, Jones CRG, Pickles A, Simonoff E, Baird G, Happé F (2010) Defining the cognitive phenotype of autism. *Brain Res* 1380: 10–21.

Courchesne E, Pierce K, Schumann CM et al. (2007) Mapping early brain development in autism. *Neuron* 56(2): 399–413.

Dale N, Sonksen PM (2002) Developmental outcome, including setback, in children with congenital disorders of the peripheral visual system. *Dev Med Child Neurol* 44: 613–622.

Geschwind DH, Levitt P (2007) Autism spectrum disorders: Developmental disconnection syndromes. *Curr Opin Neurobiol* 17: 103–111.

Guthrie W, Swineford LB, Wetherby AM, Lord C (2013) Comparison of DSM-IV and DSM-5 factor structure models for toddlers with autism spectrum disorder. *J Am Acad Child Adolesc Psychiatry* 52(8): 797–805. Epub 2013 Jun 29.

Kanner L (1943) Autistic disturbances of affective contact. *Nerv Child* 2: 217–250.

Kantzer AK, Fernell E, Gillberg C, Miniscalco C (2013) Autism in community pre-schoolers: Developmental profiles. *Res Dev Disabil* 34: 2900–2908.

Plumb AM, Wetherby AM (2013) Vocalization development in toddlers with autism spectrum disorder. *J Speech Lang Hear Res* 56(2): 721–734. Epub 2012 Dec 28.

Robins DL, Casagrande K, Barton M, Chen C-M, Dumont-Mathieu T, Fein D (2014) Validation of the modified checklist for autism in toddlers, revised with follow-up (M-CHAT-R/F). *Pediatrics* 133: 37–45.

Robins DL, Fein D, Barton M (2009) The modified checklist for autism in toddlers, revised with follow-up (M-CHAT-R/F). Self-published.

Sonksen PM, Dale N (2002) Visual impairment in infancy: Impact on neurodevelopmental and neurobiological processes. *Dev Med Child Neurol* 44: 782–791.

Trevarthan C, Aitkin KG (2001) Infant intersubjectivity: Research, theory and clinical applications. *J Psychol Psychiat* 42(1): 3–48.

Van-Rees S, De Leeuw R (1993) Born too early. The kangaroo method with premature babies. Video by Stichting, Lichaamstall, Schvenhafweg 12:1 6093 Heythuysen The Netherlands.

Waugh M-C, Chong WK, Sonksen PM (1998). Neuroimaging in children with congenital disorders of the peripheral visual system. *Dev Med Child Neurol* 40: 812–819.

Chapter 6

Non-symbolic cognition

In many developmental schedules non-symbolic cognition (NSC) is referred to as 'performance', 'non-verbal understanding' or 'eye-hand co-ordination'.

Development

At birth babies have little conceptual understanding of the functional potential of different parts of their bodies, for example of the eyes for gathering information for cognitive development, the arms and hands for reaching, manipulation and eventually creative construction, the neuromotor system for mobility etc (Sonksen 1983). In the author's view a baby's realisation of the functional potential of their own physical attributes are key cognitive advances. So too are the cognitive elements of learning, i.e. to locate touch and sound and to recognise everyday objects and routines. The inclusion of these strengthens the NSC component of test schedules for babies under a year and particularly during the first 6 months. Examples that are accessible to an assessor are discussed below together with traditional basic NSC concepts such as permanence, cause and effect, structural relationships and problem solving. The cognitive content of some other skills traditionally included in NSC (performance) scales, e.g. number of bricks held, is discussed in terms of whether the cognitive content is sufficient to justify inclusion.

Cognitive interest in looking

From birth a baby's gaze shifts around his surroundings; however it is the high inten-

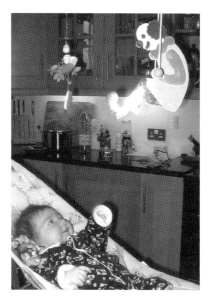

Figure 6.1 Cognitive interest in the clown is shown by the intensity of gaze and generalised excitement of this 2-month-old.

sity of gaze that accompanies fixation that characterises arousal of cognitive interest in a visual target. The target most likely to do so in the newborn period is a near smiling expressive face; indeed recognition of parents' faces is clear in many babies within days and therefore can give assessment of NSC a kick-start. Within weeks this cognitive interest can be observed for relatively large objects (12–15cm) up to a metre away – (Fig 6.1). Gradually interest is taken in smaller objects in the near distance until at 9 months a 1.2mm 'hundred and thousand' is visually fixated with interest; the relationship between size and age is well established – NDV scale, Chapter 3.

Faces, voices and hands are communicative

While primarily giving visual and auditory attention to social overtures newborn babies also assimilate the proprioceptive and kinaesthetic feedback from the tiny reciprocal movements of their own facial, speech and limb musculature. Cumulatively, the overall perceptual experience nurtures the concept that faces, voices and hands have communicative potential. The wonder of the first responsive smile heralds its arrival at perceptual level.

Hands are prehensile and at my command

Realisation that arms and hands are prehensile and under the owner's control follows a period of intense visual regard. During the first 3 months arm movements are part of

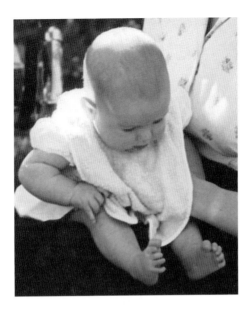

Figure 6.2 Cognitive interest in toes; having realised the potential of her hands, the 4-month-old will reach to explore them manually as well as visually.

general bodily movements, i.e. they are not purposeful or goal directed; although they pass through the visual field babies do not pay them attention until about 12 weeks when cognitive interest is suddenly aroused: initially all movement stills and the baby stares intently at his hand. Over the next couple of weeks he watches the tiny movements of his own fingers and experiments with small backwards and forwards arm movements. (Figures illustrating this are in Chapter 10). The visual information complemented by proprioceptive and kinaesthetic feedback is assimilated centrally into a construct of the functional potential of the upper limbs (Sonksen 1983). Active reaching for a dangling toy between 14 and 20 weeks is evidence of this learning. Once head and trunk control is sufficient a baby catches sight of his feet; the latter are subjected to the same intensity of gaze though now visual information is also supplemented by manual exploration of his toes – (Fig 6.2) – an essential cognitive step in learning about the functional potential of the lower limbs.

Recognition of everyday objects and routines

Babies show that they associate the visual percept and/or sound of everyday objects and routines such as their bottle, juice splashing in an any-way-up beaker, water running into the bath, keys in the front door, etc between 14 and 20 weeks by general physical and vocal excitement or more specific behaviours such as sucking movements. These responses demonstrate the formation of links between memory and NSC centrally.

Localisation skills

Newborn babies are unable to locate the source of a sound or where on their bodies they are touched. Both skills are achieved during the first year and require the construction of templates mapping sound in space relative to self and touch in relation to their own bodies. The tutor for these cognitive templates is vision (Sonksen 1979, 1983). Sound location is also underpinned by two other aspects of cognition: recognition of the physical nature of the source (voice with Daddy, jingle bells with rattle) and the permanence/substantiality of sound making objects/people. As mentioned in Chapters 1 and 4, the sequence of 'sound localisation' fits more comfortably into one on assessment of NSC than into one on hearing and speech, where it traditionally has been placed.

In the neonatal period, a baby's vision provides information about sound sources generated within her field of vision. The eye and head-turning reflex complements this learning for loud sounds generated outside her field of vision. Thus from birth collation of visual and auditory input centrally, teaches that sounds come from substantive sources (voices are generated by people, other sounds by objects), their nature (what they are – keys/rattle, etc) and their location (where they are relative to self – in front or L or R, up or down). Integrative networking of these early cognitive templates is rapid during the first few months as evinced by a baby's slow but active turn to the correct side in response to familiar sounds made outside the field of vision, to either side, at ear level, by between 18 and 22 weeks (see Chapter 4 p. 87). Between 20 and 35 weeks most babies do not turn to the side of a sound when sounds are made more than 25° above or below their ear level.[1] From 35 weeks most babies initially turn to the correct side and then look up or down as appropriate (two-stage location). By 44 weeks they look directly up or down to the sound source (one-stage location – Fig 4.4 in Chapter 4).

Q How/why is the baby able to do this?
By 35 weeks a baby is cognitively able to deduce which side a sound made above or below ear level is coming from, but not by how much it is above or below. Hence initially his eyes are directed horizontally and turn up or down once the sound source is spotted in his peripheral vision. Over the next weeks auditory and visual information are correlated centrally and the result is an integrated direct response by 44 weeks.

A parallel sequence is apparent in the ability to locate touch. A neonate does not look or move a hand towards his knee when it is tickled; he may go into a reflex withdrawal if the stimulus is unpleasant but that has negative learning value. Between 22 and 26 weeks he looks down at his knee when touched; from around 35 weeks he looks down

---

1 During this period the 'localisation' template and its connections are consolidated through everyday auditory-visual experience; processing time progressively shortens and responses become very brisk between 31 and 35 weeks.

and then moves his hand to brush the tickler's hand away; at around 44 weeks he just brushes the tickler's hand away while continuing to visually attend to his original focus of interest. He has learnt to locate touch.

Q Why is location of touch noticeably poorer on our backs?
Because we can't see our backs!

The role of vision in development of both these cognitive templates is clearly observable (Sonksen 1983). Is it surprising that blind babies fail to make progress in these areas? The cognitive elements of sound and touch localisation skills are at a higher level than the sensory and motor elements and the time frames are sufficiently 'tight' to justify inclusion in the NSC test battery.

Permanence of people and objects

Permanence is the realisation that somebody/thing still exists when no longer seen, heard or in touch. The development of permanence appears for people before objects. This is not surprising because in the first 4 months people are far more interesting to babies than objects and make excellent test material.

From as early as 16 weeks a baby beams expansively and looks around when he hears his parent's voice even though they are out of sight. This shows recognition of voices but the visual searching reflects his realisation that the parent is present even when he or she is out of sight. A favourite game in the days of coach work prams was for the mother to crawl around the pram popping up at different places, initially with a smiling 'peep bo', then silently. From about 5 months babies continued to search after the mother became silent demonstrating that they had learnt that she still existed when out of sight and sound.

Babies start to watch the trajectory of a falling object from about 24 weeks; however as soon as the trajectory passes out of view its existence appears to be forgotten. Around 35 weeks they actively search for it after it has disappeared from view demonstrating that permanence of objects (P of O) is emerging. Quite rapidly they apply this learning in more complex settings such as realising that a toy still exists when hidden under something.

Holding cubes

The number of cubes that a baby can hold in his hands features in many performance schedules. To my mind the clasping of a cube put into the hand of a 2½-month-old does not indicate a cognitive event as babies do not watch or actively participate in the operation. Reaching for a brick on a table surface or taking a proffered one (around 6 months) reflects cognitive interest in an object of this size and understanding of the prehensile function of the upper limbs. At this age a baby passively drops a brick she is holding when proffered a second one, seemingly forgetting the existence of the first and reflecting her inability to attend to more than one object at a time. Between 7½ and 8½ months both are held onto demonstrating that she can now attend to two; in fact many look from one to the other with a 'what do I do now expression?' During the following 3 months babies accept three and sometimes four cubes, which probably reflects manipulative more than cognitive progress.

Bringing two bricks together/banging them together either spontaneously or in imitation

At about 11 months babies discover that banging objects together produces noise, i.e. an aspect of cause-and-effect learning. So when a baby spontaneously bangs two bricks together enthusiastically he shows cause-and-effect understanding; if he does so after watching father demonstrate he is showing imitation – another aspect of NSC. If he brings them together without banging he is probably consolidating his learning about attending to two objects at a time (see above). This latter behaviour has also been interpreted as matching, but in my opinion it occurs too young to represent that skill.

Early problem solving

A 39-week-old is presented with a toy beyond his reach attached to a string within reach. After a few vain attempts to reach the toy he looks from toy to string several times, tentatively grasps the string and watches what happens when he tugs it. After a few thoughtful tugs he beams in triumph – the problem is solved and the toy is his. Similarly, one can watch a baby deduce 'where a ball rotating around his head is most likely to re-appear next?' In order to think in this way he needs to have P of O and to compute the visual information gained during the first two to three rotations.

Cause and effect

The first steps of most cognitive sequences involve people rather than objects, i.e. neonates find faces are more visually interesting than objects. One could make a case that 'realisation that I get mother's attention if I vocalise, smile and seek eye contact' by 2½-month-olds is the start of concepts of 'cause and effect' (C&E). Baby gyms with dangling items[2] provide a lovely learning opportunity to experience C&E from watching the parent jingle them and from the baby's own excited swipes that randomly make contact from 10 to 12 weeks. Active swipes follow with the C&E aspects being realised between 4 and 5 months. Mother shaking a rattle, bunches of keys or their bottle is another source of C&E learning through visual and auditory integration. Although a

---

2   Soft toys with jingle bells attached are more appropriate than hard plastic dangles because the noise generated by the latter is loud and harsh enough to induce startling which interferes with learning.

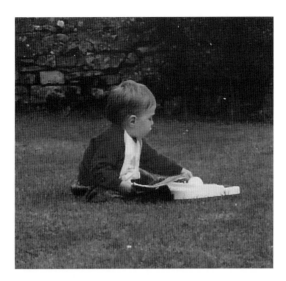

Figure 6.3 A 16-month-old demonstrates his understanding of cause and effect for a roller switch that starts his musical toy playing.

baby of 3 and 4 months closes his fingers around a rattle that touches his palm he does not look at it or seem aware that he is holding anything. A random arm movement subsequently results in hitting himself on the head with the rattle; his startled expression confirms complete surprise. He will demonstrate acquisition of the C&E aspect by reaching, grasping and shaking the rattle whilst intently watching the operation at 5 to 6 months. Banging a brick on the table for the sound effect becomes a delighted game from about 8½ months. The effect may first be realised through spontaneous excited movements or via observation of siblings. At a similar age babies eagerly grab a squeaker that the parent is demonstrating but look disappointed at the absence of a squeak as they shake or bang it; the association with squeezing is not realised until 10 to 12 months.[3] A 'light on', 'light off' game with the light switch and overhead light provide experience of the C&E of switches. Between 11 and 13 months babies experiment with opening and closing hinged lids; a music box containing a ballerina spinning to music provides visual and auditory C&E experience and concept forming information about the relationship of the component parts (lid to box).

Q Should the assessor positively score a 52-week-old for C&E, who opens and closes the box repeatedly?

---

3   Many squeakers are made of tough rather than soft synthetic material, i.e. even adults have to put effort into squeezing them!

Not unless he watches and listens entranced before he closes the box and does the same when he opens it; i.e. he is clearly motivated by the visual and auditory effects rather than the mechanics of opening and closure.

The 15-month-old in Figure 6.3 was inseparable from his light and sound toy. One of three nursery tunes played when a simple roller was spun; although absorbed in the pictures in his book his hand would reach for the roller whenever the music stopped.[4]

In modern homes C&E opportunities are everywhere, and as soon as they are mobile most babies develop an insatiable appetite to experiment with them; the switches on televisions, remote controls, mobile phones, tablets, kitchen gadgets, etc are easy to press or turn and have irresistible effects! Incidentally, Tablets are increasingly being used to entertain (or 'keep baby quiet'). The visual and sound effects of touching an icon (accidentally or intentionally) are varied and attention grabbing, but are not necessarily either meaningful or a learning experience at this age. There is a very real danger that 'Tablet babies' may become so addicted to icon touching that they deprive themselves of real-life learning experiences. In contrast the switches found on cause-and-effect toys although bigger require more strength to operate than those on modern electronic equipment, i.e. the manipulative components of most C&E toys are physically taxing for this age group and therefore not ideal for teaching or testing. Toy industry – sit up!

Relationships

Relationships between objects or between component parts of an object can be made and unmade; developmentally the latter tends to precede the former; the more components the greater the demand on cognitive processing.

Two-component relationships

A person–object phase precedes the object–object phase; the person being himself. When Andy is 5 months his father playfully leaves his vest over his face and then removes it with a smiling 'where's Andy?' Once familiar with the game Andy reaches to grab the vest off his face, beaming in triumph as he does so. Earlier responses to this activity are general tensing and a panicky breathing pattern between birth and 10 weeks and vigorously shaking the head from side to side in an attempt to dislodge the vest from 10 weeks to about 5 months.

Q Why is it important to keep describing earlier stages of sequences?

---

4 Not only did the toy provide splendid C&E experience for 12- to 16-month-olds but became a valuable part of the test battery for visually impaired infants in our Developmental Vision Clinic. We guard our residual pieces carefully, as despite our protestations, it was taken off the market. Most C&E toys are too 'busy' for typical children let alone disabled ones!

Because, as assessors become more experienced, knowledge of the nature and time scale of earlier stages gives them flexibility and freedom in assessment. For example, while assessing a 10-month-old I become suspicious that she may have severe learning difficulties. I find that she responds to the vest on her face by tensing and panicky breathing; in this respect she is functioning at less than a 3-month level. Obviously, this finding would need to be viewed in the context of other levels. One test finding does not make a diagnosis! But several that agree increase the likelihood.

Practice Point when used as a test it is essential that the interaction is presented as a game; otherwise the parents will become anxious when the assessor suddenly puts a cloth over their baby's face!

Around 8 months, when lying supine, another similar learning situation presents; Andy's stripy sock catches his visual attention; he grabs and tugs at it. One day a loose sock comes off; he has discovered an activity that will give him, if not his parents, endless pleasure while building up his templates for person–object 'relationships'.

Under 8½ months a baby treats a container and its content as a single entity (as long as the content does not protrude). Given a cup containing a toy brick he is likely to pick the cup up and shake it vigorously; if the brick flies out his startled look confirms that he had no idea that the two were separate objects and separable. From around 9 months babies grab every two-component concept building opportunity (e.g. 'wooden peg men' – 6.5cm high and 2cm in diameter standing in the recesses of a boat-shaped wooden board, saucepans or teapots with lids, wastepaper baskets full of delights). Initially a baby accidently discovers that peg men come out, or lids come off when pulled; he does not try to put them back but repeats the operation when someone else remakes it. After several weeks he demonstrates consolidation of the concept of separateness by pulling all the peg men out or all the lids off as quickly as possible; only then does he start exploring 'remaking' the relationship.

This sequence could easily be built into a testing schedule and would make a valuable addition to assessment of cognitive status during the first year. Unfortunately, although my personal experience of using these procedures is large, population data are not sufficient to yield scientifically strong age guidelines. The following average ages are a guide, based on personal experience:

- vests – *24* weeks

- socks – *37* weeks

- peg men – apart – *44*; together – *50* weeks

Consolidation at the two-component level blossoms into experimentation with three-component relationships during the first few months of the second year. This is observed in everyday routines and play with real, and with Wendy house size toys (e.g. pulling the lid off the biscuit jar to get a biscuit, putting a sock into an open drawer and pushing it shut, opening the lid of a toy box to retrieve a favourite toy).

Mechanical concepts

Unscrewing and screwing up
Removing a screw top lid from a pot or bottle requires understanding of two-component relationships; it also involves higher-level abstractions of the screwing mechanism plus motor planning to achieve it. Toddlers, who quickly pull the top off a pot or the lid off a toy saucepan, will try to do the same when presented with a pot, which has a screw top. Usually after demonstration, they grasp the lid and turn it 'to and fro'; gradually they work out that the lid must continue to turn in the same direction to come off and use this conceptual template to organise a manipulative construct to achieve it – grasp, turn hand, release, turn hand back, grasp, turn again in the first direction etc. The same applies to screwing up usually 4 to 6 weeks later.

Construction

Once a baby has motor control of grasp, placement and release, he experiments with putting bricks/blocks on top of each other, which leads to development of early concepts of construction. Between 12 and about 33 months his constructions are unidirectional/ in one plane only – vertical (tower) or horizontal (wall); the height/length increase with age. From 33 months constructions in both planes emerge; at first simple, they steadily increase in complexity through the preschool era.

Concepts of size, shape, colour and number

Size, shape, colour and number are important NSC concepts that gradually emerge between the ages of 2 and 5 years. The first or pre-conceptual stage (Level 1) is at a perceptual level and is reflected through play with one-to-one matching games (e.g. form boards and picture cards). Percepts are gradually intellectualised into concepts (Level 2) through observation and play supported by adults applying names to them; this stage was referred to as 'concept formation as an abstraction' by Cooper, Moodley and Reynell (1978). Once achieved children are ready to apply spoken words to items, i.e. point to them on request or name them, and to group objects that differ from each other in dimensions other than the target concept (e.g. colour – a yellow ball, a yellow car and a yellow brick). The age at which children in Western societies name shapes and colours has fallen over the last two decades and may reflect rising parental awareness of the importance of early development coupled with increased availability of nursery education. Nowadays naming often precedes ability to draw shapes from pre-drawn models by several months.

Concepts of size and number embody the idea of gradation and appear a little later than those of shape and colour; toddlers conceptualise 'more' as another (piece) or bigger (amount). The idea that 'two' implies 'more than one' emerges from about 30 months. The link between counting and actual number of objects 'up to four' and 'up to ten' emerges in the fourth and fifth year respectively. Games like 'one, two, three – wheee' (as the child is swung in the air) prime both the non-verbal and verbal aspects of counting; to begin with a toddler echoes 'unn, tooo, tee – wheee' without any appreciation that he is counting steps prior to being swung in the air! Similarly, a concept of size is limited to 'big and little' in 2- to 3-year-olds, after which concepts of size ordering or relative size gradually emerge.

Drawing: geometric shapes in imitation and from pre-drawn models

Drawing, like writing is a representational/symbolic skill executed by the hands to express concepts. Early in the second year toddler's realise that crayons are tools that they can use to mark paper and begin to experiment with them. Initial jabs are followed by horizontal scribble and then circular scribble; the latter two both spontaneously and in imitation of an adult. Imitation of an adult drawing a vertical or horizontal line appears around the second birthday. However Level 2 concepts of shape are required together with more advanced levels of motor planning to draw geometric shapes from previously drawn models. On average children do not reach this level until shortly before their third birthday. Two year olds often appear to be concentrating hard when 'drawing'. However when asked what they are drawing, their expression indicates that they hadn't set out to draw anything in particular. Having planted the idea that drawing is representational, some turn back and study their 'picture' before making a pronouncement. Egan's finding that only 10% of 30-month-olds attempted to "draw Mummy" supports this contention (Egan and Brown 1986).

Assessment

History

The primary history will reveal whether or not a child is at risk of NSC delay. As cognition is the central processing aspect of any task, developmental questions can be phrased so they direct the parent's thoughts into that context e.g. 'Are you happy' … 'about the interest he takes in what is going on' or 'with how he plays with toys?' Occasionally, the parent's response sets off alarm bell, e.g. 'I know all babies are different but he isn't doing as much as Sammy and Katy did'. Formulating several age-appropriate probes designed to generate a description may yield more.

- For an 8-month-old: 'What does he do with a rattle?' – 'holds it for a moment' 'bangs it on the table', 'drops it', 'shakes it', 'puts it to his mouth', 'nothing much', 'fingers the bells'.

Q Which two responses would be most age appropriate?
'Bangs it on the table' and 'fingers the bells.'

- For a 2 ½-year-old: 'How does he play with a six-piece insert puzzle?' – 'I think he has some at nursery.' 'He takes the pieces out but doesn't put them back.' 'He knows the hole for the elephant but not the others.' 'He chooses all the right holes but sometimes tries to put a piece in the wrong way round.' 'He puts them all back straight away.'

Q Which answer is expected at 2½ years?
'He chooses all the right holes but sometimes tries to put a piece in the wrong way round.'

A medical (sign) response like 'He's just like his brother John was and he's got learning difficulties – that worries me a bit' clearly requires further probing into the medical background of John and family history and the sex of those with learning difficulties.

Medical risk factors for non-symbolic cognitive delay

Risk factors are similar to other domains. Within the population who have not experienced potentially brain damaging events delay in NSC is rarely, if ever, specific. Usually, it is the least delayed of the intellectual domains, i.e. one, but not the worst aspect, of global learning difficulties, of specific language delay, of an autistic spectrum disorder or of deafness; that is why it is used as the yardstick in 'thinking in profiles'. In the past it was assumed that because adult patients suffering discrete right hemispheric damage (left hemiplegia) often experienced specific perceptual–motor and visual–spatial problems that the same would apply in children. However, studies in the 1990s suggest that individuals with right and left hemiplegia due to pre-, peri- or early postnatal insult show delays in both language and non-verbal areas compared with controls. Furthermore, although delay in language skills is greater in those (especially girls) with left-sided than in those with right-sided damage, delays in non-symbolic skills occur almost equally in both categories of hemiplegia (Carlsson et al. 1994, Khaw et al. 1994). Thus even amongst children with cerebral palsy specific delay in NSC is rare. The condition imposing the greatest constraint on NSC is profound visual impairment; in these children the other intellectual domains are variously constrained and the social-communicative domain is prone to disintegration in the second year (Cass et al. 1994, Sonksen and Dale 2002). In contrast the impact of severe hearing loss is centred on language.

Examination

Sandwiched between the sensory and motor components of skills/tasks, the intellectual components, need to be actively acknowledged, sought and documented by the examiner. If the intellectual component is the highest-level it tends to be recognised as such, but if equal or at a lower level it often fails to be considered/noticed (see Chapter 1).

> Q What are the levels of vision, cognition and manipulation of building a five or six brick tower and a six brick staircase?
> *Tower: manipulation 20 months, NSC 24 months, vision 5 months. Three steps: manipulation 20 months; NSC 54 months, vision 5 months.*

Below protocols of NSC tests are presented for newborn babies through to 4¼ years. Many schedules show baby and examiner sitting on the floor for tasks that require a surface, e.g. retrieval of a ball on a string and building a tower.

> Q Why should such tests be carried out with parent and assessor sitting opposite each other up to an adult height table with baby sat squarely up to the table on the parent's lap?
> *For several reasons – the task is more difficult for babies sitting on the floor because they have to channel a varying amount of their attention away from the main (cognitive and manipulative) aspects of the test into the gross motor domain of sustaining balance in sitting; moreover the floor is at a relatively lower level (bottom level) than the table (chest level) which further increases the gross motor demand by a need to lean forward. Individual gross motor achievement will impact on the findings and confound the age guidelines.*

In babies under 18 months assessors rely on the way a baby handles objects, toys and situations and by the thinking revealed through his eyes to access acquisition of basic non-symbolic concepts. Thereafter the language domain increasingly supports thinking and learning about more complex non-verbal concepts. The thinking of 21-month to 3½-year-olds is often externalised both in spontaneous play and test situations (e.g. 'bue un on der top' while building a three-brick bridge) and is therefore available to the assessor. Older children and adults learn to internalise the language of their thoughts though most of us find ourselves speaking out loud when tackling a particularly difficult problem!

Sources of normative data

Normative data are presented as age guidelines and age reference ranges; the distinction between the two is defined in Chapter 2, p. 38.
The data presented for each test are the age by which 50% in italics and 90% in bold

of children achieve the task; thus failure to achieve by the age in bold identifies children functioning in the lowest 10% who require further exploration through history and examination. Egan and Brown (1984, 1986) also give the age when 80% achieve the tasks, which for selection of those that need an 'eye kept on them' in primary care practice is a useful additional level.

Understanding myself and my environment

Cognitive interest in looking

The objects and their sizes, presentation, endpoint and reference ages of the NDV scale are directly applicable to this cognitive sequence, so while examining vision the assessor should note the NSC bonuses.

Protocol: Use the protocol for administering the NDV. During the newborn period the assessor's smiling face and from 2 weeks to 10 months an age-appropriate item from the scale at a distance of approximately 30cm – see Chapter 3 Vision.

Endpoint: high intensity fixation on NDV item.

Age guidelines: Face *within hours of birth–2*; 12.5cm spinning ball *4–8*; 6.25cm spinning ball *8–14*; 6.25cm stationary ball *18–22*; 2.25cm cube *21–26*; 1.25cm Smartie *24–30*; 1.2mm HT *35–42* weeks.

Faces, voices and hands are communicative

Protocol: The assessor attracts the baby's visual attention to her face, smiles and vocalises in intonated coos.

Endpoint: Baby smiles responsively and may coo

Age guideline: [Sh, GMDS] *6–9* weeks

Realisation of the prehensile potential of arms and hands

Protocol: The assessor asks the parent if she has noticed her baby 'regarding his hands' and if so at what age. With the baby supine the assessor attracts his *visual attention* to a bright toy dangling 25 to 30cm above him and observes arm movements.

Endpoint: Reaching ('swiping' movement) with one or both hands towards the ball – usually one hand leads.

Age guideline: [Sh, E, S] Finger and hand regard *13–16*; Swipe *16–20* weeks.

Recognition of everyday routines

Protocol: Initially, the assessor explores through questioning and takes any opportunity to check visual and/or auditory recognition of the baby's bottle/'anyway up cup/teacher beaker' if feeding time is approaching.

Endpoint: Clear history or demonstration of at least one.

Age guideline: [Sh, S] *14–17* weeks.

Localisation skills

Sound localisation

Protocol: This test is done following the distraction test. As hearing is no longer the main aim, sounds can be loud, cheerful and varied (e.g. a squeaker, rattle, jingle bells). The relative positions of the assessor, baby and distracter are the same. Tester presents sounds about 25 to 30° above or below ear level varying the side and sound randomly.

Endpoints: At ear level: no turn (may 'still' or look puzzled) / turns slowly / turns briskly. Above and below ear level: no turn (may move head from side to side as if scanning or look puzzled/two-stage response/one-stage response.

Age guidelines: [Sh, S]

At ear level: no turn *<20* weeks, slow *20–22* weeks, brisk *28–31 weeks.*

Above and below ear level:[5] no turn/puzzled <35 weeks; two-stage *35–39* weeks; one stage *42–45* weeks.

Practice Point The sequence is a valuable addition to the NSC aspects of a baby's development because (1) the time frame is well established and relatively tight and (2) the level of the response is a good guide to the age level of cognitive skills that need to be explored in greater depth in say a 16-month-old who only achieves a two-stage or no turn response.

Q What other domain would the assessor want to satisfy himself was normal before concluding the cause was cognitive?
Vision

Localisation of touch

Protocol: The sequence described in the development section has not been subject to

---

5   Some authors suggest that location below ear level tends to precede location above ear level by a few weeks. In my experience there may well be a disparity but just as often it is the other way round. From the cognitive point of view use the highest level observed.

scientific study so is not formally included here. It can be used to complement the view that cognition is around or below 35 weeks.

Permanence of people and objects

People

Protocol: Place the parent with baby sitting on his/her lap about 1m from a plain-backed chair; the assessor smilingly pops his face out from one or other side or above the chair with a 'peep bo' several times and then *silently*.

Endpoint: Baby eagerly searches the space indicating that he knows the assessor still exists when hidden and silent.

Age guideline: [S] *26–30* weeks for the *chair* method.

Objects

Ball dropping out of sight

Protocol: Stage 1: The assessor rolls a 12.5cm woolly pom-pom ball between his hands (about 45cm apart) to gain baby's visual interest; once gained he rolls the ball off the baby's side of the table to her left and observes whether she follows its trajectory. He repeats to her right.

> Q Why should the examiner use a woolly ball?
> *Plastic balls will make a sound as they hit the floor and may roll back into the baby's field of vision, whereas woolly balls tend to land silently and remain where they landed.*

Stage 2: He now ensures that the ball drops off one end of the table, i.e. so it disappears from view and observes whether baby bends to search for the ball on the floor.

Practice Points: Both stages are repeated two or three times. The ball is rolled at a medium pace. If the ball is rolled too slowly the baby may lose interest and look away to find something more interesting. If it is rolled too fast the baby may find it difficult to visually track and/or the ball may shoot well beyond the table edge so the 'fall' remains in view. The assessor and the parent take care not to move or search for the ball before baby's response is completed.

Endpoint: Baby bends and visually searches for ball dropped out of view.

Age guideline: [Sh, E, S] Stage 1: *26–33* weeks. Stage 2: *38–42* weeks.

Practice Point Stage 2 response confirms the acquisition of a basic concept of P of O. Stage 1 provides evidence of pre-conceptual visual behaviour only.

Toy hidden under a cloth/cup

Protocol: With a miniature car in one hand and a soft cloth (30 × 30cm²)/cup in the other, the assessor rolls the car along the table several times. Once the baby's interest is aroused he brings the soft cloth (or cup) from the other direction so the baby *sees* the car disappear under it.

Practical points: The toy that is hidden needs to be of greater interest than the object used to cover it – hence the choice of a small car. A cube is less interesting to babies of this age than a soft cloth or cup! The baby must be watching as the toy is covered.

Endpoint: The baby pulls/lifts the cloth/cup off the car: his gaze and other hand immediately latch onto the car. A baby who pulls the cloth (or lifts the cup) off and proceeds to give it his visual and manual attention before noticing the car has *not* achieved P of O at the requisite level.

Age guideline: [Sh, E, S] Cloth: *42–46* weeks. Cup *45–49* weeks.

Practice Point The cognitive component for cloth and cup is essentially the same, so the age difference is probably due to the greater demand for planning and execution of the manipulative component of the latter resulting in a shift of the child's attention away from the car. Both guidelines are given so that the assessor has a choice.

Problem solving

Retrieval of a ball by the attached string

Protocol: The assessor attracts the baby's interest to a 6.25cm plastic ball on a string by pulling it around the table surface and bouncing the ball on the table top. Once her interest is captured, he leaves the ball out of her reach with the string stretched towards her; if her attention shifts to the string as it is laid down, he taps the ball to ensure it becomes the main focus of her interest.

Endpoint: After 'assessing the situation'[6] she grasps the string and pulls the ball to her. (If doubtful about 'intentionality', repeat – intentionality is usually clearer and more decisive the second time.)

---

6 'Assessing the situation' may include reaching directly for the ball several times, then studying the relationship between ball and string, experimenting with the effect of tugging the string, etc.

Age guideline: [Sh, E, S] 39–44 weeks.

Anticipation

Q *'Where is the ball most likely to appear next?'*

Protocol: The assessor stands behind the parent's chair and introduces a spinning ball (12.5cm diameter) into the baby's R (or L) visual field from behind and rotates it in a circle (radius 30cm) several times around the baby's head at her eye level.

Endpoint: After two to three rotations the baby turns her head before the ball re-enters her R (or L) field of vision.

Age guideline: [Sh, E, S] 41–45 weeks.

Holding bricks

The cognitive elements of this sequence are less prominent than the manipulative components (see developmental section) and have already been covered by alternative tests. For those who wish to include them, holding on to a second brick is the most cognitively loaded, i.e. not forgetting the first brick when attention is drawn to a second one.

Protocol: Proffer a second brick to the 'empty' hand.

Endpoint: The baby takes the second brick, and looks from one to the other.

Age guideline: [Sh, S] 33–37 weeks.

Banging bricks together either spontaneously or in imitation

Protocol: When baby is holding two bricks, the assessor cheerfully bangs two together.[7]

Endpoint 1: Brings bricks together but not repetitively.

Endpoint 2: Either spontaneously bangs bricks together repetitively (before the assessor has time to demonstrate) or enthusiastically bangs bricks together after watching the assessor's demonstration.

Age guideline: [Sh, E, S] 1 – too indefinite to be useful. 2 – 45–50 weeks.

Cause and effect

Some of the C&E activities discussed in the developmental section do not make ideal

---

7   It is important that the assessor's demonstration is enthusiastic – I have seen so many assessors weakly pat the bricks together with an equally weak smile that conveys no enjoyment!

tests, either because population data are insufficient for age guidelines to be robust or because materials are subject to the whims of the toy industry and thus defy standardisation. Therefore three items have been selected that are secure in the above respects for the schedule. Others, such as the C&E aspect of using eye contact and vocalisation to get attention, the soft squeaker to produce the sound effect and manipulatively easy switches, are sufficiently robust to be explored through questions and/or observation by experienced assessors.

Shake a rattle

Protocol: Any rattle with an easily graspable handle (e.g. jingle bells on a stick). The assessor shakes the rattle gently as she proffers it and repeats demonstration if necessary.

Endpoint: The baby actively shakes the rattle and looks excited by the result. The cause and effect rather than the manipulative element is the endpoint.

Age guideline: [Sh, E, S] 26–**30** weeks.

Bang a brick on the table

Protocol: Tester obtains the baby's interest in a 2.5cm cube in her hand by banging it enthusiastically on the table. She then lets him pick it up, or hands it to him, with a 'now you do it'. She repeats the demonstration if necessary.

Endpoint: Baby bangs the brick up and down on the table with obvious delight at the effect.

Age guideline: [E, S,] 39–**45** weeks.

Music box

Protocol: The assessor places a music box[8] in front of the baby with the knob facing her. He opens and closes the lid fully several times, each time letting her see the ballerina 'dance' to the music. The assessor closes the lid with a 'now you do it'.

Endpoint: Baby opens the lid and looks for the 'effect'. If the assessor closes the lid baby immediately opens it again to watch the ballerina dance.

Age reference: [RZS] 54–**58** weeks.

Object relationships

Two-component apart

---

8   Specifications: Sold as jewellery boxes for little girls; Ballerina or other toy spins to music when box opened. Size: approximately 12.5 × 9 × 7.5cm. The catch is manipulatively too difficult for the age group, but is easily replaced by a small knob.

Protocol: The assessor attracts the baby's visual attention to a brick/small car in a cup or similar size pot,[9] by tilting it towards him and gently shaking it so the brick wobbles and rattles inside, then places it on the table in front of him.

Practice Point If he reaches into the cup it is OK to gently steady it for him.

Q Why is it OK to help in this way?
The manipulative aspect of the task is set at ceiling, i.e. use of one hand as executor and the other as stabiliser is only just emerging; the assistance does not affect the main (cognitive) component of the test.

Endpoint 1: Baby picks up the cup and treats it as one; the brick flies out when he shakes it but separation was not his intention.

Age guideline: [S] 37–41 weeks.

Endpoint 2: Baby puts one hand into the cup, grasps the toy and takes it out.

Age guideline: [RZS] 44–50 weeks.

Two-component together

Protocol: The assessor drops the toy into the cup and takes it out several times while the baby watches; then puts the cup and toy on the table with a 'you do it' and a 'putting in' gesture.

Endpoint: Baby puts the toy back in the cup/pot.

Q Is this test ideally designed?
No, not if the cognitive domain is the main target as actually the manipulative component is at a slightly higher level (release after placement) and may prevent some babies achieving the endpoint.

Q How could the assessor improve it?
By adjusting the endpoint, so that achievement of the cognitive component is given if the baby puts hand and toy into the cup and presses down, even if he doesn't manage to release the toy; however his intent would need to be clear.

Age guideline: [RZS, S] 52–56 weeks.

---

9   Ensure the toy fits completely inside the receptacle as protruding ones make the relationship more obvious and the task easier thus negating the age guidelines.

An alternative and manipulatively simpler way of demonstrating the separating and remaking concept is taking a lid off a container and then replacing it. Most scales use a plastic toy pot with a lid (diameter varying from 4 to 9cm) from a set of nesting pots; oftentimes the lids are a tight fit and the larger pots are too big for small hands to manage. It is preferable to use a Wendy house size saucepan[10] with lid, or toy teapot with lid, as these require a lower level of manipulative skill, i.e. the handle on the teapot and the knob on the lid make them easier to steady and grasp respectively.

Two-component–apart: two-component–together

Protocol: The assessor engages the child's interest in a saucepan with a lid *on*; takes the lid off and puts it back on several times. He says 'you do it', 'take it off' as he leaves it with the lid *on*.

Endpoint: Baby takes the lid off: Baby puts the lid on.

Age guidelines: [S,] 50–56: 54–60 weeks.

Three-component–apart: three-component – together: getting a toy out of a pot with a lid and secondly remaking it

Protocol: Apart – the assessor attracts the child's attention to watch him put something attractive into a pot with a pull off lid; he gives it a shake and places it in front of her with a 'you find it/get it out?'

Endpoint: Child pulls off the lid, looks inside and removes the toy.

Age reference: [RZS] 58–63 weeks.

Protocol: together – 'Now put it away/back'.

Endpoint: Baby puts toy in and lid on.

Age reference: [RZS] 60–65 weeks.

Practice Point If the child only puts the toy in the pot or only puts the lid on the pot he has not passed the test.

Tipping out – an early concept of gravity

Problem – 'How can I get the brick out?'

Materials: A brick and a pot. The brick should be a 'snug' fit, i.e. it should fall out when the pot is inverted but the baby should not be able to grasp it when it is inside the pot.

---

10   Purchased with 'Wendy house kitchen equipment' from toy stores or departments stores.

Protocol: The assessor holds the pot about 3in above the table and tips the brick out, while the baby watches; he reassembles and hands it to the baby with a 'now you do it.' If the baby persists in trying to grasp and pull the brick out he repeats the demonstration.

Endpoint: The baby inverts the pot and the brick falls out.

Age guideline: [S] 60–69 weeks (14–16 months)

Construction

General: The sequence spans a wide age range from 13 to over 60 months. For children under 3½ years it is better for the assessor to hold the box of bricks on her lap and hand bricks out as needed.

> **Q** Why?
> *Attention control! – see Chapter 2.*

Materials: 2.25cm wooden bricks in four colours.

Tower

Protocol: Under 2 years – The assessor places one brick on the table in front of the child and a second one about 7cm to one side, with a 'put it on the top' and gesture that suggests the second brick goes on top of the first. For those under 16 months the assessor may demonstrate building a tower of three bricks.

2 years and over: The assessor places two bricks as above saying 'lets build a tower; put it on the top'. As the child completes placement, he puts another brick to alternate sides with an 'and this one' until the tower falls.

> **Q** Why alternate sides?
> *Gives the assessor the opportunity to observe all aspects of manipulation and any difference in functional level of the two hands; these observations are manipulative bonuses.*

Endpoint: The number of bricks achieved.

Age references: [ETS] [GMDS] 2: 14–15; 3 or 4: 17–24; 5 to 7: 19–30; 8 or >, 25–37 months.

Models

The five items depicted in Figure 6.4 require a child to recreate a model from memory.

Protocol: It is *essential* that the child takes a good look at the model before it is dismantled for him to recreate. The examiner building the model behind her hands or a card results either in the child standing to peer over the top or in him losing interest and finding something else to play with. Rapport and flow of assessment are lost. Therefore the author builds the model 'in her space' chatting as she does so to hold his interest. Subsequently, she dismantles the model and pushes the bricks across to him with a 'Now you do it; make it just like mine'.

Examples of patter

- For the bridge – 'Look I'm building a bridge for the train to go through' (pushing a pencil through the bridge with a 'chuff-chuff').

- For the train – 'and that's the funnel where the smoke comes out'

- For the house – 'Now I'm making a house with a window at the top and two doors downstairs' (pointing to the gaps while speaking).

- For the steps – 'I've made steps; one, two, three (four) and jump off the top' (using two fingers to run up the steps followed by a jumping gesture).

Endpoint: model correctly built.

Q Should the child pass or fail if the bridge collapses as he pushes the pencil through?
He has passed the main aspect of the test – the intellectual one, a concept of a bridge; the purpose of the train going underneath in the demonstration is to make sure he looks at the model with interest; the collapse of the bridge is almost certainly due to his manipulative development being not quite up to the task – not necessarily abnormal, though obviously the assessor should be alert to that possibility and observe carefully for tell-tale signs of neuromotor pathology.

Practice Point The assessor should repeat demonstration if child's first attempt fails. If second attempt is almost correct it may be worth leaving the model up after a third demonstration. If he then succeeds he probably will achieve with the model dismantled within one or two months.

Age Guidelines: [ETS] [Sh] [R] [S] Bridge, 34–44; Train with funnel, 39–53; 3 steps, 52->60; House, 54–66 months; 4 steps, only 24% of Egan's sample achieved four steps by 54 months.

Q When is it worth presenting 4 steps?
Presenting 'four steps' is worthwhile in a child who has achieved the 'house' because success signals above average ability in this area.

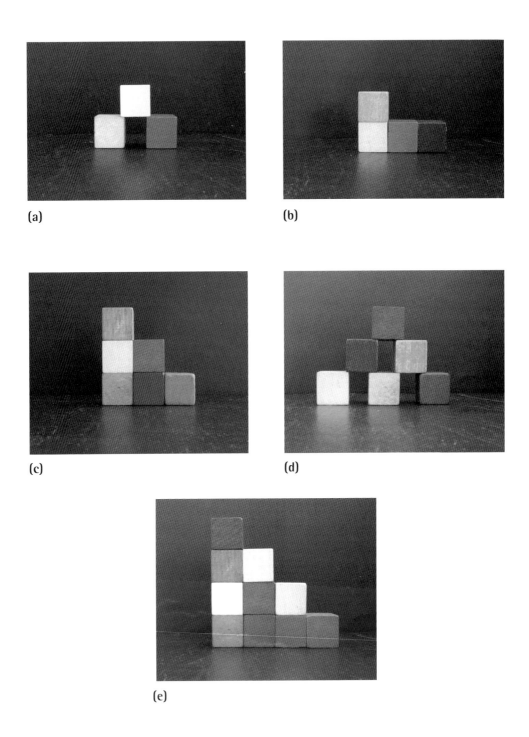

(a)

(b)

(c)

(d)

(e)

Figure 6.4a, b, c, d and e. Brick models of a bridge, train, three steps, house and four steps.

Practice Point Egan built model behind her hands and included a four-brick train but not a house; Reynell used the bridge, house and three steps.

Mechanical concepts

Unscrewing and screwing up

Protocol: With child watching, the assessor unscrews the cap of a plastic pot (3.5 to 4cm diameter), drops a reward inside, screws the cap back on (not too tight) and hands it to the child with a 'now you get it out'. If child is successful he says 'put it back and screw it up tight'.

Endpoints: Unscrewing: Successfully unscrews the cap. Screwing up: Successfully screws on the cap

Age guidelines: [GMDS, RZS, S] Unscrewing 23–25; Screwing up 25–27 months.

Practice Point Pulling and pushing are not acceptable.

Concepts of shape (geometric and letter), size and colour

Traditionally, a variety of age-appropriate non-symbolic and symbolic skills are used to access the perceptual (Level 1) and basic conceptual (Level 2) levels of shape, colour and size concepts, using one-to-one matching for Level 1 and verbal comprehension and expressive language (e.g. pointing out a shape named by the assessor or naming shapes indicated by the assessor for Level 2). Drawing is an additional way of testing shape concepts. In the test descriptions that follow the focus is NSC; the language and manipulative motor planning aspects are important bonuses.

Level 1

Shape

The following options are available.
Form boards. Many developmental scales include a series of form boards; for example the Griffith's performance scale starts with two simple shapes, round and square, and progresses through boards of three, six, nine and twelve increasingly complex geometric shapes. Essentially, the whole sequence taps into the perceptual level through one-to-one matching, which goes some way to explain why many children with learning disability achieve spuriously high scores on performance subscales heavily dependent upon

form boards. The age progression seen reflects the increasing cognitive demand of more complex shapes, the increase in number of pieces and recesses to attend to and in the levels of orientation and motor planning required to achieve the endpoint (unassisted insertion) and introduction of time-to-complete criteria for the larger boards.

Q Would you introduce time criteria that affect scoring between 18 and 42 months? What are the reasons for your choice?
The author never does; her main reason is that the attention of children of this age is so easily diverted by a small happening (the assessor speaking to the parent; child dropping a piece on the floor and disappearing under the table!) or by their own thoughts – 'Mummy, Susie got one like dat'.

Three and six-hole form boards: Assessors not using the Bus Puzzle for language may wish to include a three- and a six-hole geometric shape board for children around 24 and 30 months, respectively. A circle, square and isosceles triangle (4.5 × 4.5cm) with knobs will reduce the manipulative component to below the intellectual component, for the three-hole board and these plus a rectangle, cross and star for the six-hole board.

Bus Puzzle Test: The Bus Puzzle Test offers an alternative within a standardised screening test of language for 20- to 48-month-olds (see Chapter 8 p. 205). Nine wooden insert pieces (bus, car, dog, boy, mummy, pushchair, boy on bike, post/letter box, lollipop/traffic man) form part of an everyday Western street scene. The pieces are large with a central knob and trace the outline of the picture exactly;[11] orientation is separately scored from selection of the correct recess; no time criteria are imposed and assistance with final fine adjustment is allowed. The test is standardised and provides age references for the number of inserts correctly selected (see below).

Letter matching Sonksen logMAR Test: As explained in Chapter 3, one-to-one matching of letters is the cognitive component of the logMAR acuity test.

Q Is it a symbolic or non-symbolic skill?
Essentially letters are shapes and matching them is a non-symbolic task.

The testability data on ability to match letters provide good age guidelines. It is therefore worth noting a child's ability to letter match and to record it as an NSC bonus.

Drawing: Imitation of horizontal or circular scribble or lines following demonstration taps into Level 1 concepts of direction/shape and the level of motor planning (manipulative).

---

11   Insert puzzles available in toyshops tend not to follow the outline of the picture so closely and are often rather small and fiddly.

Three- and six-hole boards

Protocol: The assessor places the board on the table with the inserts in place with an 'I'm going to take them out …' he removes the inserts and places them in a random way between the board and the child making sure their positions don't correspond to those of the recesses ' ….now you put them back.'

Endpoint: Correct selection of recess for each insert.

Practice Point A little help to complete insertion is permitted once the choice is definite.

Q Why is help permitted with this aspect of the test?
Because the cognitive choice has been achieved; the help is with fine manipulation/ motor planning.

Age references: [GMDS] Three hole, *18–25*; six hole *27–33* months.

Bus Puzzle Test

Protocol: See Chapter 8, p. 207.

Endpoint: number of recesses correctly selected.

Age Reference: [EBPT] 3, *21–30*; 4, *22.5–31*.5; 5, *24–33*; 6, *25–34.5*; 7, *26–36*; 8, *27–39*; 9, *30–42* months.

Matching letters

Protocol: As described in the 'Training matching' section of Chapter 3, p. 57.

Practice Point Re-test any letters initially demonstrated during training.

Endpoint: All six letters are matched.

Age guidelines [SSAS] SonkLT *28–36* months.

Drawing

Protocol – under 33 months: The assessor places a piece of blank paper in front of the child. With a crayon he demonstrates the age-appropriate design scribbling and drawing freely with enthusiastic vocalisation. He puts the crayon down on the paper with an encouraging 'now you do it' – the crayon should be central with the tip pointing at the assessor.

Practice Point The assessor's scribble should occupy at least a third of the piece of A4 – little bits of neat scribble in the corner or a neat 3cm straight line are *not* suitable, as they don't represent anything the child could imitate, i.e. he won't have fine finger control yet.

Q Why is (1) a crayon used for this age group and (2) putting the crayon down on the table better than putting it into the child's hand?
(1) Because a crayon is more suited to this age groups level of manipulation and leaves them better able to focus their attention on the cognitive aspects. (2) Because the test then provides the assessor bonuses in the manipulative domain – fine manipulation and handedness.

As the child finishes the assessor takes the crayon and uses it to demonstrate the next level. Then places it as above.

Q Why should the assessor take the crayon back?
Gives the assessor the opportunity to observe manipulation and handedness more than once and prevents the child starting 'his own drawing' rather than watching the assessor's next demonstration.

Endpoint: Level of child's scribble.

Age guidelines: [GMDS] [S] [ETS] Jabs, *14–18*; Horizontal Scribble, *16–22*; Circular Scribble, *20–25*; Vertical Line, *24–29*; Horizontal Line, *25–30* months

Size

The following options are available:

Some scales use two round pots/lids of different size; saucepans are however preferable (see the earlier discussion). The Griffith's performance subscale uses a form board with one big and one small circle.

Protocol: To ensure the child understands the task the assessor presents one pot, takes the lid off and places it between the pot and the child saying 'put the lid on'. Subsequently, he presents both pots and lids so that the lids are at right angles to the plane of the pots, i.e. give no clue to which pot they belong.

Endpoint: Both lids are put on the correct pots (brief trial and error is permitted).

Age guidelines: [RZS] *17–20* months.

Colour

Level 1

Protocol: The assessor places four 2.25cm cubes of different colour (red, yellow, green and blue) in a well-spaced line in front of the child. He places a second red brick beside the first saying 'Look this one goes here'. He proffers one of the other colours with a 'where does this one go?' 'Put it with the *other* one'. If the child looks puzzled the assessor points to the correct brick saying 'it goes here doesn't it?' He avoids the word *same* as this is not understood until over 3 years whereas, *other/another* are often understood as young as 21 months. Colours proffered in random order, i.e. not the same order as in the line.

Endpoint: All 4 colours are matched.

Age Guideline: [ETS] *31–39* months.

Level 2

Drawing geometric shapes from pre-drawn models is traditional and requires Level 2 concepts, and a higher level of motor planning and organisation. Level 2 concepts can also be accessed in children of 2½ years and over through the language domain: requesting a shape by name or asking what it is called.

Shape

Drawing from pre-drawn models.

The author never presents pre-drawn models until 2 years 9 months although many scales do so (e.g. the GMDS).

> Q What might be the author's reason for not doing so?
> *The task is too difficult under the age of 2¾ years. Observation of numerous assessors presenting pre-drawn models suggests that most are unable to stop themselves gesturing over the illustrations of the horizontal and vertical lines and of the circle. Intuitively they are adapting presentation to an age-appropriate level – Level 1!*

Protocol: 33 months and over: The assessor presents a pre-prepared piece of A4 on which the shapes (circle, cross, square, triangle, and diamond – size of each approx 7 ×

7cm) have been drawn down the left hand side.[12] He points with the pencil to the circle saying 'Look I drew one like this', and 'draw one just like mine – here' as he taps the blank area beside it and places the pencil so that the tip points towards the assessor. Once the child has finished he takes the pencil gently and repeats this time pointing to the cross, etc, until she fails.

Endpoint: Shape drawn correctly (corners of the square, triangle and diamond need to be angular).

Age guidelines: [ETS] [GMDS] [S] Circle, *34–42*; Cross, *41–46*; Square, *50–55*; Triangle, *58–67*; Diamond, *64–75* months.[13]

Practice Point Whenever a child fails to achieve an adequate drawing (e.g. of a square), take the pencil, turn the page over saying 'I'll show you? Look it has four corners 1, 2, 3, 4,' – 'now you try'. The assessor's drawing should be at least 7 × 7cm in size. Success could imply that the child has the concept, but that her level of manipulative motor planning is insufficient unless facilitated by demonstration.

Q How might the assessor check further?
   Ask the child to point to the shapes on request or to name them.

Selection from name or naming.

Selection from the name usually emerges 1 to 3 months earlier than naming. Colour concepts can be assessed verbally after looking at manipulation during the peg and pegboard test, size concepts during the miniature toy test and shape during a form board or drawing shapes test.

Protocol: Tester points to a circle 'This shape is a circle' 'What is this shape called …. and this one?' pointing to each shape in turn? Only drop down to selection from naming if the child is unsuccessful.

<u>Size</u>

Protocol: 'Give me the big spoon' ….'and the little fork'

---

12   Down the right hand side if manipulation observations to date suggest that the child is left handed.

13   In Egan and Brown's study (1986) a triangle was successfully drawn by 25% at 54 months (ceiling age of sample) and a diamond by less than 10% at that age.

Colour

Protocol: 'This is a blue peg' (pointing to a blue one) 'What colour is this peg … and this one'. As for shape, go for the higher level first

Endpoints: Naming or (selection from naming) of the shape/size/colour correctly

Age guidelines: [ETS] [GMDS] [S] Materials and methodology vary between sources and impact slightly on the age guidelines.

Colour: Naming: 4 colours *36–42*; 6 colours *42–48* months. Boys were significantly worse at naming colours than girls in Egan and Brown's (1986) study.

Size: Naming: big and little *30–36* months.

Shape: Naming: round/circle *33–39*; cross/kiss/X *39–45*; square *48–54* months. Subtract between 2 months for a guide to 'selection from name'.

Comment: The design of the drawing of shapes test is not ideal as manipulation (in terms of motor planning) is too high – as high or higher than the target domain NSC. Personal experience suggests that today most children name the triangle and diamond before they can draw them, suggesting that the manipulative motor planning component is the highest level in the drawing task. Sex differences found by Egan and Brown (1986) support this contention. Boys were significantly older than their female peers in drawing the square, triangle and diamond, though this difference was *not* found when asked to name them and probably reflects more advanced motor organisational and executive skills in girls, rather than sex differences at conceptual level. Level 2 shape concepts should be explored in the future using language rather than drawing unless of course the child has a developmental language problem.

Concepts of number

General: Introduce from about 36 months; accessed through counting.

Protocol: A good time to assess concepts of number is towards the end of the peg and pegboard test, i.e. after noting the manipulative information. Initially, the assessor lines up 4 pegs in a row saying 'give me two pegs;' replaces them and asks the child to 'count the pegs;' if she counts 'unn-two-tee-tor' he increases the row to 6 and says 'how many are there now?' if she now counts 'unn-two-tee-tor-seven-ten, four is likely to be her limit'; on the other hand if she counts 'unn-two-tee-four-five-six' the assessor lengthens the row to 10 pegs.

In order to be sure the child is not counting by rote, the assessor notes whether or not her eyes and/or fingers move from peg to peg as she counts.

Endpoint: Number of pegs counted correctly.

Age guidelines: [GMDS] Four *39–45*; ten *45–52* months.

Practice Point Counting by rote does not imply any concept of number – parrots and budgerigars!

Draw a man

Dorothy Egan researched the development of drawing a man (Egan 1990, Egan and Brown 1986). Three stages were delineated – a humpty-dumpty man, an intermediate man and a mature man. The researchers found that only 1 to 2% and 10% attempt the task under 27 months and at 30 months, respectively: also that a sizeable proportion miss out the intermediate man stage.

Protocol: The assessor places a plain sheet of paper and a crayon/pencil on the table saying, 'Let's draw Mummy/Daddy – you do it'.

Endpoint: Probably the most useful endpoint is 'drawing *either* an intermediate *or* a mature man'

Age guideline: [ETS] Intermediate or mature man *48–>54*[14] months.

Comment: The test is time consuming and in no way definitive in children in the age range of this book and therefore not to be recommended.

Tables 6.1 (birth to 24 months) and 6.2 (24 to 48 months) summarise the most secure NSC tests with the ages at which 50% and 90% achieve. Select tests from the 50% column that are close to the child's chronological age and drop to a lower level if necessary; always move up to a child's ceiling as this provides the opportunity to detect a disparity between domains in otherwise above average children. On the other hand, if observations, history or referral suggest significant delay start at the level these suggest and move up or down accordingly.

---

14   At 54 months 20% had not achieved the endpoint, so the lowest 20% are 54 and > months.

Table 6.1 Non-symbolic cognition: birth to 24 months

Name of test	Achievement by	
	50% (wks)	90% (wks)
Cognitive interest in looking at increasingly small objects		
Face	Birth	2
12.5cm (spinning)	4	8
6.25cm (spinning)	8	14
6.25cm (stationary)	18	22
2.25cm cube	21	26
1.25cm Smartie	24	30
1.2mm ' hundred and thousand'	35	42
Other early concepts		
Faces are communicative	6	9
Hand regard/cognitive interest	13	16
Arms/hands are prehensile	16	20
Sounds have substantive sources voices/objects	18	20
Sound location		
Ear level – slow	20	22
Ear level – brisk	28	31
Above or below ear level - puzzled	<35	–
Above or below ear level – two stage	35	39
Above or below ear level – one stage	42	47
Permanence of people		
Silent 'peep-bo' from behind chair	26	30
Object permanence		
(Falls within sight)	26	33
Falls out of sight	38	42
Toy under cloth	42	46
Toy under cup	45	49

Table 6.1 continued

Problem solving		
Retrieves toy by string	*39*	**44**
Anticipates ball round head	*41*	**45**
Bangs bricks together spontaneously/imitation	*45*	**50**
Cause and effect		
Shake a rattle	*26*	**30**
Bangs brick on table	*39*	**45**
Music box	*54*	**58**
Object relationships		
Two-component – apart (brick/cup)	*44*	**50**
Two-component – together (brick/cup)	*52*	**56**
Three-component – apart (toy/saucepan/lid)	*58*	**63**
Three-component – together (toy/saucepan/lid)	*60*	**65**
	50% (mo)	90% (mo)
Tipping	*14*	**16**
Construction tower		
2	*14*	**15**
3 or 4	*17*	**24**
5 or 7	*19*	**30**
8 or >	*25*	**37**
Concepts of shape		
Form board – three hole	*18*	**25**
Bus Puzzle Three pieces	*21*	**30**
Five pieces	*24*	**33**
Scribble spontaneous or in imitation Jabs	*14*	**18**
Horizontal	*16*	**22**
Circular	*20*	**25**

Table 6.1 continued

Concepts of size		
Pots with lids – one big/one small	*17*	**20**
Concepts of screwing		
Unscrewing	*23*	**25**
Screwing	*25*	**27**

Table 6.2   Non-symbolic cognition 24 to 52 months

Name of test	Achievement by	
	50% (mo)	90% (mo)
Construction bricks		
Tower 5–7	*19*	**30**
Tower > 8	*25*	**37**
Bridge	*34*	**44**
Train	*39*	**53**
Three steps	*52*	**>60**
House	*54*	**66**
Shape level 1		
Three-hole board – all pieces	*18*	**25**
Six-hole board – all pieces	*27*	**33**
Bus puzzle		
Five pieces	*24*	**33**
Seven pieces	*26*	**36**
Nine pieces	*30*	**42**
SonksenLT letters		
Six letters	*28*	**36**
Shape level 2: drawing		
After demonstration – vertical line	*24*	**29**
After demonstration – horizontal line	*25*	**30**
From model – circle	*34*	**42**

Table 6.2 continued

From model – cross	41	**46**
From model – square	50	**55**
From model – triangle	58	**67**
From model – diamond	64	**75**
Shape level 2: naming		
Circle	33	**39**
Cross	39	**45**
Square	48	**54**
Size level 2: naming		
'big/little'	30	**36**
Colour level 1: matching		
Four colours	31	**39**
Colour level 2: naming		
Four colours	36	**42**
Six colours	42	**48**
Number level 2: naming		
Count 4	39	**45**
Count 10	45	**52**

Sonksen LT, Sonksen logMAR Test.

Key Points

- Think NSC.

- NSC is the yardstick of the intellectual profile.

- Assessor make sure NSC is well covered in test schedule of under 7-month-olds.

- Choose tests in which NSC component is at a higher age level than the sensory and motor components.

- Select tests with the 50% level close to the child's chronological age and rise to ceiling unless:

- Referral, history or observations suggest significant delay; in which case shift to the level indicated.

- Test findings for Level 2 concepts of shape, size and colour are more clear-cut when the response task is language rather than manipulatively mediated.

References

Carlsson GI, Uvebrant P, Hugdahl K, Arvidsson J, Wiklund LM, von Wendt L (1994) Verbal and non-verbal function of children with right- versus left-hemiplegic cerebral palsy of pre- and perinatal origin. *Dev Med Child Neurol* 36(6): 503–512.

Cass H, Sonksen PM, McConachie HR (1994) Developmental setback in severe visual impairment. *Arch Dis Child* 70: 192–196.

Cooper J, Moodley M, Reynell J (1978) *Helping Language Development: A Developmental Programme for Children with Early Language Handicaps.* London: Edward Arnold Ltd.

Egan DF (1990) *Developmental Examination of Infants and Preschool Children.* Clinics of Developmental Medicine No. 112. Oxford: Mac Keith Press, Blackwell Scientific Publications Ltd.

Egan DF, Brown R (1984) Developmental assessment: 18 months to 4½ years. The Bus Puzzle Test. *Child Care Health Dev* 12: 163–179.

Egan DF, Brown R (1986) Developmental assessment: 18 months to 4½ years. Performance Tests. *Child Care Health Dev* 12: 339–349.

Khaw CWH, Tidemann AJ, Stern LM (1994) Study of hemiplegic cerebral palsy with a review of the literature. *J Paediatr Child Health* 30(3): 224–229.

Sonksen PM (1979) Sound and the visually handicapped baby. *Child Care Health Dev* 5: 413–420.

Sonksen PM (1983) Vision and early development. In Wybar R, Taylor D, editors. *Paediatric Ophthalmology: Current Aspects.* New York: Marcel Dekker.

Sonksen PM, Dale N (2002) Visual impairment in infancy: Impact on neurodevelopmental and neurobiological processes. *Dev Med Child Neurol* 44: 782–791.

Chapter 7

Non-spoken symbolic development and imaginative play

Symbolic cognition

Humans use symbols (see Chapter 5, second paragraph) to communicate their needs, thoughts and feelings and as a medium for their own thinking at all levels. In the pre-school years the templates for spoken and gestural language and for pictorial and miniature representations are constructed and interlinked. At 5 years the human child is ready to master the challenge of written symbols. The networks and templates of spoken language are actively developing from birth.

The development and examination of non-spoken symbolic cognition (NSpSC) and imaginative play is discussed in this chapter and that of spoken symbols in Chapter 8. The two are separated in order to highlight that the delay in the understanding of non-spoken symbols and of imaginative play is a cardinal feature of autistic spectrum disorders (ASD) rather than of specific language disorders (SLD), and realisation that miniature toys and pictures represent the real object should not be equated with the comprehension of the spoken word 'chair'. Novice assessors often confuse the two.

As discussed at the beginning of Chapter 5 some symbols bear no physical resemblance, whereas others visually resemble the object they represent to variable degree. Gestures tend to mime the meaning of a communication, for example beckoning for 'come here', whereas the visual resemblance of signs to meaning in formal sign languages varies considerably from system to system. Realistic life-size pictures of common objects visually resemble the object they depict, however, in two rather than three dimensions. The degree of visual resemblance of pictograms in symbol systems designed to assist physically disabled children to communicate varies from close to arbitrary. The symbols of both speech and writing are entirely arbitrary. In all areas of normal symbolic development, understanding (comprehension) precedes expressive usage.[1]

In the human baby, the leap into all three types of symbolic understanding occurs during the first trimester of the second year, suggesting that there may be close conceptual links between these processes and that as pretend play also involves emotional and cognitive domains, it is a powerful promoter of connectivity at this age (Bergen 2002, Bergen and Coscia 2001). As the symbols of spoken language are entirely arbitrary, one might have thought that the understanding for linguistic symbols would emerge considerably later than for those that bear close visual resemblance. In fact, linguistic understanding commonly wins by a short head. Could the amount of exposure during the first year to each be a factor?

Babies are exposed to speech from birth; from the early weeks words are accompanied by gestures, facial expression and intonation intended to enhance the motive content and meaningfulness to the utterance. In contrast, exposure of babies to suitable[2] two-dimensional pictures has historically been extremely limited until the 1950s even in Western societies. Professionals realised the potential developmental value of realistic life-sized pictures of everyday objects in the years following the Second World War; 'Baby's First Book' was Ladybird Books insightful response (Lewis and Woolley 1954). Since the 1950s the demand by parents for picture books has increased and both parents and babies/toddlers enjoy looking and talking about pictures, photographs, television for toddlers and family videos. Thus, exposure to two-dimensional material between 6 and 18 months has risen exponentially in the West in the last 60 years and norms are shifting in response. In the 1960s and 70s A5-sized pictures were recommended until 2 years; babies simply did not respond to 6 × 6cm pictures of the same item. Today babies, brought up with books with four smaller pictures to the page, show recognition early in the second year. Picture books for babies and toddlers are still rare in underdeveloped countries, and the difference in the development of this aspect of symbolic understanding is very noticeable. Exposure to three-dimensional representations such as Wendy house tea set occurs between 15 and 18 months in the West and to doll's house size between 2 and 3 years. Sixty years ago exposure would have been limited to better off families and confined to a large doll and a toy pram from 2 years and maybe a doll's house (that they weren't allowed to touch), from 3 years. Nowadays, Wendy house-sized tea sets, kitchen sets, garages, push-along train sets and shopping sets are popular presents and most nurseries are well equipped.

---

1   Talking in sentences without understanding occurs occasionally in children with, for example, hydrocephalus or severe visual impairment. This type of speech is referred to as distant echolalia (learnt phrases), 'parroting' and cocktail party speech.

2   Cave paintings and a formal family portrait are hardly that!

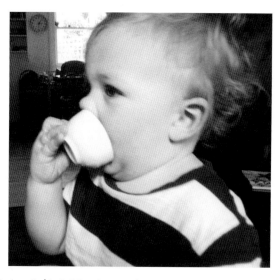

Figure 7.1 Symbolic hurdle/definition by use: In response to being given a life size cup (not his own) with a "what's this?" a 13-month-old shows that he has a concept of 'cups' by lifting it to his mouth as if drinking.

Thus the infant brain has for generations been exposed to more speech than to picture or toy representations, which may partly explain why the apparently most complex symbol system is usually 'first past the post', i.e. it is better primed as well as evolutionally older. The upward shift in norms since the 1950s and the increasing disparity between developed and underdeveloped nations confirm that exposure plays a role. Third, the near simultaneous emergence of all three types of representation suggests that they share a common prerequisite that could be described as the 'symbolic hurdle'. Around the time of their first birthdays babies show that they have conceptualised the key features and function of everyday objects, for example when given a cup (not their own) they lift it to their mouth as if drinking (Fig 7.1). This behaviour is sometimes referred to as 'definition by use'. The achievement signals readiness to understand that symbols (spoken words, two-dimensional pictures, three-dimensional toys) can be used to represent objects and people – in other words, readiness to jump the 'symbolic hurdle'.

Development

The development of understanding of two-dimensional representations (pictures) will be described first, followed by that for three-dimensional (toy) representations.

Babies recognise realistic life-sized coloured pictures of everyday objects shortly after they demonstrate 'definition by use' for real objects. A 13-month-old after gazing intently at a life-sized picture of a watch, may nod his head from side to side vocalising 'te-toch, te-toch, te-toch'.

> Q What developmental attributes is he using to indicate that he understands that the picture represents a watch?
> *Situational head gesture and situational phrase/vocalisation*

Realistic medium-sized coloured (10 × 10cm) and small pictures (7 × 7cm) pictures of everyday items are currently recognised by children in Western cultures between 15 and 18 months and 18 and 27 months, respectively – sometimes even earlier.

Toys

Definition by use (demonstrating the use of real objects on themselves) is also a prerequisite and the precursor of imaginative (pretend) play. Early imaginative play involves using a toy representation as if it was the real object. At 12 to 13 months a baby presented with a realistic large doll gazes at it with a puzzled expression and may look back and forth enquiringly at the presenter or parent before tentatively reaching out to pat the hair or face – apparently gauging whether or not it is a real baby. One is witnessing the dawn of imaginative play if, when given a real spoon, a toddler puts it to the doll's mouth rather than his own. Until 20 months dolls are carried uncaringly by the foot and stuffed unceremoniously into a pram! However, from 20 months a caring element is increasingly apparent in play with dolls/teddies, as toddlers begin to think of them as babies and themselves as mothers/fathers (Figs 7.2a and b and 7.3). Between 15 and 18 months toddlers play with the spoon and cup of a Wendy house tea set pretending to drink or feed themselves (Fig 7.4). Between 18 and 24 months they consolidate their ideas of domestic activities using child-size objects, such as the boy in Figure 7.5 is using to water the flowers. Between 20 and 24 months toddlers first recognise doll's house size cups and spoons and pretend to drink from the miniature cup. At this stage they are likely to sit the miniature doll on their own chair rather than upon the miniature. Egan (1990) referred to this type of play as self-related play (SRP), i.e. one representational item is related to a real item.

From 24 months children recognise and relate an increasing range of miniature toys to each other – tables and chairs, tea set, transport and animals. Relating miniature to miniature is known as detached from self-play (DFSP). A child's arrangement of the toys reveals understanding of what they represent. Between 30 and 42 months arrangement is steadily refined with china and cutlery arranged on the miniature table, chairs

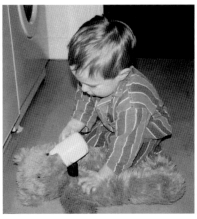
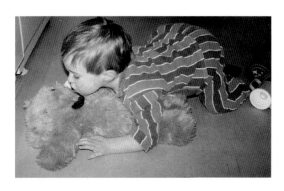

(a)   **(b)**

Figure 7.2a and b Twenty-two-month-old imaginatively and semi-caringly getting Teddy ready for bed – (a) 'last drink' and (b) a 'goodnight kiss'.

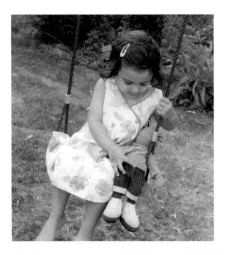

Figure 7.3 Rising 3-year-old taking care that her doll does not fall off the swing; note her motherly body language.

up to the table, dressed dolls on the chairs, naked doll in the bath and transport and animals in their own sections of the montage. It is not until 4½ years that a majority of children spontaneously indulge in sequence pretend play (SPP), e.g. pouring a cup of tea, adding milk or sugar and then drinking it or offering it to the parent or assessor. However, an increasing number do so if verbally prompted from 30 months. Boys tend to choose cars and garages rather than tea parties and tend not to play out such long tea set sequences as girls (Egan and Brown 1986). In Jeffree and McConkey's (1976) observation scheme of pretend doll play, these stages are referred to as 'self-pretending',

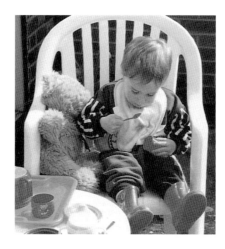

Figure 7.4 Imaginative play with Wendy House sized tea set – child feeding self.

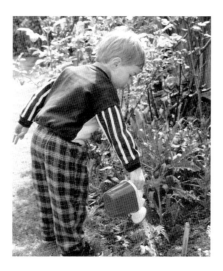

Figure 7.5 Acting through a domestic task with child-size watering can..

'decentred pretending' and 'sequence pretending'. Between 4 and 5 years imagination develops to a level where children use a tray to symbolise a shield, a necklace as a stethoscope or a pile of cushions as a house (Fig 7.6).

Q A 21-month-old was sitting on her potty when the telephone rang. Mother ran to answer it in the next room. After a minute she heard a series of 'er-erh'

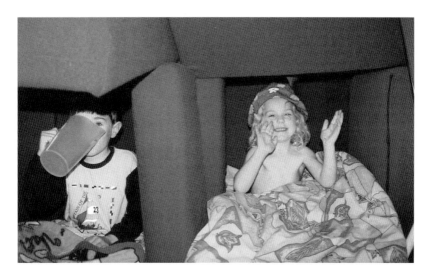

Figure 7.6 Children building their own house with cushions.

noises. As she peeped round the door the toddler picked 'Teddy' off the potty looking in to see what he had done and exclaimed 'goo ger (good girl)'!!! What type and level of play was this? What level of expressive language was she using?

Self-related play at an early level – she was Mummy, the potty was real and Teddy symbolised her 'baby'. 'Good girl' is a situational phrase (prelinguistic). Mother could hear her own intonation!

In summary, progressively smaller three-dimensional symbols are recognised between 12 and 27 months and imaginative play with each size follows quickly on recognition; play with each size is initially self-related, then decentred; the latter extends into increasingly long and more complicated sequences.

Assessment

In the context of a preliminary examination of a child exploration of the development of non-verbal symbols and imaginative play can take a back seat if spoken language development and social communication are normal. However, if they are not, or if the parent, another professional or assessor is suspicious of an ASD then this area justifies greater attention than is described here. In such cases both questions/history and examination should probe these areas more deeply.

History

Primary

The primary medical history will have alerted the examiner to general medical risk factors for developmental problems.

Secondary

Developmental
Questions are best worded to elicit a description of play. 'What does he like playing with?' 'Cars'. The assessor cannot assume any imaginative play. 'How does he play with them?' 'Mouths them'; 'pulls the wheels off'; 'crawls around the kitchen floor making "brmm-brmm" noises'; 'loves pushing them across to Daddy who pushes them back', 'lines them all up', 'loves his garage, pushes the cars up the ramps and parks them' 'stops for petrol on the way out and at the traffic lights' give the assessor an idea of the age level and normality of the play.

Medical
In addition to the primary medical history target family history of ASD and of congenital syndromes often associated with ASD (e.g. Fragile X syndrome, Rett syndrome, severe visual impairment, etc).

Examination

As a routine for a child who has not aroused concern, the assessor can regard the non-spoken aspects of toy tests as important bonuses to tests of language expression and comprehension. The rationale behind this suggestion is that symbolic play is very rarely, if ever, delayed if spoken language development is normal. Another common practice today is to request a report on this area of development from the child's nursery.

Typically toddlers and preschool children demonstrate their understanding of pictorial and toy representations in one of several ways:

• Meaningful gesture – drinking, brush to hair, feeding gesture

• Meaningful vocalisations or words – 'brmm-brmm', 'car'

• Meaningful arrangement of the items – plates and cutlery on the table; naked baby in the bath; dressed ones on the chairs; chairs pulled up to the table; aeroplane and cars at a distance from the domestic items

• Self-related play (miniature doll on their own chair), detached from self-play (miniature doll on the miniature chair), sequence play (pouring tea, then using a spoon to add sugar, stirring and offering to the parent or assessor).

Symbolic Hurdle Test

It tests readiness for symbolic understanding.

Material: A life-size child's beaker, bowl, spoon, hairbrush, toothbrush

Protocol: With an 'oooh what's this?' to attract the baby's attention, the assessor hands the baby one item and observes for 'definition by use' on self.

Endpoint: Lifts brush to own or the parent's head or takes beaker to mouth and tips it as if drinking.

Age guideline: [Sh, S] *12–14* months

Practice Point Just taking the spoon or toothbrush to his mouth and chewing on it is not sufficient evidence that he understands the function.

Picture Test

Material: Five A5-size realistic life-sized coloured pictures of objects in the everyday experience of babies with the potential for their content to be conveyed through gesture and prelinguistic vocalisation or speech. Pictures of a watch, a hairbrush, a toothbrush, a child's beaker and a car can be used.

Protocol: The assessor engages the child and hands him a picture with a 'What is it?' 'What do you do with it?' The assessor's voice and facial expression are questioning and full of interest.

Endpoint: Child conveys correct content, e.g. points to parental wrist,[3] hand to head + brushing gesture, hand to mouth + brushing movement 'tup' or 'dink' ± drinking gesture, 'brmm-brmm', etc.

Age guideline: [Sh, S] One correct *15–18*; two or > *17–22* months

---

3 Even though today's watches and clocks don't tick, watches still fascinate; the modern baby points to Mummy or Daddy's wrist when shown the picture of a watch.

Wendy House Toy Test (WHTT)

Material: Wendy house size bowl, spoon, beaker and large doll.

Protocol: The assessor places the toys on the table and observes.

Endpoint 1: e.g. Child picks up bowl and spoon and feeds self (SRP).

Endpoint 2: e.g. Child picks up bowl and spoon and feeds doll (DFSP).

*Age guidelines: 1. 15–**17**; 2. 16–**18** months.*

Miniature Toy Test (MTT)

Material: Sheridan (1976) included a set of miniature toys for assessing symbolic play amongst her STYCAR Language Test – the test was not standardised. A standard procedure was devised by Egan, which included several aspects of spoken language development in addition to NSpSC and was standardised (Egan and Brown 1986). The following age guidelines apply to Egan's adaptation.

Protocol: The assessor hands the child the toys one at a time asking, 'What's this?' and observes but doesn't interfere with the child's arrangement. Once the arrangement has been noted and the language sections completed, Egan suggests that if no sequence pretend play has been enacted, that it should be prompted in children over 30 months by the assessor saying 'Would Mummy like a cup of tea?' ± a second encouraging prompt 'Would Mummy like some milk?' if necessary. However, if the level of arrangement is typical, this stage could be left out in children in whom an index of concern regarding a possible ASD has *not* been raised, as it is time consuming.

Endpoint 1: Level of arrangement (three levels) – items placed randomly on nursery table and some SRP with spoon and/or cup; tea set on miniature table, chairs up to miniature table;all toys arranged appropriately.

Endpoint 2: Prompted sequence pretend play (PSPP); unprompted sequence pretend play (USPP).

Age guidelines: [ETS] 1. On nursery table *24*; tea set on miniature table *33–**44**; all appropriate *42* months. 2. PSPP *33–**45**;4 USPP 33% at 51 months. (Egan and Brown 1986)[4]

Practice Point The sequences played out by girls with the tea set tend to be longer and more elaborate than those of boys.

---

4   Guideline in bold is for 80% achieving.

Table 7.1 Age (mo) when 50% and 90% achieve tests of non-spoken symbolic development

Name of Test – nature of symbols	Endpoint	Achieved by	
		50%	90%
Symbolic Hurdle Test – real everyday items[a]	Demonstrates function or names item	12	14
Picture Test – realistic coloured A5 pictures of everyday items	Conveys correct content using gesture, vocalisation or naming	25	37
	One	15	18
	Two or more	17	22
Wendy House Toy Test – Wendy house-sized dinner set	SRP	15	17
	DFSP	16	18
Miniature Toy Test – Egan Test Schedule set of miniature toys	SRP with cup/spoon – NT	24	NG
	DFSP – Tea set on mini table	33	44
	DFSP – All items appropriately arranged	42	NG
	PSPP	33	45[b]
	USPP	51[c]	NG

[a]Items are real not symbolic. [b]Achieved by 80%. [c]Achieved by 33%.

Egan Test Schedule; SRP, self-related play; DFSP, detached from self-play; PSPP, prompted sequence pretend play; USPP, unprompted sequence pretend play; NT, nursery table; NG, not given.

Interpretation: The assessor considers all observations in the context of child's chronological age and the rest of the intellectual profile.

Q A 2½-year-old boy takes each toy, looks at it and puts it down on the nursery table. He does not relate them meaningfully to each other or name any of them, i.e. he has not demonstrated any understanding of what the miniature toys represent through arrangement, play or speech. How would you plan to proceed?
Present Wendy house size material and observe play. If there is still no interest or meaningful response, try everyday objects to gauge whether or not the child is ready to jump the symbolic hurdle.

Ages when 50% and 90% of children achieve age guideline levels are summarised in Table 7.1.

Key Points

- Happy 1st Birthday! – defines real objects by use; readiness to jump symbolic hurdle.

- *12–16* months – symbols come online.

  - Spoken

  - Pictures (2D) – realistic, coloured, life-size

  - Toys (3D) – Wendy house size

- 21 months – miniature toys.

- Play sequence with toys:

  - SRP → DFSP → PSPP → USPP.

- NSpSC rarely delayed if spoken language normal.

- Delayed NSpSC – think ASD or global delay.

References

Bergen D (2002) The role of pretend play in children's cognitive development. *Early Childhood Research and Practice* 16: 1.

Bergen D, Coscia J. (2001). *Brain Research and Childhood Education: Implications for Educators*. Olney, MD: ACEI.

Egan DF (1990) *Developmental Examination of Infants and Preschool Children*. Clinics of Developmental Medicine No. 112. Oxford: Mac Keith Press, Blackwell Scientific Publications Ltd.

Egan DF, Brown R (1986) Developmental assessment: 18 months to 4 ½ years. The Miniature Toys Test. *Child Care, Health Dev* 12: 167–181.

Jeffree DM, McConkey R (1976) An observation scheme for recording children's imaginative doll play. *J Child Psychol Psychiatry* 17: 189–197.

Lewis B, Woolley H (illustrator) (1954) *Baby's First Book*. UK: Ladybird Books Ltd., Series 413.

Sheridan MD (1976) *Symbolic Play Test, STYCAR Language Test*. Windsor: N.F.E.R

Chapter 8

Spoken language

The neurobiological framework for linguistic language development is primed and ready by the end of the first year. As described in Chapter 7, the ability to conceptualise the key features and function of everyday objects is the cognitive prerequisite for jumping the 'symbolic hurdle' into linguistic language.

Neural substrate

Following initial auditory processing in the auditory cortex and planum temporale, further analysis of incoming speech is undertaken in the temporo-frontal networks. In the last 15 years neuroscience team studies of the mature brain have greatly advanced the understanding of the functional roles of the component neuro-anatomical areas and their ventral and dorsal fibre track linkages, plus the temporal sequences for analysis of speech perception and for speech production (see review by Friederici 2011). Briefly, specified zones within the left temporal and inferior frontal network support basic and complex syntactical analysis; semantic analysis is less lateralised while analysis of prosodic elements is the province of the right hemisphere network. Integration of information between the two tempero-frontal networks is via the posterior limb of the corpus callosum. Similarly, specified areas of the same network and their links to long-term memory are responsible for the generation of the language and the phonological (planning and organisation) aspects of speech production. Dorsal fibre tracts from these areas transmit information to the premotor and to the face and lip areas of the motor cortex. Detailed study of a family with genetically determined severe verbal dyspraxia and another study of patients with developmental stammering have revealed the importance of the basal ganglia (caudate and putamen) and cerebellum in the selection and control of motor sequences in articulation (Vargha-Khadem et al. 1998, Watkins 2011).

Evidence suggests that the basic templates and connections including lateralisation are present at birth in the normal infant brain though may have reduced representation or functional capacity in those destined to have specific language impairments (Friederici 2006). Networking can be followed behaviourally from birth with the prosodic components of the mother tongue evident in the early days, phoneme recognition complete by 9 months, semantics dawning at around 12 months and basic syntactic awareness by 30 months. However, research suggests that during infancy the networks have the capacity to assume each other's role if the need arises, i.e. the system has a degree of plasticity not available to the adult brain. Thus speech and language problems have less potential to ameliorate when congenital or neonatal insults to the temporo-frontal networks are bilateral than unilateral.

Development

Priming during the first year

Babies quickly become attuned to the cadences and rhythms of their mother tongue and listen selectively to it. They also attend to and practice the social aspects of communication, so listening and social communicative skills are major features of development during the early months of life (see Chapters 4 and 5). During the second half of the first year parents intuitively use gesture to re-enforce the meaning of spoken communications. Within a parent–baby pair these gestures and phrases tend to be consistent to a given situation, for example the preliminary to picking up might be 'up you come' with both hands outstretched in a lifting gesture; repetition leads to understanding first of the total communication and then of the individual components – gesture and spoken phrase. The baby expresses the dawn of his understanding by reaching his hands towards his mother or father and bracing his shoulders in anticipation of being picked up, first to the total communication and then to the gesture (9–11 months) and subsequently to the phrase alone (10/11 months). Shaking the head (gesture) and the word 'No' follow a similar time sequence. Parents also use intonated situational phrases that come naturally to them during daily routines like dressing and feeding, e.g. 'arms up', 'open up' and during rhyme game routines (e.g. 'clap hands, clap hands,' or 'round and round the garden'). Babies associate the whole vocalisation with a particular activity – they are not analysing the component words of the phrase. Babies show their understanding of an increasing number of phrases between 11 and 15 months (Fig 8.1) and between 13 and 18 months use them in situational contexts (e.g. 'der-u-ar' when giving, 'or-gon' when their bowl is empty, etc.). Babies look up at the speaker when their name is called

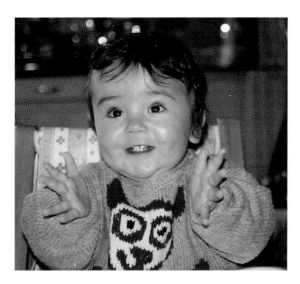

Figure 8.1 Eleven-month-old responds to mother singing "clap hands, clap hands," clapping just to the words.

from about 6 months and are rewarded by seeing the speaker gazing directly at them forming a link between their name and themselves. By 10 to 12 months the content of their visual engagement with the caller clearly says, 'Yes, you wanted me?' Under this age their response is less specific, similar to that for other incidental noises. The basic links and templates needed for speech production are also primed during the first year as babies spend time practising the musical cadences (rhythm, intonation, inflection) that their parents use when communicating with them. They experiment and practise first vowel sounds and then a range of frontal consonants like 'b', 'n', 'd' and 'm'. In some but not all babies this blossoms at 11 to 15 months into strings of sounds with the intonation and rhythm of speech known as 'jargon'.

Readiness

By around 12 months babies demonstrate that they are able to conceptualise the characteristics of common objects, for example that a cup is an object with a handle that holds fluid for drinking, or a brush is an object with a long handle and bristles for brushing hair. They do this by taking the cup to their mouth and tipping their heads back as if drinking, or the brush to their hair with a brushing motion. This is known as 'definition by use' and is a crucial sign of readiness to jump the 'symbolic hurdle' into linguistic language (see Chapter 7 and Fig 7.1). Definition by use is essentially a bridge between non-symbolic and symbolic cognitive domains; traditionally placed

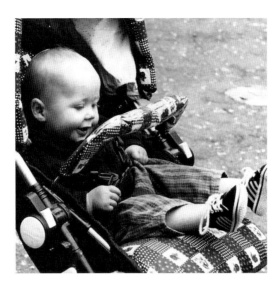

Figure 8.2 Fourteen-month-old responds to "Where are your shoes?" Lifts feet and looks at them.

in the language domain of test schedules it actually is non-symbolic as the objects are real and thus also warrants a place in non-symbolic cognition! In linguistic language the symbols are words.

At each stage of linguistic language development (understanding)verbal comprehension precedes expressive usage. Two sequences develop in parallel: meaning (semantics) and grammar (syntax). Semantics involves applying meaning, initially to mainly noun labels but progressively to other grammatical types (adjectives, verbs, prepositions, pronouns etc), and to an increasing number of key words in a sentence. Syntax involves understanding the rules that govern both word order in a sentence[1] and the effect of changing subunits of a word[2] to meaning. The two channels are more open to separate assessment on the expressive than the comprehensive side in the early years.

In the second year comprehensive vocabulary grows to around 20 words by 18 months and to 50 by 24 months.[3] Figures 8.2 and 8.3 show two babies exhibiting their comprehensive and expressive skills through gesture with or without speech The majority of these words are names of people, animals and objects, e.g. 'Mummy', 'doggy', 'spoon', 'juice', 'shoe', 'eyes', 'Teddy' plus some action words, e.g. 'kiss', 'clap hands' (without

---

1   Was the man funny?/The man was funny – often referred to as grammatical structure.

2   E.g. climb/climbed, happy/happily, car/cars – often referred to as 'morphology'.

3   In some children it may be as many as 200.

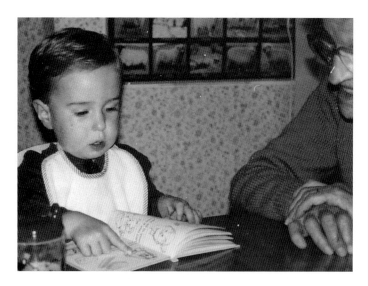

Figure 8.3 In response to "Where's the doggy?" a sixteen-month-old points at the picture saying 'dere'.

situational clues or gestures) and a few controlling words like 'no' or 'hot'. The non-noun label content contains some possessives like 'mine', demonstratives like 'dere' = there, 'dat' = that, directives like 'more' and question words like 'what'. Expressive use of each word follows once comprehension of it has consolidated sufficiently. The comprehension–expression word gap is usually short though in a few typically developing 24-month-olds with large comprehensive vocabularies, expressive vocabulary may be small; however at least 12 words should be used by 24 months.

In general children identify and assimilate two key/operative words in sentences devoid of contextual clues, e.g. 'give Mummy a kiss' 'put baby in the bath' by their second birthday; by 30 months three key words, e.g. 'Sally's ball in the garden', and by 3½ years four key words, e.g. 'give the big chocolate biscuit to Mummy' and by 4½ years five, e.g. 'bring Granny's bag and Jimmy's red shoes please'. Understanding of functional labels, e.g. 'would you like a drink?' appears from 15 to 21 months;[4] however selection of an item from its descriptive label (when there is a choice) does not appear until between 2½ and 2¾ years, e.g. 'which one do we do our hair with?' Between 2½ and 5 years children develop concepts of size, shape, colour, prepositions, pronouns, negatives, etc. and as these come online they incorporate the words for them into their receptive and expressive vocabularies. Around their second birthday toddlers begin to combine words in an effort to convey more meaning, e.g. in response to 'Where's Daddy?' they might reply

---

4   Child nods or toddles to the fridge.

'Daddy car'; they might use the same combination with a questioning inflection to ask the whereabouts of Daddy. Between 2¼ and 2¾ years sentences of three or more words containing a verb, though not necessarily grammatically correct, appear, e.g. 'me want book' or 'Mummy apple eat'. By 3½ years sentences become longer (4 to 6+ words) and are mainly grammatically correct, 'My Daddy's car is boo', 'D-ose are Donnie's wellies Mummy'. 'Where my wed ones?' By 4½ years more complex grammatical structures are appearing, e.g. past and future tenses and dependency of a second clause upon the first 'Mummy I want a biscuit, 'cos I'm hungry'.

Pragmatics refers to the social use of language and includes the rules of conversation, the impact of tone, inflection and word order on the message conveyed to the receiver and of inference, etc. Children gradually absorb these rules during their preschool and early school years. Preschool children are likely to make errors, for example asking for something in a demanding tone, barging straight into the conversation of others with their own topic, taking what someone has said literally, etc.

Assessment

History

Primary
The primary medical history will have alerted the examiner to general medical risk factors for developmental problems. In the context of spoken language development it is important to establish the cultural and language environment of the family including the number and quality of languages to which the child is exposed while taking the primary history, i.e. before starting the examination.

Secondary
Developmental: Communication with young babies involves facial expressivity, intonation, touch and gestures that mothers gradually drop as their baby's understanding of words emerges. The mothers of babies with delayed development of spoken language naturally continue these communicative strategies unaware of the number of additional non-verbal clues they are giving. It is therefore important to use definitive questions to probe both comprehension and expressive language levels; this was emphasised and illustrated with examples in Chapter 2.

When exploring first words it is essential to differentiate between babble and words used with meaning, for example 'ma-ma' (babble) and 'mamma' (as the parent's name). Fond adults eagerly equate their 10-month-olds babbled 'dad-dad-dad' 'nan-nan-nan' with the child calling them. Why else do the words for close relatives in so many languages contain the babbling phonemes mamma/mammi, dadda/daddi, nanna/nanni, baba/babi, gaga/gagi? Jargon and imitation are also commonly misconstrued, by parents, as 'talking'. A father once reported that his 10-month-old was putting two words together. When asked to give an example he picked her up, engaged her attention and then said 'Hallo Daddy" with exaggerated intonation. She watched his mouth intently and replied slowly "AH – oh – aah – ee"; a good example of imitation. Suppose the parent of a 2-year-old, in response to your question 'When were his first words?' replies, 'He started talking at about 10 months but then stopped'. Are you dealing with regression? Hopefully not – it is much more likely that he babbled, jargoned or imitated (words that an adult had just stressed) and has not yet moved forward into linguistic expressive language, i.e. jumped the symbolic hurdle. However, you won't know until you explore the words used and in what circumstances they were used. If the word was 'nana' it would be babble if executed while playing and not eye referencing Granny; imitation if the parent had just said 'here's Nana' and linguistic language if as Granny walks into the room the child points and/or looks at her saying, 'Nana'. If the word were 'car' or 'poon' ask whether Mother had just said, 'Here's your car?' (imitation) or whether the baby referenced a car and then said 'car' spontaneously. Random utterances often sound like words and tend to be interpreted as such, for example while playing quietly a baby jargons 'de-de-di-dar': he is surprised when fond granddad thrusts a car into his hands saying 'he wants his car'!

Medical: Specific secondary medical history should enquire into

• concerns about hearing – current or past;

• family history of sensorineural or conductive deafness (serous otitis media/otitis media with effusion) in childhood;

• family history of specific developmental language delays or disorders (phonological–receptive–expressive) or of dyslexia;

• family history of ASD. The extent and pattern of language delay/disorder seen in ASD is extremely variable but some degree of delay/disorder is commonly present;

• family history of learning disorders.

Practice Point Either or both aspects of language development are frequently more delayed than other aspects of development in children with global learning disorders, both syndromic and non-syndromic.

Table 8.1   Examination of prelinguistic receptive and expressive behaviours that underpin the development of spoken language

Protocol	Endpoint receptive	Age guideline receptive (wks)	Endpoint expressive	Age guideline expressive (wks)
Cradle, smile and coo gently to engage the baby socially	Attends briefly (several seconds)	*3–6*	Response contains little 'aahs' grunts or other vocalisations	*3–6*
Listen for spontaneous vocalisations Socially engage and vocalise to baby[a] – pause – repeat	Listens attentively (>10 seconds)	*14–18*	Tuneful cadences of vowel sounds, e.g. 'aaah' 'ahoo' 'er-rooh' – may pause while adult vocalises	*18–20*
Listen for spontaneous vocalisations Socially engage and vocalise to baby[b] – pause – change adult vocalisation Note attentiveness and range of vocalisations	Listens attentively >15 seconds	*16–20*	Single c/vs 'ba' 'ma' 'ger' – turn takes	*28–33*
			Strings of c/vs combinations 'da-da-da' – turn takes	*35–39*
			'dad-dad-dad → nan-nan-nan' (imitates changes)	*48–56*
			Jargons (spontaneously)	*54–63*
Ask the parent about S Ph's that he understands[c] and uses Ask the parent to demonstrate[d, e]	Baby shows understanding of:		S Ph usage 'or gon' 'der-u-are' 'der-i-is"	*78–90*
	Words with gestures and physical prompts	*44–48*		
	Words with gestures	*48–54*		
	Words alone	*54–58*		
Object concepts: Present several real everyday objects and observe what he does with them Readiness to *'jump the symbolic hurdle'*	Baby shows that he has a structural and functional concept of the object – 'defines by use' e.g. takes brush to hair	*54–60*		

[a]Coo and talk tunefully.

[b]Use consonant/vowel combinations that typically emerge in the first year 'ba-ba', 'da-da' and 'ma-ma' between 5 and 9months; talk with tuneful inflection to 9 months and over.

Table 8.1 continued

c e.g. 'up you come', 'clap hands', 'pat-a-cake', 'wave bye-bye', 'no', 'shall we do row, row, row the boat'

d Baby 9 months or less: for wave bye-bye. Suggest mother gestures and voices exactly as she does at home but doesn't physically help the baby to wave. If the baby doesn't respond to words and gestures encourage mother to start him off by waving his arm a few times; this avoids any sense of failure – indeed if the baby is only 8 or 9 months it is entirely age appropriate.

e Baby 10 month or over: Ask mother to voice exactly as she would at home only leave out hand gestures and physical prompts. If the baby doesn't respond to words alone, ask her to add her own gesture, e.g. to wave as she says 'bye-bye' and then if necessary to start him off.

c/v, consonant/vowel combinations. jargon, strings of sounds with the intonation, rhythm and cadences of speech; S Ph, Situational phrase.

Examination

Prelinguistic

Table 8.1 summarises the assessment (protocol, endpoints and age guidelines) of prelinguistic receptive and expressive behaviours that underpin the development of spoken language. It is an essential element of assessment of babies under 15 months but also of older ones who fail to score at linguistic levels of language.

Linguistic

There are a number of standardised developmental language scales – the Reynell Developmental Language Scales (RLDS), The Derbyshire Language Scheme, British Picture Vocabulary Test, etc. – for assessment of spoken language in the preschool years. The RLDS, first developed by Joan Reynell in the 60s, is widely used and respected across the world; a fourth revision has recently been re-standardised by the Granada Learning Group on UK children – the New RDLS (NRLDS) (2011). Full scales are time consuming in the context of preliminary assessment.

Two schemes that can be used are described with the intention of giving the reader insight into the practicalities of assessing spoken language and hopefully enabling them either to choose which method is most suited to their personal practice and level of skill or to appreciate more deeply the content of the screening procedures/language tests that they already use routinely.

The author worked with Joan Reynell from 1972 to 1977 and Scheme A owes much to the latter's wisdom. It uses real objects, miniature toys and realistic coloured pictures of everyday activities. Many of the age guidelines are derived from the RLDS, others from Dorothy Egan's adaptation and standardisation of Sheridan's Miniature Toy Test (Egan and Brown 1986) and others from years of personal experience using miniature toys to explore verbal comprehension and expressive language in depth. The strength of Egan's standardisation lies in provision of age guidelines for NSpSC and for expressive verbal labels for the 14 miniature toys.

Scheme B uses the Egan Bus Puzzle Test (EBPT) designed to screen early language development (Egan and Brown 1984). Apart from language domains the test explores recognition of shape – an NSC sequence that helps put language findings into a wider context. The test was standardised on a representative sample of the UK population aged between 18 months and 4½ years and norms are presented as centile charts. Productivity has never been formally researched. Children younger than 24 months can be tested using the set of real objects from Scheme A.

Tables 2.2 and 2.3 are particularly relevant to delivering the language section of a developmental assessment; some readers may like to re familiarise themselves with them before continuing.

Practicalities

- Materials: The choice includes Mummy, the baby, real everyday items, a large doll, Wendy house size or doll's house size (miniature) toys, pictures of single items, plurals, actions and everyday scenes and the Bus Puzzle. Choose materials well within the symbolic competence of typical children of the testee's age; otherwise it will be difficult to decide whether failure is due to delay in spoken language or not appreciating what the test object represents.

- A child's best language levels will be revealed if child and examiner are engaged in an interesting and mutually enjoyable dialogue centred on the play material. This is hard work for the assessor as she is multitasking – selecting and delivering age-appropriate tasks, noting the child's responses, holding their attention and helping 18- to 36-month-olds to shift it back and forth between the assessor and materials while maintaining rapport. The age group will be quick to grab any opportunity to 'do their own thing' with the miniature toys, subsequently rejecting and reacting negatively to adult attempts to direct their play.

- Judging the moment to switch attention back to oneself and issue the next instruction takes practice but is crucial; aim for the moment that the current command is completed and before the child has a chance to switch his attention to something of his own choosing.

- Opportunities to engage a young child in dialogue outside the test format is usually rewarded with a few linguistic pearls.

Table 8.2 Verbal comprehension: number of key words, examples and age guidelines

Operative words	Sample instructions	Age guidelines (mo)
1a	'Where's <u>Mummy?</u>'[a] 'Give it to <u>Daddy</u>'[a] 'Give Mummy (indicating Mummy) a <u>kiss</u>'	*12–15*
1b	'Where's Mummy's (indicating Mummy) <u>nose?</u>' Give me[b] the <u>shoe</u>' 'Where's the <u>spoon?</u>' '... and the <u>car?</u>'	*17–23*
2	'Put <u>dolly</u> on[c] the <u>chair</u>' 'Put the <u>baby</u> in[c] the <u>bath</u>' 'Give me[b] the <u>cup</u> and the <u>plane</u>' 'Put the <u>spoon</u> in the <u>cup</u>'	*24–30*
3	'Put <u>doggy</u> <u>under</u>[c] the <u>table</u>' 'Put the <u>baby</u> in the <u>bath</u> and give me[b] the <u>chair</u>' 'Give me[b] the <u>big</u> <u>spoon</u> and the <u>teapot</u>'	*30–46*
4	'Put the <u>spoon</u> in the <u>cup</u> and the <u>baby</u> in the <u>bath</u>' 'Put the <u>doll</u> on the <u>red chair</u> and give me[b] the <u>car</u>' 'Give me[b] the <u>plane</u>, the <u>bath</u>, the <u>spoon</u> and the <u>baby</u>'	*42–52*
5	'Put the <u>little</u> <u>spoon</u> in the <u>cup</u> and give me[b] the <u>white</u> <u>chair</u>' 'Put the <u>dog</u> <u>under</u> the <u>table</u> and give me[b] the <u>plane</u> and a <u>plate</u>' 'Give me[b] a <u>plate</u>, a <u>spoon</u>, a <u>cup</u>, a <u>car</u> and the <u>bath</u>'	*54–60*

Key words are underlined.

[a]Prime Mummy/Daddy not to move; [b]Examiner holds hand out in a 'give me' gesture being careful not to direct it towards the named object. [c]Prepositions in and on are not being tested as the relationship is the obvious one; under is being tested as child could put the dog on or beside the table.

N.B. The names of familiar adults (Mummy, Daddy, Johnny {brother}, Anita {daytime carer} Granny) and words for activities they participate in are usually understood before the names of objects, hence division of one operative word into 1a and 1b

Practice Point Pausing to 'think up' the next instruction or to praise children under 42 months gives the child ample time to turn her attention elsewhere. All this necessitates that test content and age-appropriate instructions are at the assessor's fingertips.

Scheme A

Table 8.2 provides examples of the number of key/operative words of an adult directive that typical children can assimilate at different ages. Table 8.3 gives samples of length and content of utterances used by typically developing children at different ages. Both tables provide age guidelines for the tests described here.

Real objects

Age: 12 to 24 months.

Aspects of language: Equally good for expressive language and verbal comprehension

Materials: A teaspoon, a cup or small mug, a baby's hairbrush, a toy car (10–12cm) a large doll, a ball (12cm), a bowl, a baby's shoe. For body parts – Mummy herself or the large doll (hair, nose, eyes, teeth, feet are usually the earliest).

Number of items: The ideal number of items for children to choose from is 3 under 16 months, 4 between 16 and 20 months, 5 between 20 and 24 months, 6+ at over 24 months. The limit is an intellectual one.

Protocol: Babies under 21 months sit on the parent's lap up to an adult height table; the assessor keeps objects on her lap or beside her. As babies tend spontaneously to name objects shown to them expressive language is explored first. The assessor proffers one at a time with an 'oooh what's this?' – if the child doesn't speak she continues 'it's a … pause for response …' If not named the assessor observes for definition by use. The assessor gently removes the object and repeats with the next, … etc.

For verbal comprehension the assessor lays an age-appropriate number of objects in a line on the table, captures the child's attention and makes either a single or a two key-word request, e.g.

- 'Where's/Give me the shoe?' (Assessor holds out her hand in a 'give me' gesture but is careful not to point to the object.)

- At the two-word level she either asks for two items or to relate two together, e.g. 'put the spoon in the cup'

- 'Give Mummy a kiss' is a two-component alternative, though the assessor needs to

Table 8.3   Expressive Language: examples of typical utterances in different situations and age guidelines

Number of words	Sample utterances	Age guidelines (mo)
1a	'Daddy' {sp} 'gannie' (Grannie) {sp} 'oggy' (doggy) {sp}	*14*–**18**
1b	'baby' (doll) {obj} 'poon' (spoon) {obj} 'tar' (car) {obj} 'bra' (brush) {obj} 'boar' (ball) {obj}	*18*–**22**
1c	[a]'car, boy, wor-er' {AP} [a]'oggy, dirl, boy, mummy, {AP}	*20-26*
2	'dirdie gone' (birdie gone) {sp} 'tup boke' (cup broke) {sp} 'daddy car' {AP} 'dirl ridin' {AP} 'boy cook' {AP}	*23*–**28**
3	'daddy gone work' {sp} 'moo see car' {sp} 'mummy bed make' {AP} 'oggy dink moock' (dog drink milk) {AP} 'dirl ridin orsey' (girl riding horsey){AP}	*30*–**36**
4	'Mummy riding Johnny's bike'{sp} 'I got a pink duvet'{sp} 'the boy and girl making a cake' {AP} 'boy give doggy a dink' {AP}	*42*–**51**
5 or >	[b]'The cat drinking milk cos he's dirsty'{AP} [b]'Daddy washing the blue car and Johnny put poliss on' {AP} [b]'Children hanging-up clothes so they dry' {AP}	*58*–**64**

[a] The earliest response to activity pictures is to name people or objects, i.e. a list of noun labels as separate utterances - enumeration. b The first and last sentences are complex because the second clause depends upon the first. The second sentence is not complex because the two parts are separated by the conjunction 'and' which effectively turns it into two separate short sentences. {sp} typical spontaneous utterance; {obj} typical response when shown object; {AP} typical response when shown activity pictures

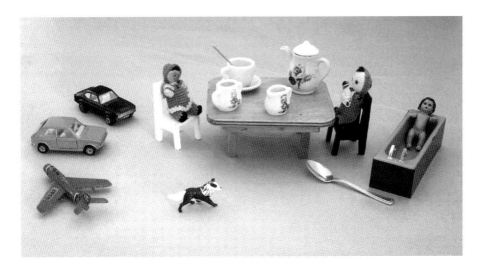

Figure 8.4 A set of miniature toys: a wooden table (7 × 5 × 3cm), two chairs (two colours), a bath, a naked doll, two sitting dolls (dressed), two spoons and two forks (size 5cm and 7cm), an aeroplane, two cars (different colours), a dog, a standing cat, a sitting cat, a china tea set (plate, two cups and saucers, teapot with lid, jug and sugar bowl). For Egan's test schedule, a ship and a knife (5cm) are included.

prime the parent first not to lean forward with 'kiss-kiss' expression, but to remain still until the baby initiates his response.

If the correct object is picked up, the assessor takes it with a 'thank you' and replaces it/back on the table before continuing to request the others in random order. If the wrong or no choice is made she requests another item. If the child is unsuccessful the assessor gives a toy to the child saying 'Give it to Mummy' (having first primed mother not to move before the child's response is complete). Alternatively she tries body parts – 'That's mummy's mouth' pointing to it. 'Where are Mummy's eyes?'....

The assessor records examples of expressive language.

Age guidelines – see Tables 8.2 and 8.3.

Miniature Toys

Age: 21 months to 4 years.

Aspects of language: good for verbal comprehension across age range and for expressive language in children under 2¾ years. However a set of activity pictures is often needed to access higher levels of syntax and language usage in children over 3 years.

Materials: Figure 8.4 illustrates some of the toys used to explore basic levels of representation in miniature, verbal comprehension and expressive language.

Protocol: The child sits at the nursery table and the assessor again retains the box of toys. The test is designed as an expanding and flexible package, so start at the beginning and cease when the child's ceiling is reached. Although the early section may be below the expressive language age level of over 3-year-olds, it has the benefit of relaxing the child into conversation with the assessor and allows the assessor to observe the level of NSpSC.

Expressive language: Explore early expressive language as toys are presented. Start with the miniature table and chairs as this ensures that the child has a choice of tables on which to arrange the cutlery and crockery. The assessor proffers one at a time with a 'look, what's this?' – if the child doesn't speak she adds 'it's a …' *pause for response.* Whether or not it is named the assessor gives the toy to the child and lets him arrange it.

(Q) Why should the assessor do this?
  Because arrangement of toys is part of the assessment of NSpSC.

If he continues to hold it in his hand, the assessor asks, 'Where – are you going to put it/does it go?' A more natural dialogue is created by interjecting Dorothy Egan's seven questions as the child names the relevant item and engenders sentences, rather than single word utterances.

- Plane: 'Yes. Where do we see aeroplanes?'

- Knife: 'What does Mummy do with a knife?'

- Jug: 'What does Mummy put in the jug?'

- Bath: Point to the taps 'What comes out of the taps?'

- 'Why do we have two taps?'

- Teapot: As the child places the lid 'Why do we put a lid on the teapot? What's the lid for?'

- Ship: 'Where do you see ships?'

More importantly these questions tap into the level of a child's ability to use language as the medium for thought. Interestingly, the questions all contain the same number of operative words, yet Egan's normative data indicate that the two why questions tap into a higher level of conceptual and verbal reasoning than the five where and what questions.

Throughout, the assessor observes and notes labelling, spontaneous comments and spontaneous arrangement of toys

Verbal comprehension: Once all the toys are 'in play' the assessor may need to undo some of the child's arrangement in order to test verbal comprehension. Introduced with 'let's put dolly here for a minute and the spoon here' the assessor's rearrangement is usually accepted. The assessor starts with an age-appropriate command.[5] Examples together with age guidelines are given in Table 8.2. If the full instruction is carried out the assessor either gives a second at the same level or moves up a level. If only part or none of the instruction is carried out she drops to a lower level.

An assessor should always ensure the following:

- Children under 3 years are looking at her, i.e. giving her their full attention before giving a command. For example, if Johnny is an 'eager beaver' she says 'Johnny', and as he looks up she gently places her hands over his, issues the instruction and then withdraws (see Attention control, Chapter 2).

- She does not give non-verbal clues such as looking at or pointing to the target items. In an effort not to give clues some assessors become rather 'expressionless', resulting in loss of rapport.

- She never includes a toy the child is already holding in the command.

  Q Why is this?
  The number of operative words is effectively reduced by one because a child does not have to select an object already in his hand.

- The full command is given before the child has started to carry it out.

  Q Why is this?
  Because the second part of the instruction effectively becomes a new short one. This does not mean the command is spoken rapidly but that it is at her fingertips and completed while she still holds the child's attention.

- The instruction is sensible; some children will be puzzled if the command requests that they relate objects in an unnatural, or at home 'forbidden' way, e.g. 'stand dolly on the table'.

- For higher levels of instruction, i.e. three, four or five operative words, the dialogue contains one or two concept words of colour, size or position as this makes it more

---

5   Unless her examination to date indicates a lower level of NSC; if it does she goes in at that level and moves up or down as indicated by the child's responses.

Table 8.4   Miniature Toys Test: number of toys named[a]

Number of toys named	Age achieved by	
	50% (mo)	90% (mo)
2	21	33
6	27	36
12	36	48
14	45	NA

[a] Extrapolated from Egan and Brown (1984); NA, not available.

natural/interesting than a list, e.g. 'Give me two cars and put the little spoon in the cup', rather than 'Give me the car, the spoon, the cup, the bath and the chair'. However the assessor must be sure that the child has these concepts before using them.

- Prepositions are concepts of relative position. 'in' and 'on' are the everyday relationship of spoons and cups, cups and tables and dolls and chairs. Using 'in' and 'on' in two-component commands (put the spoon in the cup) therefore does not test understanding of 'in'. 'Behind' and 'in front' present difficulty for 2½-year-olds, e.g. 'put the dog behind the aeroplane'. Children who have a concept of behind may place the dog on the far side of the plane relative to themselves rather than relative to the back of the plane. Use of these prepositions as key words in tests for children under 4 years is therefore not advised. 'Under' on the other hand is relevant (e.g. 'put the dog under the table') because even if the child puts the dog under the nursery, rather than the miniature table, he has demonstrated comprehension of both the word 'under' and the three-component command. This developmental phenomenon may have impacted on Egan's findings in relation to comprehension of prepositions.

Record: Expressive language and verbal comprehension findings.

Age guidelines: See Tables 8.2 verbal comprehension, 8.3 expressive language and 8.4 MTT expressive verbal labels from Egan and Brown (1986), 8.5 additional language concepts and constructs for flexible experienced assessors.

A set of activity pictures constitute a useful follow-on test of expressive language for 3- and 4-year-olds who have not yet produced age-appropriate sentences (see below).

Table 8.5   Understanding the usage of other language constructs with examples

Concept/construct	Comprehension	Expression	Achieved by Average age (mo)
Possessives		'Mine'	20
Plurals	'Give me the spoon<u>s</u>'	'Flower<u>s</u>'	24
Prepositions	'Put the cat <u>under</u> the table'		33
Size	'Where's the <u>little</u> fork?'	'It's a <u>little</u> cup'	33
Colour	'Where's the <u>red</u> chair?'	'Daddy's car is <u>boo</u>'	33
Pronouns		'Me' ('You'), ['Him, Her']	24 (33) [36]
Negatives	'... spoon <u>not</u> in the cup'		38
Descriptive labels	'... do we <u>do our</u> hair with?'		38
Past tense		'I jump<u>ed</u> in ...'	39
Future tenses		'I <u>will</u> go tomorrow'	48
Use of language as medium for thought[a]			
What?/where?			30–36 (range)
..do with knife, out of taps, put in jug, aeroplanes, ships			
Why? two taps, lid/ teapot			47

[a]From Egan and Brown (1986). N.B. Any sensible answer also conveys comprehension of the question as well as the level of expressive language, but the age guidelines reflect the level of ability to use language as a medium for thought.

Set of activity pictures

Age: 21 months to 4½ years

Aspects of language: Good to access expressive language across the age range; mainly used to explore higher levels of syntax and language usage in the children of 3 years or 4 years.

Materials: Six *realistic* coloured pictures (size A5) that depict everyday childhood experiences (e.g. shopping, feeding the dog, making a cake, washing the car, playing in a park). Assessors should collect their own set, making sure that the pictures are realistic, clear and uncluttered.

Protocol

- The assessor presents the picture with a 'Look – what's happening/going on in my picture?'[6]

- If the response is less than age appropriate, the assessor encourages more with 'yes, anything else?'

- The child may be reticent to speak or a little uncertain of what is wanted, with the first picture, so if the assessor thinks this is the case she says 'they're cooking a cake for tea, aren't they' and then presents another picture with a 'and what's happening in this one?'

- Three or four pictures usually suffice to get an adequate sample of expressive language.

Record: The assessor notes the length, content and construct of the highest-level examples.

Age guidelines: see Tables 8.3 and 8.5.

Scheme B

Egan Bus Puzzle Test

Age range: 21 months to 4 years

Aspects of intellect: The test explores the development of expressive language, verbal comprehension and the non-verbal skills of recognition of shape and spatial orientation.

Materials: A colourful wooden inset puzzle (45 × 29 × 1.2cm) depicts an everyday Western street scene with nine lift-out pieces: a boy with a letter, a Mummy with a baby in a buggy, a boy on a bike, a dog, a bus, a car, a post box and a lollipop man – Figure 8.5.

The test is divided into five sections:

1. Expression – verbal labels for lift-out pieces

2. Comprehension – of verbal labels for lift-out pieces

---

6 'What's happening' and 'what's going on' tend to induce longer utterances than 'what can you see' or 'what are they doing'. 'What can you see' tends to induce a list of noun labels and 'what are they doing' just a present participle, e.g. 'washing up'.

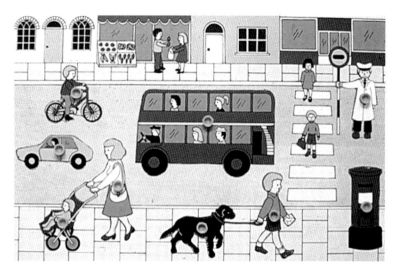

Figure 8.5 Egan Bus Puzzle Test.

3. Non-verbal – Recognition of recess for each lift-out piece

   • Orientation of each piece for insertion

4. Six questions about situations illustrated

   • Comprehension

   • Expression – level of expressive response

5. Objects in Mummy's handbag

Protocol: The protocol is summarised here as the test comes with a detailed manual (Egan and Brown 1984).

Expressive verbal labels (EVL): With 'I've got a puzzle for us' the assessor places the puzzle on the nursery table facing the child and says 'What's this?' as she points to the dog. Once named the child is asked to 'take it out and put it' on the table to his left – the assessor indicates where he is to put it by tapping the table. If the child remains silent or her answer is not the proper name, e.g. the child says 'horse' for the dog, the assessor says 'I call it a dog' or 'yes, it's a dog isn't it?' i.e. she feeds back the correct name. Each piece is presented in turn. Many of the younger children may not use the proper name giving instead a generic or functional name, e.g. for the lollipop man 'lollipop' or 'traffic' or 'crossing' man would be proper, farmer, policeman or milkman would be functional and daddy or man would be generic names – scoring 3, 2 and 1 respectively.

Comprehension of Verbal labels, Recognition of Shape and Orientation of the Pieces are carried out concurrently. 'Where's the bus?' – 'yes' (as they pick it up) – 'put it back' or 'where does it go' (indicating the puzzle generally but not pointing to the recess). The assessor notes choice of piece, selection of recess and orientation of piece to recess.

Comprehension of verbal labels (CVL): The assessor always uses the proper name. If the child picks up the wrong piece she takes it gently and puts it back on the table, gets his attention and repeats. The assessor starts and finishes with an item from earliest vocabulary – car or bus or dog or bike. The lollipop man should come in the middle because he is the most difficult and if he is left to last the child does not have to make a selection.

Recognition of shape (RS): Some trial and error is allowed and the child can be encouraged to 'look all round' but the assessor should take care not to indicate the correct recess.

Orientation of pieces (OP): The pieces are irregular in outline so once the child has the correct general orientation the assessor may help nudge it in, to avoid the child getting cross with it!

Six questions about situations illustrated in the street scene: The questions are asked in the order presented below. The child's attention is drawn to each scene by pointing, though care needs to be taken not to inadvertently gesture the answer to the question, e.g. by running ones pointing finger up the stairs or from the letter to the slit in the post box![7]

The six questions are as follows:

1. 'Why do we have steps on a bus' – 'what are the steps for?'

2. 'What is Mummy doing?'

3. 'What is he (boy with letter) going to do with it?'

4. 'What is he (boy with letter) doing with this hand?'

5. 'What is this boy (boy on bike) doing?'

6. 'What is the lollipop man doing?'

Comprehension of Questions (CQ) embraces understanding of the spoken question and of the situation depicted; a positive score is dependent on an acceptable expressive response.

Expressive responses to Questions (EQ): there are three levels of expressive response to questions (1) gesture, e.g. child gestures upwards (Q1) or noun label (2) present partici-

---

7   Attention is drawn to the letter by pointing to it and asking what it is. If the answer is purse or piece of paper say 'it's a letter isn't it?'

ple or two or more words without a verb and (3) three or more words including a verb.

Objects in Mummy's Handbag: 'What do you think Mummy has in her handbag?' Unlike the other questions the answer is not illustrated; i.e. the child cannot see what is in the handbag so she needs to shift her thinking from the illustration to experience of handbags. This is a higher level of abstraction that comes online between 4 and 5 years. Although only 38% suggest one item at 48 months, a 3-year-old who does so is providing a very favourable developmental marker. However the assessor needs to be careful not to actively direct the child to think about his own mother's handbag.

Age references: Age references are provided in the manual as centile curves for the following aspects of the test – EVL, CVL, RS, OP, CQ and EQ; the 10th, 20th and 50th centiles are depicted.

Interpretation: Children falling to the left of the 50th centile are functioning above average for age, those to the right of the 10th require more in-depth assessment and those between the 10th and the 20th certainly warrant ongoing observation. The centile charts not only allow the assessor to compare the testee with children of the same age, but highlight disparities within the child's profile, e.g. between verbal comprehension and expressive language.

> (Q) What would you use to test a 16-month-old's verbal comprehension?
> *Real objects and a doll and or Mummy – at 16 months a toddler is unlikely to see miniature toys as being representative of the real objects and appreciation of Wendy house size will be tenuous in many. Similarly life-size realistic pictures will be recognised by some but not all at this age so real objects are the most age-appropriate choice.*

The two schemes differ in how well they test the various aspects of language development. Although Miniature Toys are excellent for the noun labelling level of expressive language and generate some spontaneous comments in 2½ to 4½-year-olds, the latter tend to be less expansive than if asked 'What's happening?' when given pictures of everyday scenes or when questions like those used by Dorothy Egan in both her version of the Miniature Toy Test and the EBPT are added.

On the other hand Miniature Toys in the same age group are better than Pictures or the questions level of the Bus Puzzle for assessing higher levels of verbal comprehension, because the child is required to demonstrate his assimilation of each of the key/operative words of the assessor's instruction by physically carrying it out; in the Bus Puzzle his comprehension of a spoken question is judged on his expressive language level, which is short of ideal, as in typical development expressive language trails behind verbal comprehension and expressive language is likely to be considerably worse than verbal comprehension in many children with language delays/disorders.

Table 8.6 Advantages and disadvantages of the Miniature Toy and Bus Puzzle Tests

Advantages	Disadvantages
Miniature Toys	
Egan version has a standard protocol	Egan version only partially standardised
High inherent interest	Flexible protocol not standardised
Clear levels for comprehension of key words	Very 'playable' with. Therefore attention control more difficult to manage
Includes early levels of non-spoken symbolic development and imaginative play	Risk of the assessor confusing non-spoken symbolic understanding with verbal comprehension
Flexibility (experienced assessor) to probe language in greater depth particularly VC	
Bus Puzzle	
Designed as a screening test and standardised	Limit of EL – three-word level
High inherent interest	Both aspects of NSC peak at 30 to 33mo
Management of AC easier than for miniature toy	VC for questions dependent on EL response

EL, expressive language; VC, verbal comprehension; AC, Attention Control; NSC, Non-Symbolic Cognition.

Another advantage of the Miniature Toys and Picture Tests is that they can be expanded by more experienced assessors to explore language development in greater depth to reveal a wider perspective of the growth of semantics, syntax pragmatics and the use of language as a medium for thought (Table 8.5). The relative advantages and disadvantages of the Miniature Toy Test and the Egan Bus Puzzle Test are summarised in Table 8.6.

Delayed and disordered language development

For her studies of intervention strategies for children with specific language disorders (SLD), the admission criteria used by Joan Reynell (1972) were that either or both aspects of language were less than two-thirds that of NSC, i.e. that there was a major difference between language and non-verbal areas of intellectual ability. The wisdom behind her choice of criteria was supported by a large population study of 3-year-old children in the UK screened for language and or behavioural delay; 37% of those with language age less than two-thirds chronological age had similarly delayed NSC levels

(Stevenson and Richman 1976). Whenever language delay is found the assessor's first step is to compare the level with that of NSC as this will separate out those with global developmental delay. Comparison of levels of verbal comprehension and expressive language will clarify whether either or both are specifically delayed and may signpost hearing impairment if the latter is slightly higher than the former. Even when it is not, the findings of the hearing assessment need to be carefully looked at in all cases of SLD. Concomitant delay in NSpSC may point to the likelihood that the language delay is part of an ASD; in the context of ASD Tomblin et al. (1997) point out that children with SLD rarely have joint attention difficulties, so referring back to the joint attention findings in the social communication domain provides another valuable piece of the jigsaw when formulating a quality plan of action.

Aetiology. Epidemiological studies confirm that there are genetic influences and that prevalence of SLD is higher in boys than girls (between 3 and 4:1 (Stevenson and Richman 1976, Tomblin et al. 1997). In a paediatric study of children referred to The Wolfson Centre language research programmes, Sonksen (1978) found that sex differences were even greater when children were divided into primary/constitutional (no causative agent identified) and secondary (causative agent identified – brain damaging event, hearing impairment, adverse environmental circumstance) aetiological groups. Eighty-five per cent of the primary group were boys, which suggests that constitutional disorders are genetically determined and sex-limited; there were five times as many boys as girls in families with and without positive family histories, suggesting that sex limitation operates throughout the primary group. Familial relationships suggested polygenic origin with incomplete autosomal dominant transmission; the occurrence rate was 1 in 3.4 amongst male and 1 in 15 amongst female siblings irrespective of the sex of the index child. In the secondary group the number of boys and girls was equal; 2% were found to have anomalies of the sex chromosomes; metabolic screening did not provide any aetiological pointers. At the time rubella serology was pertinent amongst the hearing impaired subgroup (Sonksen 1978). Recently, the *FOXP2* gene has been implicated in a family with severe verbal dyspraxia (Liegeois et al. 2011) and pre-, peri- and neonatal complications have been confirmed not to play a significant role in the aetiology of SLD (Whitehouse et al. 2014).

Associated neurodevelopmental difficulties. In The Wolfson Centre study neurodevelopmental difficulties other than language occurred in over 80% of SLD preschool children and were multiple in up to 45%; their range, pattern and severity were very variable and bore no absolute relationship to aetiology, language profile or sex. Behavioural disturbance was present in 50% to 60% of all aetiological subgroups, in some children as part of the primary disorder, in others secondary to the language problem or to a mixture of both. A trend for delay in gross motor and manipulative development, with children shifted towards the lower end of the normal range, was common; however, positive neuromotor signs were confined to the secondary group; neuromotor delay was most marked for skills where a child needs to adjust his movements to a moving environment, e.g. catching, throwing (Sonksen 1978). Preschool children with delay mainly in expressive language tend to experience fewer learning and behaviour difficulties in school than those in whom language is initially disordered or both receptive and expressive aspects are delayed.

Landau–Kleffner syndrome, otherwise known as acquired receptive aphasia of childhood, although rare, deserves special mention (Landau and Kleffner 1957). The condition affects as many girls as boys and presents after a period of apparently normal language development with the onset of deep receptive aphasia and seizures; the latter may appear concomitantly or shortly after the aphasia, though occasionally no seizures are apparent. However, sleep electroencephalographic studies reveal underlying electrical status epilepticus in sleep (ESES), and a correlation study suggests that language and behavioural outcomes may be favourably influenced by timely medical or surgical treatment of ESES (Robinson et al. 2001). Often the depth of the aphasia is such that the clinician initially suspects acquired deafness unless pure tones are used.

The question of screening for SLD is still going round in circles 40 years after Court (1984) debated the topic and the scientific specifications for doing so were defined by Rose (1978). A systematic review of screening for SLD was carried out for the US Preventative Task Force and concluded that evidence was still inadequate and inconclusive on all fronts (Nelson et al. 2006). Buschmann et al. (2008) provide evidence that screening language development by community personnel at 24 months identifies children who justify a diagnostic workup. Their screening protocol, like those mentioned in Chapter 5 developed for screening autism, identifies children with the target disorder (SLD) plus those with other developmental delays and disorders that will benefit from diagnostic workup and intervention.

Key Points

- The foundation stones of language development are laid during the first year.
- Readiness to jump the symbolic hurdle is heralded by 'definition by use'.
- Parents tend to overestimate comprehension.
  - Observe for non-spoken clues in parent–child interaction.
  - Probe to establish between words used with meaning, imitation and babble.
- Testing
  - Have commands at your fingertips.
  - Ensure child is attending when instruction given.

- Complete full instruction before child starts.

- Ensure instructions are sensible.

- Keep instructions interesting – use concepts not lists

- Beware of giving non-spoken clues.

- Do not include an item already in child's hand in the instruction.

- Interpretation of verbal comprehension for prepositions is not clear cut.

- Outside the test situation the effort of engaging young children in dialogue is usually rewarded with a few linguistic pearls

- Construct language profile and consider it in context of other aspects of intellectual profile, sensory and motor findings.

References

Buschmann A, Jooss B, Rupp A et al. (2008) Children with developmental language delay at 24 months of age: Results of a diagnostic work-up. *Dev Med Child Neurol* 50: 223–229.

Court SDM (1984) Meaning and method in child health surveillance discussion paper. *J Roy Soc Med* 77: 863–865.

Egan DF, Brown R (1984) Developmental assessment: 18 months to 4½ years. The Bus Puzzle Test. *Child Care Health Dev* 12: 163–179.

Egan DF, Brown R (1986) Developmental assessment: 18 months to 4 ½ years. The Miniature Toys Test. *Child Care Health Dev* 12: 167–181.

Friederici A (2006) The neural basis of language development and impairment. *Neuron* 52: 941–952.

Friederici A (2011) The brain basis of language processing: from structure to function. *Physiol Rev* 91: 1357–1392.

Landau WM, Kleffner F (1957) Syndrome of acquired aphasia with convulsive disorder in children. *Neurology* 7: 523–530.

Liégeois F, Morgan AT, Connelly A, Vargha-Khadem F (2011) Endophenotypes of FOXP2: Dysfunction within the human articulatory network. *Eur J Paediatr Neurol* 15: 283–288.

Nelson HD, Nygren P, Walker M, Panoscha R (2006) Screening for speech and language delay in preschool children: Systematic evidence review for the US Preventive Services Task Force. *Pediatrics* 117: e298–e319.

New Reynell Developmental Language Scales (2011) GL Assessment. UK

Reynell J (1972) Language handicaps in mentally retarded children. In ed Clarke ADB, Lewis MM, editors. *Learning, Speech and Thought in the Mentally Retarded*. London: Butterworth.

Robinson RO, Baird G, Robinson G, Simonoff E (2001) Landau-Kleffner syndrome: Course and correlates with outcome. *Dev Med Child Neurol* 43: 243–247.

Rose G (1978) Epidemiology for the uninitiated: screening. *BMJ* 2: 1417–1418.

Sonksen PM (1978) The neurodevelopmental and paediatric findings associated with significant disabilities of language development in preschool children. MD Thesis, University of London, UK

Stevenson J, Richman N (1976) The prevalence of language delay in a population of three-year-old children and its association with general retardation. *Dev Med Child Neurol* 4: 431–441.

Tomblin JB, Records NL, Buckwalter P, Zhang X, Smith E, O'Brien M (1997) Prevalence of specific language impairment in kindergarten children. *J Speech Lang Hear Res* 6: 1245–1260.

Vargha-Khadem F, Watkins KE, Price CJ et al. (1998) Neural basis of an inherited language disorder. *Proc Natl Acad Sci USA* 95(21): 12695-12700.

Watkins KE (2011) Developmental disorders of speech and language: From genes to brain structure and function. *Prog Brain Res* 189: 225–238.

Whitehouse AJO, Shelton WMR, Ing C, Newnham JP (2014) Prenatal, perinatal and neonatal risk factors for specific language impairment: A prospective pregnancy cohort study. *J Speech Lang Hear Res* 57: 1418–1427.

Chapter 9

Gross motor development

For over half a century gross motor development has been, and for many still is, the primary yardstick of infant development; understandably for parents because each motor milestone – sitting, crawling, walking, running – is so visible and such a joy bringing event. However, professionals who are satisfied that development is normal based on motor milestones give an impression of having never actually thought seriously about child development. Man's facility for *complex thought* rather than *movement* is what separates *Homo sapiens* from the rest of the animal kingdom; gross motor development is a relatively poor predictor of intellectual status – some children with autism and severe learning difficulties are frighteningly agile; others quite the reverse. Certainly the likelihood of disabilities in cognitive and/or sensory domains is greater in babies with abnormal than with normal neuromotor development. Over the millennia man's neuromotor and musculoskeletal systems have adapted in remarkable ways, to the demands of his enlarging brain (e.g. to walk and run on two legs, to perform complex and intricate skills with the upper limbs and with the speech apparatus). Cognitive growth of a species is dependent on the possession of a movement system that is responsive to demand and has the capacity of continuous adaptation.

The voluntary and involuntary neuromotor systems are involved in every aspect of life; some of the latter, like heartbeat and peristalsis, are never subject to voluntary control whereas others such as bladder and bowel control are learnt. However, the systemic neuromotor systems that mastermind gross motor, manipulative and speech development are the focus of this and the next two chapters. These systems provide postural stability; mobility; eye movements (see Chapter 3); manipulation (see Chapter 10) and speech (see Chapter 11).

Collectively they provide the physical means to do the following:

- Learn about 'how the world works and how I work' through gross motor, manipulative, visual and tactile exploration in the first year

- Care for oneself and others

- Develop behavioural independence, self-esteem, confidence, creativity, etc.

- Develop social and communicative skills

- Process information at increasingly higher levels

- Participate in sporting/leisure activities

- Be employed and earn a living, and much more

The developmental consequences of disorders of neuromotor development on other areas are wide ranging and the effects are cumulative.

Thinking may not involve any movement, but in order for one individual to know what another is thinking, requires the latter to initiate some voluntary movement. Thus voluntary movement, however minimal, conveys the content of the testee's response to the assessor in all developmental testing, for example stilling, turning head and eyes, pointing, carrying out the conditioned response task in tests of hearing. Thus, homing in on the level, range and nature a child's motor attributes early in an assessment is as important as tuning in to her level of attention control, because if a neuromotor problem constrains her ability to respond to tests exploring other domains, the assessor can identify and use a motor response that is available to the child.

Neurological substrate

The neurological substrate of the systemic motor system at birth is made up of primary motor templates and connections at cortical, subcortical and spinal levels and of primary connections with non-motor sensory and cognitive templates. The configuration is species-specific (evolution) with individual variations the consequence of genetic influences and intrauterine climate. Fetal movements in utero probably play a role in shaping these primary neuromotor templates and their connections. Postnatal development is dependent on (1) the quality, quantity and variety of visual, auditory and tactile experiences to trigger cognitive interest in, for example motor exploration of objects, movement and mobility and (2) processing of proprioceptive, kinaesthetic, labyrinthine and visual feedback from the musculoskeletal system. Over time the most useful inter- and intratemplate connections are selected and strengthened, while less favourable ones are discarded. Further modification of these secondary templates and connections continues in response to changing and more challenging environmental opportunities and demands. At a behavioural level babies are observed to consciously practice new motor actions until they are sufficiently well controlled to 'go on automatic'. Are they selecting and strengthening the subcortical templates, for example of the cerebellum, destined to subconsciously mastermind stability and flow of movement? Throughout, genetic, motivational and environmental influences contribute to variation in competence between individuals. The earlier outline is in tune with the Neuronal Group Selection Theory (Edelman 1989) that brought together and transcended the Neuro-maturational and Dynamic Systems theories of motor development of the middle third of the last century, whilst acknowledging the 'nature' aspects of the former and the 'nurture' aspects of the latter within a much broader neurobiological framework of influences. The hallmark of the Neuro-maturational theory is that motor development is tied to the biological clock of myelination; the latter starts in the third trimester, is most rapid in the first 2 years and follows a set sequence that results in a cephalo-caudal pattern of gross-motor development; the primitive mass movements and primitive reflexes of the neonate are replaced by voluntary controlled movements as a consequence of maturation and cortical inhibition of subcortical nuclei. The Dynamic Systems theory has a broader and more interactive framework and emphasizes interaction between innate motivators (emotional, cognitive and physical), environmental opportunity, sensory feedback from the musculoskeletal system and biomechanical factors (Thelen 1995). Both theories failed to give sufficient status to the process of neuronal selectivity and connectivity. For further reading see Hadders-Algra's (2000) overview of theories of motor development. We still have a lot to learn about the developments in neurocellular physiology that occur through the era of neuronal connectivity and template formation.

Gross motor development

The tension in a muscle at any moment is known as *tone*; it fluctuates constantly during movements and in response to changes in posture. Tone in the muscles powering a movement (agonists) will be higher than in the muscles that oppose it (antagonists); for movement to flow smoothly the tone in agonists and antagonists must constantly change in unison but in opposite directions; similarly, tone needs to fluctuate accordingly in the muscle groups providing stability/fixation for the action. This requires a highly tuned system of *reciprocal innervation*.

Evolution has seen the brain of *Homo sapiens* become relatively larger than that of other mammals; growth is very rapid during gestation and by 9 months fetal head size is maximal in terms of successful passage through the birth canal. Thus a top-heavy baby is born with a relatively immature neuromotor system compared to other mammals – a system that lacks adequate strength and stability for independent mobility. The newborn human has minimal intrinsic stability and requires almost total body support in all postures – the most stable posture is side lying; resting tone is higher in flexor than in extensor muscles; movement control is rudimentary with no ability to voluntarily differentiate or dissociate the movements of joints or limbs; integration of sensory feedback from muscles, joints, labyrinths or eyes is minimal; functionally the reciprocal innervation system is unprimed. Thus, when startled or crying, jerky mass movements occur – the trunk, head and limbs all flex or extend at the same time. All the earlier aspects of the gross neuromotor system need to develop and integrate at neurological level before, for example, a baby can sit unsupported and move an individual limb. Whatever the static or dynamic skill, the movement template is not fully mature until the action flows smoothly and is carried out without consciously monitoring and planning every component. Movement development is therefore a continuous integrative process influenced by genetic endowment, maturation, environmental opportunity and demand – the latter representing motivational links with visual, behavioural and cognitive domains. Sugden and Wade (2013) review theoretical considerations and recent research into typical development of movement and of movement in motor impairment.

Priorities in the newborn period and early months are to do the following:

- Address the imbalance of resting tone to one more suited to independent motor development – flexor dominance may have been advantageous for the foetus but not out in the big wide world!

- Shift distribution of weight in prone and supine postures caudally so that the head, arms and finally lower limbs are free to move and thus enhance opportunities for visual and manual exploration en route to mobility.

- Develop postural stability of the head, pectoral girdle, trunk, and pelvic girdle so that movements of the head and limbs can be dissociated from those of the trunk and subsequently from each other.

- Myelinate cortical pathways to advance control of tone and movement cephalo-caudally and to inhibit the subcortical nuclei that govern a set of primitive reflexes of dubious biological import.

- Develop online mechanisms for postural control and for protective actions when balance is lost, that depend on sensory feedback from the musculoskeletal, labyrinthine and visual systems – known as *equilibrium/balance* and *saving* reactions, respectively.

The traditional sequences of early gross motor development in static and dynamic postures, two horizontal and two vertical – prone, supine, sitting, standing – are widely known and form part of the basic training of paediatricians and paediatric therapists; they have been well documented and well-illustrated for three-quarters of a century (Gesell 1940, Illingworth 1962, Sheridan 1973, Piper et al. 1992). They are therefore summarised diagrammatically and age referenced in Table 9.1. The following descriptions are an attempt to give the reader a more qualitative gestalt of postures and of patterns of movement development, the importance of repetition/practice in selection and strengthening of secondary motor templates, the dependence of cognition and social communicative development on movement, the interplay of cognition and personality with motor development and the role of the special senses particularly vision in this process. From birth vision provides a baby with a vivid, exciting and enticing 3D perspective of the world that spans time and fuels his innate 'drive' and motivation to become mobile, explore and learn through closer visual inspection. It provides precepts of the way humans move and of the structure of the surroundings, from which concepts of his potential for movement and of the floor as a base to move across are founded. Vision tutors proprioceptive and labyrinthine feedback in development of equilibrium responses and is actively employed to monitor every stage of learning new movements; once mastered visual feedback continues at a less conscious level and forewarns of changes in the environment (Sonksen et al 1984).

From birth to walking

When placed in prone or supine the top-heavy neonate with his flexor dominance of tone turns his head to one side and weight is distributed through the head.

Prone
In prone the legs are flexed under the abdomen and the pelvis is high and tilted posteriorly so there is a risk of toppling. By 8 weeks the balance of tone has become more even and weight distribution has consequently shifted caudally. A typically developing baby now actively tries to lift his head and then brace/stabilise his shoulders and push his chest off the floor on bent forearms. At 4 and 5 months with head and chin raised to about 80° an attempt to look around or reach with one arm causes him to topple over onto his back – his startled look confirms that it was not an intentional roll; however, after several such 'accidents' the potential of rolling as a form of mobility dawns and cognitively triggers him to practice rolling prone to supine. Push up in prone becomes more stable between 5 and 6 months with weight distributed through a flat pelvis and extended legs; he now looks straight ahead supporting his head and chest on extended arms. At this stage many babies experiment with pivoting around the pelvic axis. They also attempt to draw first one and then the other knee under the pelvis. Initially, the knee and thigh are three-quarters flexed and the hip partially abducted, so the pelvis is nearer the floor than the shoulders. Many babies repetitively rock backwards and forwards in this position, presumably priming reciprocal innervation and hip stability.[1] Most are fully on hands and knees by 9 months; this is the ideal starting position from

---

1 These and other repetitive movements such as bouncing up and down on the parent's lap are common between 4 and 7 months; persistence into the second year is concerning and requires more in-depth examination.

which babies can work on becoming effectively mobile and moving into and out of other stable postures (e.g. crawling and moving into or out of unsupported sitting and pulling to stand). All these actions require increased pelvic girdle stability, better control of shifts in weight, more functional balancing and saving reactions and reciprocal innervation. Nine to twelve-month-olds concentrate hard on gross motor development, and carefully monitor every aspect with their eyes. Certainly they are great believers in *practice makes perfect!*

Supine
As in prone a neonate placed *supine* turns her head to one side, the trunk turns with the head and she tends to settle most stably in side lying. By 6 weeks weight is distributed more evenly through the trunk (rather than the head), the pelvis is in neutral, arms and legs more gently flexed and consequently a supine posture is sustainable. In supine the limbs are not needed for support and babies can see and learn about their hands and their surroundings without lifting their heads; thus the limbs are freed up earlier in supine than in prone to move independently of the trunk – the upper ones for specialised (non-gross motor) development of reach grasp, etc.

The development of head control in supine is vital in the development of sitting unsupported and standing. If support is given in a sitting position (by holding the forearms) most neonates maintain the head upright very briefly; this gradually improves to fully sustained by 3½ months. When picked up and held upright most neonates brace the shoulders momentarily; mother should not feel that her baby might slip through her fingers. There is still considerable head lag on pull to sit at 2 months but the mother should no longer need to support her baby's head when she picks her up at 4 months; by 5 months a baby braces her shoulders and lifts her head as she is grasped.

Equilibrium mechanisms

Righting and saving responses are of critical importance; without them any action that requires a shift in centre of gravity (e.g. leaning out from a sitting position to reach a proffered toy) will result in falling. Righting responses are adjustments in tone of the muscles of the neck and trunk to compensate for the displacement and provide stability for active movement, i.e. they are in the opposite direction to the displacing force. Saving responses are movements of the limbs to counter falling, for example extending the arms towards the ground when tripping; they are in the same direction as the displacing force. Saving reactions come into play when righting responses fail to maintain equilibrium. Babies with profound visual impairment, who are otherwise neurologically normal, are very slow to develop equilibrium responses (Sonksen et al. 1984, Sonksen and Stiff 1991). Unlike their sighted peers, they are unable to use changes in the visual coordinates of their environment, e.g. door and window frames or the 'upright' of their father as he lifts them above his head to tutor the interpretation and integration of

Table 9.1 Prone and supine development – birth to 6 months

Prone	Birth	1mo	2mo	3mo	4mo	5mo	6mo
Ventral suspension							
Placed prone							
==> Prone mobility							
Supine							
Placed supine							
Pulled to sit							
Held sitting							

==> towards

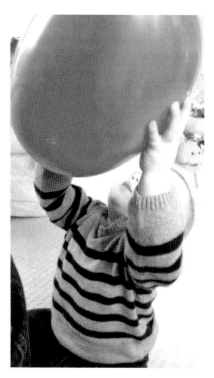

Figure 9.1 Secure truncal righting for reaching above his head: in that position he is compensating for the backward tilt of his 'heavy' head.

inputs from the labyrinths and proprioceptive receptors in the development of righting responses. Similarly, learning that floors provide a solid continuous surface for 'saving' is difficult if vision is very severely impaired. Vision continues to have a major role in monitoring and coordinating equilibrium responses throughout life – simply close your eyes and walk around your own home or on sloping uneven ground!

Righting
The head of most neonates held in vertical suspension and tilted gently sideways or forwards will flop. By 10 to 12 weeks some active curvature of the neck is seen to bring the position of the head back towards the vertical. At 9 to 12 months a baby held around the pelvic crests and tipped sideways or forwards curves his thoracic as well as his cervical spine towards an upright posture. In sitting unsupported similar adjustments are seen first when reaching forwards at 8 months then sideways at 10 months and finally above and behind at 12 months (Fig 9.1). A similar sequence of increasing pectoral, then truncal and finally pelvic balancing reactions provide the stability for four-point kneeling to progress to crawling. In order for standing to become dynamic, reactions

that stabilise the pelvic girdle and individual limb joints are necessary, first when weight is distributed through two legs (standing to crawling or standing to sitting) and then through only one (walking, standing on one leg, hopping, running, kicking, skipping etc.) from 11 months through to 4 years.

Saving

Saving reactions emerge once babies have developed a concept of the floor/ground, as a solid and continuous surface beneath them, commonly between 5 and 6 months. First to appear are the 'downward' and 'forward' parachute – the baby abducts his legs and spreads his feet in anticipation of touching base when rapidly lowered towards the bed during a bouncing game (7 months); this is followed shortly by the 'forward' parachute – the baby actively extends his arms towards the floor and spreads his fingers when tipped forwards. In sitting, saving forwards appears at 6 to 7 months and to either side at 8 to 9 months and finally behind at 10 to 12 months. As babies pull up to stand and cruise along the furniture the lower limbs participate in saving reactions; when balance is in jeopardy the non-supporting leg is quickly moved into a more favourable position to share weight-bearing and restore equilibrium; these are sometimes referred to as 'staggering' reactions. Equilibrium reactions continue to become faster, more finely tuned and more efficient through childhood and beyond, as new and varied physical challenges present. Age guidelines are found in Table 9.2.

Sitting

Sitting unsupported like many motor skills matures through several stages; the stage needs to be specified or described when reporting or researching. The stages essentially reflect increasing trunk stability, righting and emergence of saving responses.

Stage 1: Baby sits for a brief period when placed; the back is rounded and any movement results in 'disaster' or slow collapse; head stability is good, upper trunk moderate and lower trunk minimal, upper limb saving reactions typically emerge between 5 and 7 months (Fig 9.2).

Stage 2 (static sit): Baby sits securely with straight back holding or transferring toys from hand to hand; tends *not* to lean out to reach or shift centre of gravity; lower trunk stability is good; righting responses and forward propping are emerging, though neither strong nor brisk enough to prevent tumbling when shifts off balance – typically between 7 and 9 months (Fig 9.3).

Stage 3 *(dynamic sit):* Baby sits securely, leans and reaches out confidently in all directions and moves into and out of crawling posture; truncal stability and righting responses are brisk and effective, as are upper limb saving reactions that typically emerge between 9 and 11 months (Fig 9.4).

Table 9.2   Age guidelines for equilibrium responses

Response	Average (mo)	80% (mo)
Righting		
Head (held vertically and tipped to either side)[a]	*1*	**2.5**
Trunk in sitting		
Reaching forwards	*8*	**10**
Reaching sideways	*10*	**11**
Saving		
From held vertically[b]		
Downwards (legs/feet)	*7*	**9**
Forwards (arms)	*8*	**10**
From sitting		
Forwards	*7*	**8**
Sideways	*8*	**9**
Backwards	*10*	**11**
Staggering from standing		
Forwards, sideways	*11*	**13**
Backwards	*12*	**14**

[a]Held vertically around the chest under the armpits. [b]Sometimes known as forward and downward/leg parachute responses, respectively.

Crawling

Babies achieve a crawling posture, on hands and knees, typically between 7½ and 8½ months usually through the prone route or from sitting. Once achieved many rock backwards and forwards, some even pushing themselves backwards before mastering forward progression

Walking

Walking requires maintaining balance while the legs are alternately off the ground. Babies actively take weight through their feet at 6 to 7 months and most 7- to 8-month-olds delight in bouncing up and down on laps. Pulling themselves to stand using low furniture or cot sides and standing on the floor holding their parent's hands are achieved between 9 and 10 months. For the next 2 or 3 months babies take every opportunity to

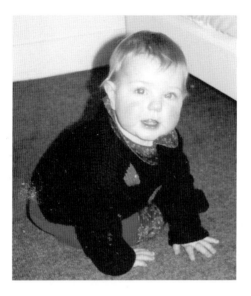

Figure 9.2 Sitting: Stage 1 – note rounded back and effort to prevent collapse by 'propping'.

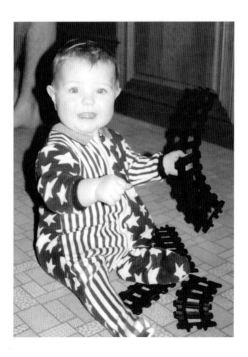

Figure 9.3 Sitting: Stage 2 – confident sit with straight back; able to give attention to the toys and the photographer.

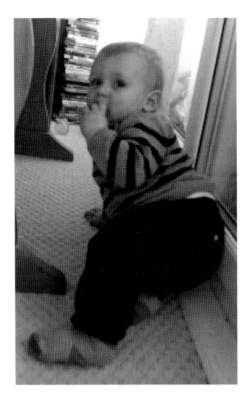

Figure 9.4 Sitting: Stage 3 (dynamic) – moving from crawling to sitting and vice-versa.

progress towards walking without support – walking crabwise along the sofa, stepping forwards with both, and then with only one hand held – relinquishing support gradually as their equilibrium reactions improve. Standing free usually precedes first steps by 1 to 2 weeks (Fig 9.5).

Stage 1: gait is characterised by abducted extended arms (for balance) with widely based, short 'staggering' steps of variable speed and a flat foot strike (Fig 9.6).

Stage 2: Through the second year gradually the arms relax towards the trunk, the stride lengthens and the variability of speed and bouts of instability lessen (Fig 9.7). Figure 9.8 of the same child on the same day illustrates how children revert to an earlier stage when confronted with an unfamiliar surface – in this case, slippery – and emphasises the need to consider the appropriateness of clinical facilities when using them for developmental assessment.

Stage 3: Between 2 and 4 years the base narrows, heel strike and heel–toe shift replace whole foot strike; reciprocal movements of the arms are established and gait becomes smooth, even and stable.

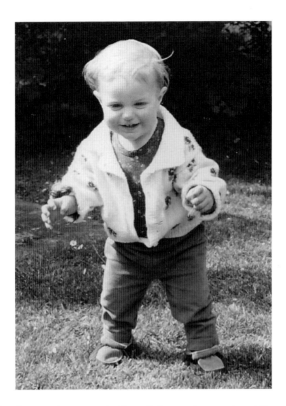

Figure 9.5 Standing free: note concentration all focused on motor skill, wide stance and wide elevated arms.

Running Stage 1 tends to be achieved at 6–7 months after walking Stage 1.

Robson (1984) studied a normative sample of children from a London district and found that the age of walking varied from 9 to 28 months. However, when grouped according to pre-walking patterns of motor development and general tone, clear differences emerged. Eighty-three per cent of typically developing children crawl, 6% stand up and walk, 9% bottom shuffle and 1% creep or roll before they walk. Tone in the latter two groups tends to be at the lower end of the normal range, whereas it tends to be in the middle and at the higher end in crawlers and stand up and walkers. A higher proportion of babies of Black African than European origin walk under 12 months of age. Crawlers and stand up & walkers tend to walk significantly earlier than creepers or rollers and bottom shufflers. Table 9.3 gives ages when different groups achieve sitting, crawling and walking (Robson 1984).

Since Robson's study, opportunity to develop in prone has fallen as mothers world-

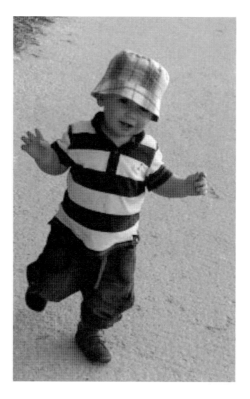

Figure 9.6 Walking: Stage 1 – note distribution of weight and maintenance of balance now alternates through one leg; assistance still required from wide elevated arms.

wide are advised to place their babies in supine for sleep.[2] Newborn babies sleep for 16 or more hours a day and nowadays their waking hours are spent either cradled in an adult's arms or lying supine on 'cushions'. They quickly become so accustomed to the supine position, that when placed in prone they struggle and cry, and so are immediately turned back or picked up and cradled. The opportunity to learn and integrate the lessons of prone development (see the earlier discussion) with those of supine is thus put 'on hold' and, in my experience, impacts negatively on the ages at which sitting becomes dynamic and both crawling and walking are established. Although first rolls from prone to supine tend to be 'accidental' they tutor concepts of rolling and mobility and kick-start the sequence; on the other hand 'accidental' rolling from supine to prone is a physical improbability so babies deprived of prone experience are doubly disadvantaged. Moreover, low-toned babies are less likely to attempt or to achieve rolling from supine to prone, than their higher toned peers. The urge to visually explore the excit-

---

2   To reduce the incidence of cot death.

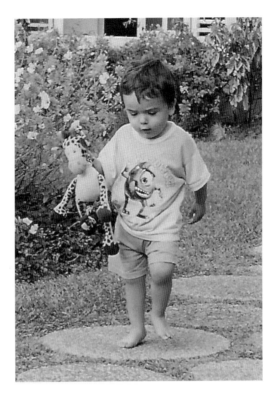

Figure 9.7 Walking: Stage 2 – note gait is stable with hands low and swinging freely while carrying a toy – new territory so visually monitoring where he puts his feet.

ing environment into which they have been born is a potent stimulus for babies to lift their heads and push up on their forearms. Parents should be advised to give their 0- to 4-month-old babies as much supervised prone experience as possible during waking hours, for example, communicatively interact or present colourful mobile lures while baby lies prone on the bed/sofa with mother kneeling on the floor.

Bottom shufflers

Bottom shuffling is considered a normal variant that occurs in 9% of western populations and tends to run in families. These babies tend to have low muscle tone (benign hypotonia), lax joints, flat feet and a dislike of being placed in prone, weight bearing or bouncing during the second half of the first year. Characteristically they 'sit on air' when lifted vertically. Sitting unsupported and walking are noticeably delayed compared to the rest of the population, excepting the few that roll and then creep/commando crawl.

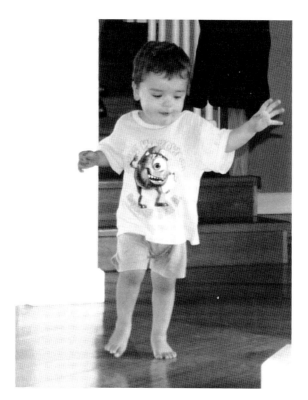

Figure 9.8 Same child as in Figure 9.7, on the same day – note the effect on gait of the challenge of a slippery surface – reversion to an earlier stage.

Rollers and creepers/commando crawlers
Characteristically, the 1% that roll and then creep/commando crawl have low tone and poor core strength and roll into prone later (at 8 to 10 months). They initially achieve mobility by rolling or creeping/commando crawling with the abdomen on the floor. Crawling on hands and knees and walking are delayed until core strength, truncal tone and balancing reactions are sufficient for four-point kneeling and unsupported standing to become dynamic.

Additional upright dynamic skills between 12 and 54 months

As competence in standing and walking improves children attempt, practice and integrate additional skills into their motor repertoire (e.g. walking up and down stairs, sitting themselves in a chair, running, walking on tip toes, standing on one foot, jumping, hopping, skipping, etc.). As with gait there are several stages in the development of each skill that need to be defined if they are to be used as developmental markers. The characteristics of these stages are outlined in Table 9.4 together with age guidelines.

Table 9.3 Ages (mo) when 50% and 90% (or 97%)[a] achieve sitting, crawling and walking according to pre-walking behaviour

Skill/Level	Crawling		Standing up and walk		Bottom shuffling		Rolling and creeping	
	50%	90% (97)%	50%	90% (97)%	50%	90% (97)%	50%	90% (97)%
Sitting Stage 1	6	7						
Sitting Stage 2 (static)	7	(9)	7	(9)	12	(15)		
Sitting Stage 3 (dynamic)	9	(10)						
Crawling	9	(11)					12	(17)
Walking Stage 1	13	(18)	11	(14)	17	(28)	18	(27)
Walking Stage 2	24		24					
Walking Stage 3	36		36					

[a]Numbers in brackets are from Robson's (1984) study that gives the age when 97%, rather than 90%, of children have achieved the skill/level.

Girls tend to achieve hopping, skipping and galloping skills earlier than boys (Keogh 1968). Obviously the acquisition of these skills will be influenced by age of walking so the age guidelines are typical of crawlers and stand up and walkers, and not of bottom shufflers or rollers and creepers.

Adults all envy a toddler's ability to squat on his haunches with his feet flat on the floor without falling over backwards and rise to standing without assistance from his hands – Figure 9.9.

Q Why then do you think that he undertakes the following precarious and complex manoeuvre in order to sit himself in a nursery chair – climbing forwards onto the seat, standing up, turning around before plonking himself down into the seat?
He clearly has the stability to lower himself into the seat; the manoeuvre more likely reflects difficulty in conceptualising his relationship to the chair when he is not facing it, i.e. when he can't see it. Once the concept of the world behind him consolidates and is linked into motor planning he will start to practice backing up to sit.

Table 9.4 Development of additional dynamic skills once walking is achieved in babies who crawl and those who stand up and walk

Going upstairs	Age range, mo	Going downstairs	Age range, mo	On toes	Mo	Standing on one foot	Age range, mo	Hopping	MAge range, mo
Crawls	11–17	Sitting bumps or creeps backwards	14–20	Balances momentarily but lowers prior to stepping	24–29	Tries but unable (cheats[a])	24–29	Tries but jumps with both feet	30–41
Walks two feet/step, hand(s) held	18–21	Walks two feet/step, hand(s) held	21–27	Walks but heels touch floor often	30–35	Succeeds momentarily ⇑ to 1 or 2 seconds	30–36	No of hops on the spot ⇑ from 1 to 6, girls earlier than boys	42–59
Walks two feet/step holding rail	22–32	Walks two feet/step holding rail	28–44	Walks up on toes	36–44	3–6secs	37–53	Progresses forward while hopping	60 and >
One foot/step holding on	33–39	One foot/step holding on	45–53	Runs on toes	45 and >	>6secs	54 and >		
One foot/step (no hands)	40 and>	One foot/step (no hands)	54 and >						

[a]Holds on to the examiner's hand or a piece of furniture; Age guidelines are derived from Griffiths Mental Developmental Scales (2006) and Sonksen, MD Thesis (1978) and given as the age range when the method described is the most common. ⇑, increasing.

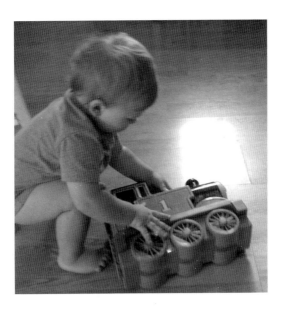

Figure 9.9 Toddler squat.

Motor skills that involve adjustments to environmental motion or movement of 'objects' within it – visuomotor skills
Avoiding collision with moving 'objects' (people, animals), catching or kicking a moving ball or jumping onto or off an escalator require conceptual understanding of the activity, of relative speed, fast processing and high levels of motor planning/timing. Throughout the first year babies experience people and pets coming towards and avoiding them; despite this passive experience the need to adjust their own pace and direction to avoid collision is slow to dawn after they start walking; the adult instinctively continues to be the one to take avoiding action. Several months after first walking and after beginning to avoid stationary objects toddlers stop in their tracks as a person approaches; several seconds pass while they think and motor plan how to take avoidance – the observer can literally 'see the wheels go round'. Smoothly flowing 'passing' generally takes another 18 months at least.

Similarly, the development of catching, throwing and kicking involves continuous integration and constant adjustment to a moving and changing scene, challenging the motor planning and execution frameworks of movement. A description of stages in development of catching, throwing and kicking with age guidelines are presented in Tables 9.5, 9.6 and 9.7, respectively (Sonksen and Mifsud 1976, Sonksen 1978). Catching requires

Table 9.5 Development of catching

Stage	Description	Age range; age for concern (mo)
Stage 1 Direct throw[a]	Tense stance with hands together at chest level. Gazes at hands or nowhere in particular. No movement until 2 or more seconds after ball has bounced off hands onto ground.	13–30; **33**
Stage 2 Direct throw	Stance more relaxed; gaze on thrower. Opens and closes arms in effort to clasp ball to chest; rarely successful.	31–46; **53**
Stage 3 Direct throw	Arms relaxed at sides; gaze on thrower. Tracks terminal part of ball path and moves hands to clasp ball. Catches 30–40%.	47–58; **70**
Indirect throw[b]	Initially similar but fails to turn, move arms to the side or clasp until ball has passed behind them.	
Stage 4 Direct throw	Tracks most of ball flight and moves hands into position for catching earlier. Succeeds >70%.	59–70; **82**
Indirect throw	Anticipatory movements earlier but usually too late and too rushed to succeed.	
Stage 5 Indirect throw	Eyes, arms and body are smoothly co-ordinated to catch most balls.	71–>84; NA

[a]Direct throw: gentle underarm throw of woolly ball aimed to land centre chest. [b]Indirect throw: gentle underarm throw of woolly ball aimed to one or other side. Age range, age when the stage described is the most common.

NA, not available (84mo is the upper age limit of sample).

judgement of the speed and direction of an approaching ball. A toddler initially learns to grasp at the right moment, then to time movement of their arms and trunk as necessary and finally to run and position themselves to receive a ball not thrown directly to them.

Although the ball is always stationary at the point of release in throwing, detailed motor planning and execution are required. Throwing to someone who is running requires additional computations of his speed, and of its impact on trajectory and power require-ments. Casting is initially a baby's way of practicing release. The exaggerated extension of the releasing fingers seems to be facilitated by strong extension of the elbow and the

Table 9.6   Development of throwing

Stage	Description	Age range; age for concern (mo)
Stage 1 "Duck pond"[a]	Stance – 'square' to receiver. Truncal movement predominates. Propels self more than ball – see text.	**28**[a]
Stage 2	Movement mainly at the shoulder: arm extended for over-, side- and under-arm deliveries. Release at any point; trajectory highly variable.	12–26; **42**
Stage 3	Elbow now flexed; elbow extension assists shoulder movement. Stance still 'square' in majority.	27–52; **57**
Stage 4	Release now better timed and flexion of a 'cocked' wrist improves control of direction and height. *Ipsilateral* leg often brought forward to receive weight.	53–78; **NA**
Stage 5	Arches body forwards with weight shift onto the *contralateral* leg; shoulder drops prior to delivery. Individual finger movements at metacarpal-phalangeal and interphalangeal joints. Precision timing of release ensures perfect trajectory, speed and distance.	71->84; **NA**

[a]The percentage of children in stage 1 was never sufficient for it to be typical of the age range. Age range, age when the stage described is the most common.

NA, not available (84mo is the upper age limit of sample).

concept of throwing is probably born at this time (11 to 13 months). Toddlers expend a great deal of energy to little effect. The main movement is truncal. Most hold the ball mid-chest in both hands with elbows flexed, stoop, then heave the body forwards as they straighten and release the ball, most commonly with minimal if any arm movement or with sudden extension of the elbows. Substitute a lump of bread for the ball and a duck pond for the lawn and the chances are that there will be a splash!! Generations of parents have instinctively held onto reins or coat collars while their toddlers enthusiastically 'feeds the ducks'.

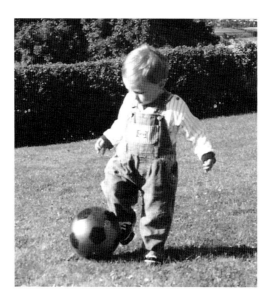

Figure 9.10 Kick: Stage 1 – walks into the ball.

Some toddlers hold the ball as above, look at the catcher's hands, stoop and straighten but then toddle towards the receiver with their hand(s) outstretched.

Q Which aspect(s) are not yet fully primed?
They demonstrate an understanding at a conceptual level but cannot yet fully plan, sequence and execute the final motor aspects of the task.

A small proportion hold the ball in one hand, arm extended and abducted; truncal rotation is the main movement with release of the ball at any time, leading to highly variable trajectories. In under arm and over arm throws the arm moves in an arc and trajectory is determined by the position in that arc that the ball is released; fine tuning of trajectory requires fine finger control of release.

In the early stages a toddler is likely to walk into, or step onto, a ball he wishes to kick (Fig 9.10). He learns first to strike a stationary ball from standing, then from running, and eventually to adjust his own pace of movement to that of an approaching ball, so that the ball is precisely dispatched in a planned new trajectory, i.e. the level of skill and complexity of motor planning advance in parallel.

Table 9.7   Development of kicking – including sex differences

Stage	Description	Age range; age for concern (mo)
Stage 1 Stationary ball	Toddles towards and into the ball displacing rather than kicking it or pauses near the ball, lifts one leg and steps onto ball; may lose balance	All: 13–24; **28**
Stage 2 Stationary ball	Runs to ball, stops, adjusts own position or that of the ball and then kicks it	Girls: 25–57; **65** Boys: 25–42; **51**
Stage 3 Stationary ball Oncoming ball	While running anticipates placement of supporting leg accurately and swings kicking leg all in one movement Misjudges the placement of supporting leg	Girls: 58–>; NA Boys: 43–66; **69**
Stage 4 Oncoming ball	Now integrates own and the ball's movement accurately	Boys: 67–84+; NA Girls[a]

[a]Only two had reached stage 4. Age range, age when stage described is the most common.

NA, not available (84mo is the upper age limit of sample).

Assessment

History

The primary medical history alerts the assessor to children at risk of neuromotor disorders.

Developmental history

Explore current gross motor abilities and concerns. Parents are less likely to voice concern about the early motor development of their first than of subsequent babies as many may not have experienced how typically developing young babies feel when handled; second time round they notice floppiness, unusual postures, etc. However, examination as indicated below, rather than reliance on history, is advised for all babies in the first year. Grandparent concerns should be taken seriously. In babies and toddlers with developmental co-ordination disorder (DCD), responses to questions about gross motor and visuomotor milestones, equilibrium responses and tone, tend to be atypical rather than definitive. Questions containing the words 'co-ordination' or 'clumsy' such as 'Would you say he is well coordinated or a bit clumsy?' focus the conversation on the qualitative aspect of movement and lead naturally to requests for description. If replies raise the examiner's index of concern familial trend and social circumstances should be explored.

Examination

Milestones are but one, somewhat arbitrary, stage on a continuum. The first staggering steps of a toddler are undoubtedly a triumph – that is written all over her face and reflected in her parent's expressions – but she still has quite a few steps to go on the walking continuum before walking is 'automatic'. In light of the multiplicity of factors influencing motor development it is hardly surprising that the age range for emergence of traditional motor milestones and motor sequences (stages in the development of motor skills) are often too wide for them to stand alone as markers of normality or abnormality of motor development. For assessment, milestones and stages need to be set in a more qualitative framework of observation and to be supported by neurological examination during the first 4 months and whenever tone, skill levels, movement patterns, postures or quality of movement raise the assessor's index of concern. Low-tone babies, creepers and sitters on air/bottom shufflers should always be examined neurologically as up to 10% have a degree of cerebral palsy. In an effort to define stages within the continuum of progress towards a mature skill, professionals extract multiple aspects of movement from their observations of a population of children and group those that occur concurrently together; these constellations when sequenced in time define 'stages', which become the subject of normative studies of variable scientific strength. Structural aspects predominate in texts describing stages, rather than more qualitative components, such as smoothness, directness, economy of effort and level of motor planning. However, the latter are equally important in evaluating normality and although advances in their measurement are being made, current schedules such as the Infant Motor Profile (Heineman et al. 2008) are too long and too specialised to be part of preliminary assessment. Assessors should increase their gestalt of the qualitative aspects of movement at different ages through thoughtful observation of babies and preschool children playing on the beach or in the park, as they are a valuable indicator of status. Alternatively the internet provides some authoritative developmental sites which illustrate movement development with videos (e.g. *http://library.med.utah.edu/pedineurologicexam*).

Age guidelines

Age guidelines are given in Tables 9.1 to 9.8. Provision of precise age guidelines is frequently difficult as three or four stages may span several years (e.g. the kick). Age ranges not only are very wide but often overlap considerably. In these circumstances mean and median ages are not particularly informative.

- From 5 to approximately 21 months, the month during which the skill/stage is typically achieved is given in *italics* and the age for identifying the lowest 10% in bold.

- As age ranges widen and increasingly overlap, the age range during which a stage is typical (used by at least 50%) is given in regular text, together with the age for identifying the lowest 10% in bold.

Table 9.8 Primitive reflexes

Reflex	Typical age range (concern if persists)	Alarm bells if
Moro	Birth to 4mo (6mo or >)	Absent in neonate Asymmetrical
Standing	Birth to 4mo	Asymmetrical
Walking	Birth to > 2mo	Asymmetrical
Stepping up	Birth to > 4mo	Asymmetrical
ATNR	Birth to 5 (>6mo)	Asymmetrical

ATNR, asymmetric tonic neck reflex.

Ages in bold are given to alert the assessor to children who require fuller examination or continued observation, i.e. are in the slowest 10%.

Gross motor guidelines are based on the following sources:

Illingworth (1962), Keogh (1968), Sheridan (1973), Sonksen and Mifsud (1976),[3] Sonksen (1978), Robson (1984), Frankenburg et al. (1992), Griffiths Mental Development Scales (2006), Sharma and Cockerill (2008), Noritz et al. (2013).

Protocols for different age groups

Initially, the assessor facilitates and notes the level and quality of age-appropriate static and dynamic postures and skills in four positions: supine, prone, sitting and standing. Traditionally, this is undertaken in a 'back to front' cycle, i.e. starting in supine and progressing through prone. Obviously once a child is mobile the order may change!

The first 4 months

Protocol: For this age group the assessor places a non-slippery mat on the examination table or floor (if no table height surface is available), chooses a time when the baby is awake and alert but not crying; clothing should be minimal (naked or nappy

---

3   The sample size for the catch throw and kick study was 261 (137 boys; 124 girls), 12- to 84-month-olds, attending nurseries and primary schools in central London, UK

only). She observes posture and spontaneous movements through the back to front sequence – placed supine → pulled to sit → supported sitting → supported standing → placed prone. The assessor then adds ventral and vertical suspension as they inform truncal tone and in vertical suspension tilts the baby to each side to look for neck righting.

Age guidelines: See Table 9.1

Primitive reflexes: Observation of the core primitive reflexes is advisable even in babies in whom the earlier examination is normal. Their elicitation is part of standard neurological examination so is not re-iterated here. Timing of their appearance/ disappearance and symmetry strengthen the examiner's view of the intactness or otherwise of the neuromotor system.

Age guidelines: Table 9.8 shows key primitive reflexes with their normal time scale.

From 5 months to walking

Materials: A non-slip mat on the floor, a nursery (>18 months) or an adult (<18 months) table and chair and a couple of attractive toys.

Protocol: While formally assessing other areas the assessor observes the baby on parent's lap, noting how much support she gives him, whether righting responses occur when he reaches out for toys, how mobile he is on her lap, etc. Subsequently on a gym mat the assessor targets age-appropriate skills within the back to front sequence, encourages positional shifts and mobility using strategically placed attractive toys and observes the manner, symmetry, quality of movements. In other words she takes each baby to his highest level whilst being ever ready to intercept any loss of balance and to stabilise any piece of furniture being used for support. Equilibrium responses are formally tested at age-appropriate level. For example neck and truncal righting can be observed in a sitting baby by encouraging him to reach out for a favourite toy, held just beyond his reach to either side at his shoulder level; if absent he simply abducts his extended arm without shifting his centre of gravity; if present he reaches and leans compensating for the shift by curving his spine. Checking for pelvic stability may induce anxiety. Success is greater if displacement is incorporated gradually into an action nursery rhyme such as 'Ride a Cock Horse' – initially the assessor sits the baby across her thigh and supports his trunk while gently bouncing him up and down on her knee; once his confidence and enjoyment grows she gradually slides her hands down so that support is at the junction of pelvis with thigh only, and introduces small excursion tilts to one and then the other side, or forwards and backwards. She gradually increases the excursion and observes the level of righting, being ready to reduce the excursion if baby shows any alarm. Saving responses require an unexpected displacement; it is therefore wise to explain what will happen to parents, to vocalise cheerfully 'whoops' and to ensure a saving arm is strategically placed.

Age guidelines: See Tables 9.1 to 9.3.

<u>Walking and beyond</u>

Materials: An attractive toy and a woolly pom-pom ball of 12 to 15cm in diameter.

Protocol: While fetching the child and mother from the waiting area, the assessor observes and mentally notes the patterns and quality of the child's rise from the floor or a chair, walk/run down the corridor, etc. If these have not been observed, she sets the stage to do so at the beginning of the motor assessment. First, she observes and notes the characteristics of his gait – position and tension in arms, wideness of base, type of foot strike and balance – Table 9.3 for stages. She chooses age-appropriate skills from the skill sequences – Table 9.4 and demonstrates and joins in the activities, as this helps under 4-year-olds to understand the instruction and renders them less self-conscious.

Although the age ranges for the stages are wide with considerable overlap, the assessment of catching, throwing and kicking is valuable because, being a familiar and popular play activity, anxiety about being expected to 'stand on one foot' or 'walk on your toes' rapidly dissipates into free flowing motion and thus provides an excellent opportunity to observe qualitative aspects of movement. Another reason for including these skills is that they are likely to be more delayed than those in Table 9.4 in children with specific developmental language delays/disorders (Sonksen 1978). The assessor and child stand 2 to 3m apart facing each other (2m for catch and throw and 3m for kick). The assessor uses a large woolly pom-pom ball.

Q Why?
Because it will not hurt if it hits a younger child's face or chest and is unlikely to damage the clinic room if kicked or thrown by an overenthusiastic 4- to 5-year-old!

Catch: The assessor throws the woolly pom-pom ball in a gentle vertical arc into the child's outstretched hands. If he achieves stage 2, she throws the next three or four balls slightly to his right or left side; the assessor should look at the child and not to the side of the throw – Table 9.5.

Throw: The assessor encourages the child to throw the ball back to her after each attempted catch; if he persistently throws it under arm she encourages him verbally and by gesture to throw over arm – Table 9.6.

Kick: The assessor places the ball half way between herself and child. She stands with legs well apart as a 'goal' and encourages the child to run and kick the ball into the goal. If child achieves Stage 3 with a stationary ball, the assessor rolls the ball towards him asking him to run and kick it while it is still moving – Table 9.7.

Age guidelines: Gait – Table 9.3; Stairs through hop – Table 9.4; Catch, throw and kick – Tables 9.5, 9.6 and 9.7.

Typical developmental levels and quality of movement suggest the absence of neuromotor disorder and can simply be considered in the context of the whole profile. However, delay in levels of skill, suspicion of asymmetry, abnormal tone, abnormal posture or of disordered quality of movement should raise suspicion that a neuromotor, dyspraxic or muscular disorder may be present; the findings then need to be viewed in the context of the presence or absence of signs of neuromotor pathology and/or delay/disorder in other developmental domains, i.e. a more extensive neurological, paediatric and developmental examination should be undertaken.

Movement disorders – outline

Conditions associated with abnormal patterns or delay of gross motor and manipulative development fall into three broad categories : cerebral palsy, DCD and muscular dystrophy; approximately 0.25%, 5% and 0.03% of western populations respectively are so affected. The epidemiology, incidence, impairments and risk factors of cerebral palsy were summarised by Odding et al. (2006). Very low birth weight babies are a high risk group for cerebral palsy and The American Academy of Pediatrics recommends that they should receive a structured examination of neuromotor function at least twice during the first year; the effectiveness of current test techniques has been evaluated by Spittle et al. (2008). The neuromotor hallmarks of babies and young children with cerebral palsy are abnormalities of tone (hyper/hypo-tonicity), of movement (voluntary/involuntary) and of posture, persistence of primitive reflexes and asymmetries. The Gross Motor Function Classification System (Palisano et al. 1997, Rosenbaum et al. 2008) has revolutionised the classification of cerebral palsy. A wide and variable range of mild to very severe learning, attentional, cortical visual disorders and sensory impairments feature in at least 70% of babies and young children with cerebral palsy.

In contrast DCD tends to run in families, is more common in boys than girls and among the poorer socio-economic groups, and is often the presenting feature of chromosomal disorders (e.g. Fragile X syndrome and Down syndrome), and of neurodegenerative and neuromuscular disorders (Noritz and Murphy 2013). Clumsiness, poor co-ordination, poor sensory integration and motor planning difficulties characterise young children with DCD and comorbidity of DCD with other developmental disorders such as autistic spectrum, specific language, phonological and attention deficit disorder is strong and has recently been reviewed by Kirby et al. (2014).

Duchenne muscular dystrophy is an X-linked condition affecting boys and characterised by weakness. For many years mild learning difficulties, particularly of non-symbolic cognition, have been thought to feature in some boys with DMD. A recent study correlating mutations along the dystrophin gene with neuropsychological findings has further clarified the situation (D'Angelo et al. 2011). The authors found that full-scale IQ was on average 1SD below the population mean for the whole group ($n = 42$) and that those with Dp140 mutations were overall more effected than those with mutations at the proximal end of the dystrophin gene. Those with Dp140 mutations featured specific impairments of visual memory and of both visuospatial and syntactic processing; in contrast in the group with proximal mutations visual memory and visuospatial processing appeared intact and syntactic processing was less affected. As weakness is often not noticed until boys are over 3 years of age, it is imperative to check *rising from the floor* in all preschool boys presenting with mild to moderate delay in non-symbolic cognition or specific language delay.

The understanding and management of motor disorders have increased enormously during the last decade and the following books by Hadders-Algra (2010), Dan et al (2014), Seal et al (2013), and Sugden and Wade (2013), are recommended reading.

Key Points

- Movement development is a complex process requiring a continuum of integration at multiple levels of the nervous system between multiple domains.

- Milestones are an inadequate description of motor ability and require more precise definition of levels and qualitative parameters.

- A neurological examination should be done in all bottom shufflers and creepers and rollers.

- Delay in levels of skill and/or concerns about quality of movement require a full neurological examination.

- Weakness on rising from the floor should be tested in boys presenting with cognitive or language delays – risk of DMD.

References

Dan B, Mayston M, Paneth N, Rosenbloom P (Eds) (2014) Cerebral Palsy: Science and Clinical Practice. Clinics in Developmental Medicine, ISBN: 978-1-909962-38-5, London Mac Keith Press.

D'Angelo MG, Lorusso ML, Civati F et al. (2011) Neurocognitive profiles in Duchenne muscular dystrophy and gene mutation site. *Pediatr Neurol* 45: 292–299.

Edelman GM (1989) *Neural Darwinism. The Theory of Neuronal Group Selection.* Oxford: Oxford University Press.

Frankenburg WK, Dodds J, Archer P, Shapiro H, Bresnick B (1992) The Denver II: A major revision and restandardization of the Denver Developmental Screening Test. *Pediatrics* 89: 91–97.

Gesell A (1940) *The First Five Years of Life*. London: Methuen.

Griffith's Mental Development Scales – Extended –Revised: Birth to 8 years (2006) London: Hogrefe,

Hadders-Algra M (2000) The Neuronal Group Selection Theory: A framework to explain variation in normal motor development. *Dev Med Child Neurol* 42: 566–572.

Hadders Algra M (2010) Examination of Children with Minor Neurological Dysfunction, 3rd edition. Practice Guide. London. Mac Keith Press.

Heineman KR, Bos AF, Hadders-Algra M (2008) The Infant Motor Profile: A standardized and qualitative method to assess motor behaviour in infancy. *Dev Med Child Neurol* 50: 275–282.

Illingworth RS (1962) *An Introduction to Developmental Assessment in the First Year*. Little club clinics in developmental medicine 3. London: William Heinemann Medical Books Ltd..

Keogh JF (1968) *Developmental Evaluation of Limb Movement Tasks*. Technical report 1–68, Los Angeles, USA: University of California at Los Angeles

Kirby A, Sudgen D, Purcell C (2014) Diagnosing developmental coordination disorders. *Arch Dis Child* 99: 292–296.

Levitt S (1982) *Treatment of Cerebral Palsy and Motor Delay*, 2nd ed. Oxford. Blackwell Scientific Publications.

Noritz GH, Murphy NA, Neuromotor Expert Screening Panel (2013) Motor delays: Early identification and evaluation. *Paediatrics*. Originally published on line May27, 2013. http://pediatrics. aappublications.org/content/early/2013/05/22/peds.2013-1056.

Odding E, Roebroeck ME, Stam HJ (2006) Summary of "The Epidemiology of cerebral palsy: Incidence, impairments and risk factors." *Disabil Rehabil* 28: 183–191.

Palisano R, Rosenbaum P, Walter S, Russell D, Wood E, Galuppi B (1997) Development and validation of a gross motor function classification system for children with cerebral palsy. *Dev Med Child Neurol* 39: 214–223.

Piper MC, Pinnell LE, Darrah J, et al. (1992) Construction and validation of the Alberta Infant Motor Scale (AIMS). *Can J Public Health* 83(Suppl 2): S46.

Robson P (1984) Prewalking locomotor movements and their use in predicting standing and walking. *Child Care Health Dev* 10: 317–330.

Rosenbaum PL, Palisano RJ, Bartlett DJ, Galuppi BE, Russell DJ (2008) Development of the Gross Motor Function Classification System for cerebral palsy. *Dev Med Child Neurol* 50: 249–253.

Russell DJ, Rosenbaum PL, Wright M, Avery LM (Eds) (2013) Gross Motor Function Measure (GMFM-66 and GMFM-88) 2nd edition. London Mac Keith Press.

Seal A, Robinson G, Kelly A, Williams J (Eds) (2013) Children with Neurodevelopmental Disabilities: The Essential Guide to Assessment and Management. Practice Guide. ISBN: 978-1-908316-62-2, London. Mac Keith Press

Sharma A, Cockerill H (2008) *Mary Sheridan: From Birth to Five Years.*: Abingdon, Oxon: Routledge.

Sheridan MD (1973) Motor development. In: *Children's Developmental Progress from Birth to Five Years: The STYCAR Sequences*. Windsor, Berkshire: NFER Publishing Company.

Sonksen PM (1978) The neurodevelopmental and paediatric findings associated with significant disabilities of language development in preschool children. MD Thesis, University of London, UK

Sonksen PM, Levitt SL, Kitzinger M (1984) Identification of constraints acting on motor development in young visually disabled children and principles of remediation. *Child Care Health Dev* 10: 273–286.

Sonksen PM, Mifsud A (1976) The development and assessment of three visuo-motor skills – catching, throwing and kicking. Presentation to 10th international group on child neurology and cerebral palsy. Oxford, UK

Sonksen PM, Stiff B (1991) Show *Me What My Friends Can See: A Developmental Guide for Parents of Babies with Severely Impaired Sight and their Professional Advisors.* London: The Wolfson Centre.

Spittle AJ, Doyle WD, Boyd RN (2008) A systematic review of the clinimetric properties of neuromotor assessments for preterm infants during the first year of life. *Dev Med Child Neurol* 50: 254–266.

Sudgen D, Wade M, editors (2013) *Typical and Atypical Motor Development.* Clinics in Developmental Medicine. London: Mac Keith Press.

Thelen E (1995) Motor development: A new synthesis. *Am Psychol* 50: 79–95.

Chapter 10

Upper limb development

The neurological substrate of the systemic neuromotor system was discussed in Chapter 9.

Development

In humans the upper limbs are highly specialised for prehension and fine manipulation, though earlier in evolution mobility and stability would have been their primary function. Today the upper limbs still play a major role in gross motor progress from totally dependent in the newborn period to stable stance and mobility on two legs. Prehension *(reach, grasp, release, manipulation)* develops alongside allowing the individual to feed his intellect through feel and close visual inspection, to use tools effectively and creatively and to communicate emotions, such as tenderness, through touch.

General

Position and degree of comfort have a marked effect on both posture and quality of arm movements in the newborn period. For example, the arms tend to rest in slight flexion at the elbow and loose flexion of the fingers around an adducted thumb in a supine and content baby; in contrast, the vigorous crying of a neonate, not appreciating the experience of being taken out of the bath, will be accompanied by tight flexion of the elbows and fingers and jerky, erratic movements of small excursion at the flexed joints. Tiny movements and intricate postures of the fingers are seen in response to social engagement; these are more likely to reflect activity within and links between fetal networks for social communication and fine finger movement rather than, as has been suggested, 'imitation' – the cognitive ability to imitate is not evident until 7 to 8 months.[1] Similarly, the large rhythmic arm movements engendered by the sight of the parent during the first 2 months, probably reflect links between motive[2] templates and primary motor networks already present at birth, rather than purposeful reaching. Another motive trigger is suckling, expressed through ecstatic tiny movements of the toes. During this period repetitive scratching and grasping movements of their own or their parent's clothes are common. Generally both arm and fine finger movements are bilateral and the thumb is opposed to the palm when the hand is closed.

In previous chapters the importance of arousal of cognitive interest in looking, and its critical role in the manipulative development has been emphasized. During the first 10 weeks the arm and finger movements of a baby with visual impairment are similar to those of a sighted one; between 10 and 14 weeks a sighted baby catches sight of his hands as they move within his visual field, he alerts and intently studies his hand visually; over a number of days he watches the small movements of his fingers and small 'too and fro' excursions of his hands; some also look back and forth with great interest from one hand to the other (Figs 10.1a and b). At this age the arms and hands of a supine baby with visual impairment tend to fall back to their shoulders with their fingers aimlessly opening and closing. The sighted baby is learning through his vision about his upper limbs and realising cognitively their potential for prehension and manipulation; without the tutoring effect of vision the baby with visual impairment has failed to appreciate the functional potential of his arms and hands. Once a sighted baby achieves this cognitive level the stage is set for development of voluntary control.

Aspects of development

Shoulder, elbow, wrist, core and even lower limb musculature participate to varying extent in every upper limb activity (reaching, viewing, drawing, switching, throwing, threading) to provide stability and to fine-tune position and power. *Reach, grasp, manipulation* and *release* develop during the first 18 months and in the context of assessment it is worth thinking about them separately for this age group. Concomitantly, specialisation of one hand as executor and the other as stabiliser, in tasks that require two hands to perform co-operatively but in different ways, is gradually established. Although fingertip grasp and release develop within the first 18 months, fine manipulation of grasped objects within the fingers tips of one hand does not emerge until the third and fourth year.

Reach
The stages in the development of reach between 3 and 6 months were discussed in

---

1   Imitation of babbling sounds made by an adult during proto-conversations.
2   Reflecting excitement aroused by recognition of the parent.

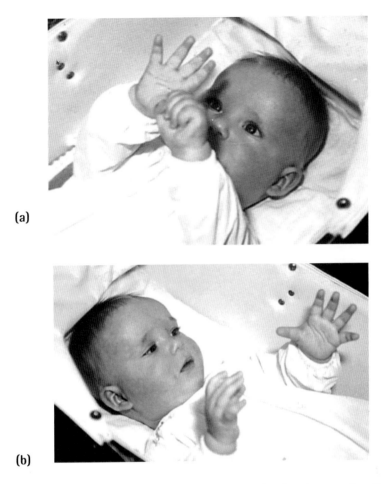

(a)

(b)

Figure 10.1a and b Fourteen weeks. Dawn of concept that hands are prehensile (a) studying finger movements (b) 'actually I have two hands!'

detail in Chapter 1. After 5 months and still under the tutelage of vision the quality and coordination of reach in sitting becomes more accurate and more fluid; orientation and shape of the hand for grasping is increasingly adapted to the shape and orientation of the object and each arm increasingly acts independently of the other. A baby with visual impairment still has toys pressed into his palm; unfortunately as sensory feedback from the palm about the nature or shape of the object is inferior to that from vision or the tips of his fingers, his learning experience is increasingly jeopardised and he is at risk of becoming tactile defensive – after all most of us find it is hard to prevent drawing back when someone says 'shut your eyes' while pushing something into our palm. In sighted

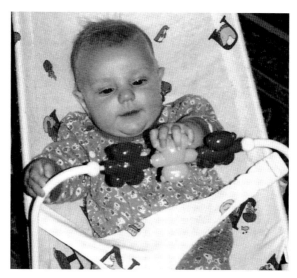

Figure 10.2 Four-month-old in reclining seat: Basic palmar grasp. Note convergence and visual interest.

development reach and orientation for grasping in sitting are usually smoothly enacted by 10 to 12 months; however, they will be less so in standing.

Q Why might that be?
Because the baby is giving so much attention to co-ordinating his postural mechanisms.

Q When will reach and hand orientation for grasping in standing become fully mature?
When postural control in standing is 'on automatic'.

Grasp
The grasp reflex appears between the fourth and sixth month of gestation and disappears between 2 and 4 months post term. The reflex induced by exerting pressure on the palm may have helped our infant forebears not to 'fall' as their parents traversed the canopy.

In the following description babies are supine or fully cradled. A baby's fingers actively close around their parent's finger or a toy between the second and third and third and fourth months, respectively. The thumb does not participate in gripping, though is usually outside the palm. Figure 10.2 shows a 4-month-old well supported in a reclining seat. Her visually directed swipe made contact; her grasp is palmar with no radial dominance.

Grasping brick/cube size (2.25cm) toys or larger on a table surface: The hand of a 5-month-old baby is open as his palm makes contact with a cube: he then makes raking movements with all four fingers trapping the cube within the palm (palmar grasp). Over the next weeks the raking and grasping movements are increasingly made with the middle and index fingers (radial palmar grasp); from 6 months the index finger increasingly leads the approach to both cube size and smaller items and the thumb helps trap the item between the three radial digits; thus the radial palmar grasp becomes radial digital by 8 months. At 9 months the side of the terminal phalanx of the thumb closes to the side (scissors grasp) or to the palmar surface (inferior pincer grasp) of the middle phalanx of the index finger; around the first birthday the cube is gripped between the tips of the index (+ or – middle) finger(s) and thumb (pincer grasp). The mature/fine pincer grasp (tips of index finger and thumb) is reserved for smaller objects and appears in the first 2 months of the second year.

Grasping smaller objects – Smartie (1.2cm) to hundred and thousand (1.25mm): Once babies are cognitively interested in looking at objects of these sizes (5/6 months and 9 months, respectively) they tend to attempt pickup using the current level of their grasp for a brick/cube-sized object. Thus, a 6-month-old baby is likely to use the same grasping technique (radial–palmar) for both a cube and a raisin and is more likely to succeed in picking up the bigger item. However, supervised opportunities to pick up smaller items motivate a baby to refine his technique. Success in picking up an hundred and thousand is limited before a baby's pincer grasp is fully mature, i.e. 12 to 14 months.

Release
In the first 6 months release is not an active movement; it occurs as a child's grip relaxes (passive drop), for example as his interest is attracted to something else or as part of general relaxation.

Release and transfer of brick/cube size (2.5cm) or larger toys: Six- and seven-month-olds transfer from one hand to the other by pulling the toy out of the holding hand with the receiving hand, rather than active relaxation of grip. In my experience active release is first evident into the mouth at around 7 months. A baby of this age with a banana held in a palmar grasp lifts it to his mouth and bites or sucks off successive pieces. With the last piece within his palm he 'thinks' 'how do I get this bit in?' He presses his fist against his mouth and extends all five digits; first active though rather messy release achieved! Some active relaxation of the fingers of the holding hand is noted during transfer between 9 and 10 months, indicating the beginning of active participation in release and using the two hands co-operatively (Figs 10.3a and b).

From 10 months babies reach towards an adult who holds out a hand in a 'give' me gesture; however the adult has to grasp the toy and pull it gently from the child's hand, i.e. the baby cognitively wants to give but hasn't the manipulative skill yet to do so. Elev-

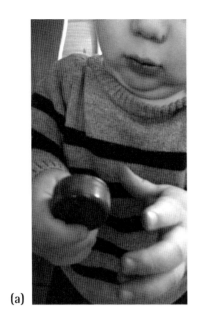 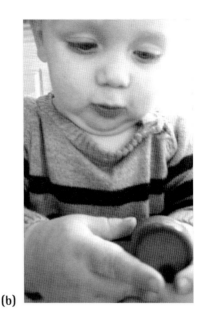

(a)   (b)

Figure 10.3a and b 10-month-old transferring toy: (a) note orientation of the receiving hand for grasping (b) note a degree of active relaxation/release of the original hand.

en-month-olds watch intently as they actively extend all five digits to release a toy into space; at this stage there is no attempt to place the object on a surface before its release, consequently it usually lands on the floor; this behaviour known as 'casting' probably represents *practice* of movement patterns[3] rather than any desire to irritate their parents[4] – attempts to place onto a surface before release are made by 12-month-olds; first the toy is firmly pressed on the adult palm several times but then withdrawn with the toy still in the baby's hand. One day between 12 and 14 months the toy though still firmly pressed will be released onto the palm with the now familiar exaggerated extension of the fingers. Over the next few weeks the movement is enacted with less pressure, more smoothly and more economically.

Release and transfer of smaller objects (≤1.25cm): Active release of small items occurs from each level of pincer grasp; however the less mature the pincer grasp the less efficient and clumsier the release. For example the release of a Cheerio held in a scissor or an inferior pincer grasp into the mouth begins by pressing the gripping digits on the lips, then simultaneous extension of the fingers causing the Cheerio to fall into the palm[5] or

3   To consolidate networks and templates.

4   Babies don't yet have negative agendas!

5   In which case success is achieved via palmar pushing, c.f. the banana

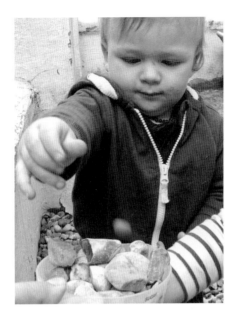

Figure 10.4 Fourteen-month-old practicing pincer release.

onto the floor! A successful neat release into the mouth occurs shortly after the pickup is pincer or mature pincer, i.e. at 12 to 14 months. The success and neatness of release into a small pot is similarly linked to the level of pincer grasp and follows a similar timescale. Transfer of Cheerio held in a scissors or inferior pincer grasp is enacted by the receiving hand and pulling. Once the grasp is pincer or superior pincer the transfer is facilitated by active relaxation of grip. Figure 10.4 illustrates a 14-month-old 'practicing' pincer release of pebbles into a bucket. The aspects of development between 5 and 14 months are summarised in Table 10.1.

Placement and release both mature during the second year and babies experiment with different combinations and degrees of wrist extension/flexion and elbow pronation/ supination to better enact and monitor activities. For example in building a tower of bricks the following stages are seen.

Stage I: From 12 to 24 months (Figs 10.5a and b)

- Arm posture – the elbow is pronated and the wrist flexed throughout (limits visual monitoring)
- Placement – is characterised by over-push (threatens stability)

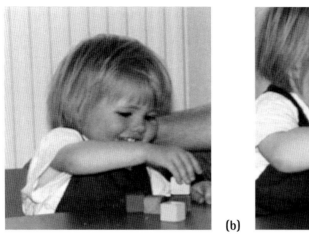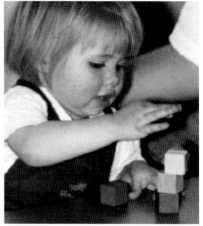

(a) (b)

Figure 10.5a and b Seventeen-month-old building tower: (a) Stage 1- placing hand is pronated and obscures her view of base bricks and (b) top brick shifts as a consequence of over-push and asymmetrical release.

- Release – is asymmetrical, i.e. the relaxation of the fingers and thumb are not fully synchronous (threatens stability)

Stage II: From 2 to 3 years

- Arm posture – a quarter to half supination of the elbow and partial extension of the wrist increasingly occurs during the activity (facilitating visual monitoring and control)

- Placement – the amount of over-push decreases (increasing stability)

- Release – becomes increasingly symmetrical (increasing stability)

Stage III: 3 years and over

- Wrist in neutral, fine adjustment of placement occurs through rotation at the elbow (pronation ⟺ supination); release is symmetrical.

As a consequence towers stand steady and tall.

Executor and stabiliser
During the first 4 to 6 months purposeful movements such as reaching are made with

both arms and reflect the generation of bilaterally synchronous messages from primary cortical and subcortical templates. Efficient exploration and use of objects requires each arm and hand to enact different movements whilst acting co-operatively. This requires the brain to coordinate a continuously changing flow of different messages to each limb; the messages are the consequence not only of planning at cognitive and motor levels but ongoing assimilation of sensory feedback from the visual and motor systems. In most tasks one limb positions and stabilises the object whilst the other explores and operates the moveable parts; in others the limbs may alternate executor and stabiliser roles.

The first sign is the development of a leading hand between 4 and 6½ months – the non-leading hand does less rather than a different action (e.g. in reaching for a toy and later during the early active shake of a rattle). Shortly afterwards, while visually inspecting a toy held in the leading hand, a baby brings his second hand to feel the moving parts and a little later to grasp and pull it from the holding hand (transfer). Until two-handed mid-line play and one-handed across mid-line reach have been established for several months, the leading hand does not really provide clues to future handedness. During the last trimester of the first year babies help themselves drink from a beaker by employing the second hand to assist tipping; however, while playing with toys on a table or on the floor they tend to use one hand only for example to take the toys out of a box or take a lid (with a knob) off a pot.[6] Using the second hand to pick up and hold a pot in order to pull the lid off occurs around 15 months. Holding objects stationary on the table surface with the non-executive hand is only occasionally evident before 2 to 2½ years, e.g. the base of a peg men boat, the paper in pen and pencil tasks. Unscrewing requires a concept of the mechanism (cognitive) and the physical prowess to grip, turn, release, turn hand in other direction, re-grip and turn in the original direction, etc. Under 20 months most babies just pull; between 20 and 24 months most turn the lid back and forth without releasing and re-gripping; between 24 and 28 months most manage to unscrew the lid.

Q What are the three responses teaching us?
The 20-month-old clearly does not have the concept but is likely to have the manipulative ability to grip and turn; the 24- to 28-month-old clearly has the concept and the manipulative skill; the 20- to 24-month-old certainly understands that turning is necessary, but it is not yet clear whether she appreciates that the lid should continuously be turned in the same direction. If she does then presumably this understanding is not yet fully integrated with motor planning.

Overall the task reveals more *cognitive* than manipulative information. Consider the complexity (cognitive and motor) of the task of spreading butter on toast. Both the

---

6   This is so, even in babies who are well supported, so it is not because of a need to prop in order to maintain their sitting posture.

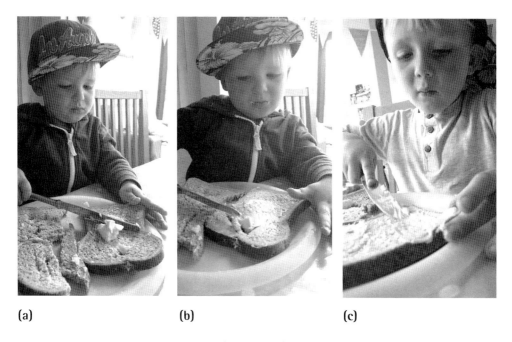

(a)   (b)   (c)

Figure 10.6a, b and c. The two-year-old (10.6a and b) gives all his attention and effort to control movement of the knife; he even tries to steady the plate. He spreads away from himself with a somewhat erratic sweeping gesture exerting uneven pressure. The 4-year-old's efforts (10.6c) are more 'controlled' and more effectively planned. He has spread towards himself (fairly smoothly) and is controlling the pressure on the knife with his index finger.

2-year-old in Fig 10.6a and b and the 4-year-old in 10.6c need to give the task all their concentration. Execution and motor planning are at a higher level in the 4-year-old; even so the motor and (cognitive) modules in his cerebellum clearly require further conditioning to recognise inputs from higher levels increasingly early, for execution to shift from 'controlled' to 'automatic' and to require only a minimal amount of his attention (Ramnani et al. 2006).

Fine manipulation
Fine manipulation is the intricate and coordinated movements of the fingers to control the position of objects within the hand. Although the index finger approach heralds fingertip grasp and release, it is not until between 3½ and 5 years that children can control movements of the interphalangeal joints of individual fingers to reposition small objects (e.g. pegs) held within their fingertips or to effect fine movements, for example, of a pencil tip. Such movements differ from the wide variety of exploratory movements of fingers witnessed in the early months because a feeling hand is *not* also grasping.

The movements of held objects during the first two to three years, such as 'taking to the mouth', 'transfer to the other hand', 'shaking', 'banging', scribbling', 'insertion of a peg into a pegboard' occur at the shoulder, elbow and wrist rather than at the metacarpal-phalangeal and interphalangeal joints.

Crayon/pencil and paper
By 15 to 18 months babies realise (cognitive) that crayons can be used to mark paper. At a younger age they may pick up a crayon, but are more likely to take it to their mouths or bang it than attempt to scribble, though some will do so if encouraged by an adult. The cognitive aspect of imitating and then copying increasingly complex geometric shapes (horizontal scribble to a diamond) has already been discussed in Chapter 6, p. 147. The motor aspect is the modus operandi to grasp the pencil and to control movement of its tip; both gradually mature so that small as well as large movements of the tip can be effected. Rosenbloom and Horton (1971) delineated three stages; Erhardt (1982) subdivided Rosenbloom and Horton's Stage 1 into two, hence four stages are described here.

Stage 1 – palmar supinate or palmar pronate: Typically between 14 and 21 months grasp is either palmar supinate or palmar pronate and the business end of the crayon may or may not point towards the paper (motor planning). Movement all takes place at the shoulder joint with the whole arm moving as a unit (Fig 10.7).

Stage 2 – digital pronate: Between 21 and 27 months the shaft of the crayon/pencil is grasped by the fingers with the elbow pronated and the wrist slightly ulnar deviated. Movement is enacted by the shoulder and elbow.

Stage 3 – static tripod: Transition to an immature and static tripod grasp occasionally occurs as early as 2½ years, but more typically between 3 and 4 years. The shaft is grasped between thumb, index and middle fingers somewhere along its length. The hand moves as a unit. In other words, no movements occur across the metacarpo-phalangeal and interphalangeal joints. Gradually, as children realise that control is easier when the pencil is held close to the tip they shift their grip distally by pushing or pulling the pencil through their fingers with the other hand.

Stage 4 – dynamic tripod: Typically between 4 and 6 years the pencil is grasped close to the tip, precisely between the tips of the thumb and first and second fingers; the wrist is slightly extended and the elbow less fully pronated; stabilisation of the metacarpo-phalangeal arch allows the interphalangeal joints to effect small controlled movements of the pencil tip.

The templates of the motor system are now primed for writing.

Pegs (1.5 × 0.75cm). Putting small pegs into a pegboard is a fun and educational play activity from 21 months but needs to be carefully supervised (not for children who put everything into their mouths).

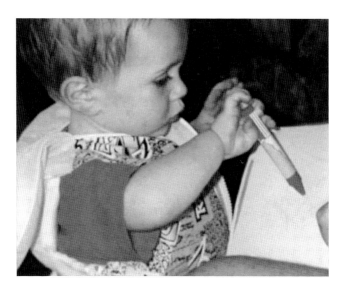

Figure 10.7 Fifteen-month-old: Early Stage 1 grasp of crayon. His grasp is palmar at the proximal end of the shaft; the forearm is pronated, making his efforts to mark the paper ineffectual.

Stage 1: The peg is grasped in a pincer grip with pronated or partially pronated elbow and slightly flexed wrist. If the tip of the peg points straight out from the finger tips a child is likely to adduct his arm at the shoulder to position the peg over the hole and then push it in ; he may push too hard and/or release 'asymmetrically' so that the peg 'jumps' out. If the peg protrudes at 90° to the line of his fingers he is likely to abduct and internally rotate the shoulder to position and insert the peg. Stage 1 is typical between 21 and 30 months.

Stage 2: Adjustment of pegs for insertion is effected in one of two ways:

- By loosening grasp and rolling the peg against another surface (own shirt front or the table surface) and then re-grasping.

- By transferring to the other hand and then re-grasping.

Release tends to become more synchronous and hence the pegs remain in the board. These methods are typical of 2- and 3-year-olds.

Stage 3: From 48 months adjustment of pegs is increasingly carried out through collaborative, coordinated movement of the thumb, index and middle fingers of the ipsilateral hand (intradigital manipulation)[7]. Note that in order to rotate the peg within the fingers without dropping it, the thumb and one of the other digits need to be lightly gripping at every point in time. Agonists and antagonists acting synchronously results in smooth insertion and release of pegs.

Handedness

In the first 6 months movements of the upper limbs are usually synchronous and bilateral. Gradually, between 4 and 6 months one hand, though not always the same one, increasingly tends to lead (e.g. when swiping at a dangling toy). Between 6 and 8 months a leading hand is a common feature of reaching from a supported sitting position. In reaching tasks, the leading hand tends to be the one on the same side as the toy. In tasks that are ultimately carried out predominately by one hand as executor, such as feeding with a spoon, brushing hair or writing, children initially experiment with both right and left hand; gradually a definite preference emerges for each task. The hand in the executor role commonly ends up the same for each task, though *not* invariably. Handedness or hand dominance is usually allocated with respect to eventual handedness for writing, drawing and painting tools, though dominance for other tasks is sometimes taken into account. Hand dominance for drawing and writing tends to become established between 4 and 6 years. However, 6% of typically developing children spontaneously change handedness for writing in either direction between 6 and 10 years. Ten to fifteen per cent of typical individuals are left handed. The incidence of left handed individuals in a sibship increases directly with the number of parents who are left handed (i.e. genetic influence); the increase in incidence amongst brain injured populations is a feature of the distribution of handedness within the normal population – assuming an equal number of right and left hemispheres are damaged.

Assessment

History

The primary medical history – see Chapter 2, p. 34 – alerts the assessor to children at risk of neuromotor disorders.

Developmental history
A question such as 'Do you think he is good or clumsy with his hands?' channels the conversation into upper limb skills? If the parent answers 'clumsy', frame some questions to identify the skills she is concerned about and the nature of the difficulty; also why she is concerned (e.g. is it because of comparison with performance of older siblings or

---

7   Some individuals utilise the tip of the ring finger as well.

peers). Older children with developmental coordination disorder (DCD) often voice their dislike, whereas preschool children may simply 'run off', do something else or throw a tantrum, when drawing or getting dressed are suggested. If the primary history does not suggest a neuromotor problem upper limb function is more effectively assessed through observation of structured play activities than developmental questioning.

Examination

Except during the first 10 to 12 weeks, assessment of upper limb function is linked to that of non-symbolic cognition (NSC) because young children demonstrate this type of understanding mainly through upper limb movements. Many of the NSC tasks are ideal for the examination of manipulation so these are picked out in the following paragraphs and expanded as necessary. (The reader can refresh his or her memory of the NSC protocols in Chapter 6.) Novice assessors will find it helpful to observe and note the cognitive aspect(s) and then the manipulative ones, allocating each to their own section of the record sheet. A small peg and pegboard test is added to facilitate observation of fine manipulation.

General practicalities

- Observations are made with a baby cradled in his parent's arms or supine during the first 12 weeks, supine from 12 to 22 weeks, sitting on the parent's lap up to an adult height table from 5 to 18 months and at a nursery table from 18 months onwards.

- The assessor ensures that the child is sitting squarely up to the table with his weight evenly spread through the buttocks; babies between 5 and 10 months may need some support around the trunk. Sitting slightly twisted away from the table reduces the likelihood of a child voluntarily using his second hand and even if he does, the manipulative levels are likely to appear lower than those of the first hand, giving a false impression of asymmetry – even raising unwarranted concern about hemiplegia

- Babies have *two* upper limbs, so there is a risk of missing hemiplegia unless a point is made of observing both. If a child leans on his left arm and persists in reaching across with the right hand to bricks/pegs proffered to his left, the assessor gently places her left hand over his right hand and lightly touches his left hand with a 'this hand's turn'. This usually succeeds in getting him to use each hand.

- Several trials are essential to judge whether or not, in the context of a specific task, the roles of executor and stabiliser, hand preference or handedness are emerging or clearly established.

Age guidelines

Manipulative milestones suffer from the same problems as gross motor milestones and lack the qualitative content so vital to identification of developmental motor disorders (see Chapter 9, p. 238). Modern schedules for looking at qualitative aspects are again too long and too specialised for preliminary assessment (Heineman et al 2008).[8] Age ranges for sequences (e.g. in development of pencil control) are similarly wide with considerable overlap between stages. Age guidelines for manipulative development are therefore presented in a similar format to those for gross motor development – see Chapter 9, p. 238-239.

Ages in bold are given to alert assessors to children who require fuller examination or continued observation.

Protocols for different age groups.

Protocols for different age groups are given in this section; these are drawn from a selection of the sequences mentioned in the previous section on development.

First 12 weeks

Protocol: At this age the assessment is part of the general examination of the motor system; so the assessor observes

- General posture

- Posture and movements of arms and fingers

- Distribution of tone

- Presence/absence of palmar grasp

Endpoint

In the newborn period

- Flexed

- Flexed, fingers closed over thumb most of the time; large erratic arm movements when excited or upset or startled.

- Tone higher in limbs than trunk

- Elicitable

---

8   Preliminary assessors can complement their gestalt of the qualitative characteristics of upper limb movement at different ages and stages through active observation of typically developing babies and preschool children, in the flesh or on web sites.

From 6 to 12 weeks

- Less flexed

- Fingers more often open, though when flexed thumb is usually apposed; scratchy movements of fingers

- Limb tone lower; neck and truncal tone/control increasing

- Elicitable

12 to 20 weeks

The assessor dangles an attractive toy over a supine baby. Once visual interest is gained she observes arm movements.

Endpoint: Reach: Large bilateral swiping arm movements when excited by a visual lure; hands tend to stay closed with thumb inside during 'excited' arm movements

Age guideline: 14–18 weeks>

When a baby's hand is naturally open the assessor gently strokes the under surface of his fingertips with her own or with the handle of a rattle.

Endpoint: Baby closes fingers and grips for a few seconds. Release by passive relaxation

Age guideline: finger *10–12* weeks; rattle *14–16* weeks

5 to 15 months

Materials: Jingle bell stick or ring rattle, 2.5cm cube, 1.2cm Smartie.

Rattle

The assessor places the rattle on the table; observes and notes characteristics of the following:

- Reach (symmetry, directness, smoothness, pre-grasp orientation)

- Grasp

- Exploration with other hand

- Transfer to other hand

- Release to the assessor

Age guideline: – see Development section of this chapter

Cubes

The assessor places a cube on the table directly in front of the baby with, 'and that's for you' and observes

- reach (symmetry, directness, smoothness, pregrasp orientation);
- grasp – nature (palmar/pincer) and level/stage;
- release including transfer – passive relaxation, active (onto table surface or examiner's hand) and level/stage.

From 8 months, she also observes grasp and release of a Smartie at the end of the vision test.

Endpoint: stage achieved

Age guidelines: – [Sh] [S] (Erhardt 1982, 1994) – see Table 10.1.

Practice Point A rattle gives more information on explorative movements of the contralateral hand than a cube. Although a cube is standard equipment for the assessment of reach, grasp and release, a Smartie better demonstrates the level of pincer development; thus both should be used from the age of 6 months.

12 to 36 months – Tower

Protocol: See protocol for building a tower – Chapter 6, p. 158. The assessor places the cubes one by one on the table alternately to right and left side of the base brick with a spoken and gestured 'put it on the top'.

Q Why should the assessor do it this way?
As this gives the assessor the best opportunity to observe the levels of grasp, placement and release for each hand, and in a context of (a) hand preference noting small disparities and (b) neuromotor disorder noting large ones.

She observes grasp and arm posture for pickup, placement and release.

Endpoint: Stage achieved. For stages see description under development, p. 253, and Table 10.2.

Age guidelines: [S] – see Table 10.2.

Assessment of fine finger control:

12 months onwards

Table 10.1 Development of 'manipulation' for a 2.25cm cube/brick and 1.2cm Smartie through year 1

Reach	Grasp	Transfer Placement	Release	Achievement (mo)	
				Typ	AC
Approach swiping with leading hand open	Palmar rake		Passive relaxation	5	7
Smoother and more direct	Radial palmar rake		Passive relaxation	6	8
Smoother and more direct	Index leads -radial-palmar	Transfer – other hand grasps and pulls	Active extension of fingers[a]	7	9
Smoother and more direct	Radial-digital Thumb helps trap cube	Transfer – other hand grasps and pulls	No active relaxation when adult takes toy	8	9
Direct and smooth	[b]Scissors	'ditto' + some active relaxation of fingers	Some active relaxation when adult takes toy	9	11
Direct and smooth	[b]Scissors or inferior pincer	Equally in transfer	Active extension of fingers in casting	10	12
Direct and smooth	[b]Pincer	Reaches and withdraws	Casting	11	13
Direct and smooth	[b]Pincer	Places on adult hand, pushes and withdraws	Cube not released	12	14
Direct and smooth	[b]Fine pincer for Smartie	Places cube with several pushes	Active extension of the fingers to release onto adult hand	13	15

Typ, typical child uses this method; AC, age for concern if not present by this age; [a]To push into mouth – only observe this if item suitable (e.g. a piece of banana); [b]A Smartie is used to assess grasp and a cube to assess release onto a hand.

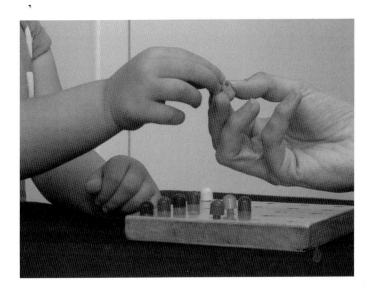

Figure 10.8 By being proffered the pointed end of the peg, the child has to alter its position within her fingertips in order to insert it into the pegboard.

Crayon/pencil

Protocol: See protocol for geometric shapes – Chapter 6, p. 163 and 165. The assessor uses a crayon with children under 30 months, and a pencil with those over 30 months. She places the crayon/pencil on the table in the child's mid-line with the business end pointing away from the child and gently extracts it from the child's hand between each item using it to demonstrate or to point to the next item.

Q Why?
So that sufficient evidence is accumulated to judge not only the child's stage of manipulation but also his/her **handedness.**

In order to be sure of witnessing the highest level of fine manipulation of children of 3 years or over she draws some 'teeny-tiny' circles for the child to copy or asks him to draw 'tiny buttons' on the shirt of an outline drawing of a man. The stages are described fully in the development section, p. 257, and summarised in Table 10.3.

Age guidelines: see Table 10.3 (Rosenbloom and Horton 1971) (Erhardt 1982, 1994).

Table 10.2   Stages and age guidelines in placement of bricks on top of each other

Stage and description	Age range; age for concern (mo)
Tower	
1. Pincer grasp; elbow pronated; wrist flexed; over-push; asymmetric release	12-24; **27**
2. Pincer grasp; elbow ¼ to ½ supinated; wrist partially extended; less over-push; increasingly symmetrical	25-36; **42**
3. Pincer grasp; elbow as above; wrist in neutral; no over-push; release symmetrical	37 onwards; NA

Age range, age when the stage described in most common. NA, not available as upper age limit of sample too low.

21 months onwards

Small pegs and pegboard

Protocol: The assessor places a 25-hole square wooden pegboard directly in front of the child. For children under 36 months she says, 'Look my peg goes in the hole' putting one into the middle hole and 'Now you put this one in here' as she places one peg on the table to the child's right of the board and points to a hole. The assessor observes grasp, placement and release then places the next peg to the child's left and subsequent ones alternately right and left. After two or three to each side she proffers one with the 'sharp end' protruding from her finger tips Figure 10.8; consequently the rounded end protrudes from the child's fingertips and he will need to adjust its position for insertion – perfect for observing his level of fine finger control. Repeat several times to each hand. The stages are described fully in the development section, p. 258, and summarised in Table 10.3.

Age guidelines: See Table 10.3 (Sonksen, unpublished data).

One advantage of the peg test is that Stage 2 adjustment of grasp involves quite small and controlled movements of the fingers, for example 'rolling the peg up his shirt or along the table surface' before re-grasping in a good position for insertion – it also provides an opportunity to observe a child using tactile (as opposed to visual) monitoring. Fine finger control at the intradigital and metacarpal-phalangeal joints (Stages 2 and 3) develops at a younger age than for pencil skills and is therefore more manipulative-

Table 10.3 Stages and age guidelines for manipulation of pencils and pegs

Stage and description	Age range; age for concern (mo)
Pencil	
1. Palmar pronate or supinate	15-21; **27**
2. Digital pronate	22-41; **45**
3. Static tripod	42-57[a]; **64**
4. Dynamic tripod	58 and over; NA
Pegs	
1. Pincer grasp; pronation of elbow; abduction of shoulder; partial flexion of wrist; over-push; asymmetrical release	21-27; **30**
2. Adjust grasp by rolling on table or shirt, or transfer back and forth; less over-push; release more synchronous	28-48; **54**
3. Adjust grasp by intra digital manipulation; smooth insertion and release of pegs	49 and over; NA

[a]In Rosenbloom and Horton's (1971) study the static tripod was never typical of any age group probably due to a combination of the age distribution within a relatively small sample. Age range, age when the stage described is most common. stage; NA, not available due to upper age limit of sample.

ly definitive for children in the preschool era. Qualitative differences between the two hands are frequently apparent in typically developing children who use the same stage with each hand; unfortunately longitudinal data on qualitative differences are not available but could perhaps provide a way of predicting handedness, for tasks that require fine manipulation. Pencil tasks – drawing geometric shapes inherently inform the NSC domain, whereas the cognitive component of putting a peg in a hole is not in anyway definitive (at a 12 month level); however the peg test offers high level cognitive bonuses after manipulation is assessed. Consequently, it is better to use both tests.

Q What are the high level cognitive bonuses offered after manipulation is assessed?
Colour and number.

Q Apart from observation of the function of each hand, handedness, etc, what developmental factors lie behind the recommendation to take the pencil back after each item and to give out the pegs one at a time?

Management of attention control – children under three will immediately 'do their own thing' with the pegs if allowed to help themselves from the pot or from a pile in front of them. Taking the pencil/crayon away helps the assessor transfer the child's attention back to her for the next, instruction.

Q How does the assessor judge whether failure of a 36-month-old to build a tower of more than six bricks is cognitive, or motor?
If manipulative, the height of the tower is likely to vary more than it would if cognitive; the child would either be in Stage 1 or exhibiting qualitative or neuromotor signs. If cognitive the tower tends to reach the same height on each occasion. Further observation and viewing the findings in the context of his profile should clarify the most likely reason(s).

Six- to eight-month-olds tend to passively drop a held brick when a second one is proffered to the other hand; by 8 to 9 months they hang on to both.

Q Which of the three domain categories is responsible for the advance and what aspect of it?
The advance is cognitive not manipulative– permanence of objects. At 7 months babies immediately 'forget the existence' of the first brick when their attention shifts to the second.

Manipulation disorders

Apart from congenital upper limb deformities and injuries, for example of the brachial plexus, manipulation problems feature as part of more generalised motor disorders (e.g. cerebral palsy and DCD). Therefore the discussion of movement disorders and references at the end of Chapter 9 are pertinent to this section. Severe involvement of the upper limbs in cerebral palsy seriously constrains learning potential, especially in the NSC domain. The psychological impact of disordered manipulation in DCD often escalates during the first two years of Primary school as the emphasis on writing and drawing, and the need to tie laces and do up buttons increase. Self-esteem and self-confidence drop and may be expressed as a variety of negative behaviours and sadness. The demoralisation tends to worsen unless the therapy plan addresses the psychological as well as the motor problem.

Key Points

• Upper limbs are anatomically highly specialised for manipulation. hence essential for learning and physical creativity.

- Progress is highly dependent on intact vision.

- Reach, grasp, release and manipulation come on line in order and then refine side by side.

- On average fine finger control is accessed younger using the peg than the pencil task.

- Handedness

  - Most children experiment with both hands before hand dominance for a task is established.

  - Hand dominance for executive tasks is usually, but not always, uniform.

  - Six per cent of children change handedness for writing at >6 years.

- Entering school puts physical and psychological demands on children with DCD that need addressing before they become entrenched.

References

Erhardt RP (1982, 1994) *The Erhardt Developmental Prehension Assessment (EDPA)*. Maplewood MN: Erhardt Developmental Products.

Heineman KR, Bos AF, Hadders-Algra M (2008) The infant motor profile: A standardized and qualitative method to assess motor behaviour in infancy. *Dev Med Child Neurol* 50: 275–282.

Ramnani N, Behrens TE, Johansen-Berg H et al. (2006) The evolution of prefrontal inputs to the cortico-pontine system: Diffusion imaging evidence from Macaque monkeys and humans. *Cereb Cortex* 16: 811–818.

Rosenbloom L, Horton ME (1971) The maturation of fine prehension in children. *Dev Med Child Neurol* 13: 3–8.

.

Chapter 11

Speech sound production: articulation and phonological processing

The articulation of speech is a highly complex and finely tuned neuromotor skill requiring extremely rapidly co-ordinated activity of respiratory, laryngeal, oropharyngeal, lingual and labial musculature, i.e. it is the motor execution of both centrally generated expressive language and phonological processing. Phonological development is included in this chapter as impairments of both the phonological and articulatory system lead to disordered speech sound production (SSP).

Neural substrate

In the adult brain specific areas of the temporo-frontal networks, with links to long-term memory, are responsible for the generation of the language and the prosodic and phonological aspects of speech perception and production. On the expressive side the latter includes recall, planning and organisation of phoneme sequencing, within both individual words and sentences. Subsequently, links with the premotor and motor frontal cortices, the basal ganglia (caudate and putamen), olives and the cerebellum lead to finely tuned and precisely controlled activation of the speech musculature. In terms of SSP, lateralisation issues have a degree of flexibility in the infant's brain, unless insults (genetic or physical) are bilateral (Watkins 2011). At birth a basic expressive network is present and responsive: connectivity and template consolidation is reflected behaviourally first in prosodic, followed by phonemic, then semantic and finally syntactic aspects of expressive language. The generation of the latter as speech requires phonemic retrieval and organisation (phonological processing) followed by transfer to the musculature of the speech apparatus for execution – the phonetic (articulatory) aspect of speech production.

Observed development

The sciences of phonology and phonetics refer to SSP in *words* rather than in *non-meaningful vocalisations*/protophones. However, it is pertinent to remember that the sensory – cognitive – motor circuits of both systems are being primed from birth.

A wide variety of apparently spontaneous silent movements are visible in the oro-facial musculature of newborn babies; these movements generate sensory (proprioceptive and kinaesthetic) feedback and set in motion building a network and store of movement patterns that can later be used in goal-directed speech production and communicative facial expression. Spontaneous unformed emotive vocalisations, such as crying and little coos of contentment, add auditory feedback to the developing template. The first communicative smiles at around 6 weeks are often accompanied by moist coos. Prosodic and phonemic experimentation with vowel sounds is witnessed from 3 months. By 4 months the cadences of the parent's vocalisations are reflected in a baby's side of proto-conversations and active experimentation with airflow and labial movements are in evidence – 'raspberry blowing'. By 6 months consonant–vowel sound combinations are experimented with first singly – 'ba' and by 8 months in strings – 'ba-ba-ba'. Between 9 and 12 months babies experiment with consonant–vowel–consonant (CVC) and VCV combinations, e.g. 'mam', 'ama', 'eewoo' at the same time playing with cadence and loudness. Although by 9 months babies are believed to recognise all the phonemes in their mother tongue, they can only produce a limited number of CVC combinations (babble); the latter are not true words, i.e. the baby is not using them as symbols to represent an object or person. The templates dedicated to semantic processing, their links with the phonemic working memory bank and phonetic motor repertoire are sufficiently primed between 12 and 16 months for meaningful utterances in the form of situational phrases or single words. At first the listener relies more upon the cadences (prosody) and vowel sound content than the consonant content, to fathom meaning. For example the cadence and the vowel sound content of a parent's 'up you come' as she picks up her baby are clear in his utterance 'uh-ooo-um' whereas the consonants are not. The challenge of subsequent years is to increase the number and complexity of phonemes (single consonants, consonant clusters and more complex vowels) that can be summoned up, sequenced (phonological processing) and articulated (motor competence) in the service of a phenomenal expansion of the language base between 1 and 8 years of age.

The phonological and articulatory systems develop side by side and responsively each to the demands of the other and to those of expressive language. The best way to become familiar with typical patterns of SSP in preschool children is to take every opportunity to listen to them talking amongst themselves and with their caregivers and digest the SSP content in the context of age. Clearly, significant degrees of hearing loss, learning difficulties and specific language delays/disorders will impact on the development of both systems. The nature of the first language will influence the repertoire of phonemes. As phonological processing is the precursor of articulation in the generation of speech, it is discussed first.

Phonology

Phonological processes on the expressive side mature gradually through the preschool years. Until recently, the patterns of sound production heard in the speech of typically developing preschool children were frequently referred to as phonological 'errors'. The use of the word *error* to describe a normal process was unfortunate as it gave parents and professionals the impression of abnormality. Normal cognitive–manipulatory processes, such as non-realisation by a 7-month-old that a toy he has just seen being hidden under a cloth still exists (permanence of objects) or the palmar grasp with which he picks it up once it is exposed to view again, are not labelled as errors/abnormalities because they differ from adult performance. Why therefore were phonological processes labelled in this way for so long? Their normality recognised, they are now commonly referred to as phonological 'simplifications' used by young children (Williamson *http://www. speech-therapy-information-and-resources.com/phonological-processes.html*); 'typical patterns in phonological development' are preferred to 'simplifications', but both will be used.

Articulation

Refined rapidly co-ordinated control of the musculature of the vocal tract from lips to voice box and of the muscles of respiration is required to articulate clearly the 20 vowel sounds, 24 single consonants and 20 consonant blends/clusters of the English language. Vowels are referred to as *open* sounds as they do not involve closure of the vocal tract; consonants on the other hand do and hence are referred to as *closed* sounds. Consonant sounds are defined in three ways:

1. Where in the vocal tract they are made – *place* – bilabial, labio-dental, dental, alveolar ridge, postalveolar, palatal, velar and glottal

2. How they are made, i.e. the type of contact that is effected – *manner* – plosives, nasals, fricatives, affricates, approximants

3. Whether or not the *vocal cords* are activated – voiced or voiceless

The complexity of movements demanded of the muscles of the speech apparatus parallels the intricacies of phonological demand. The motor demands of some phoneme sequences and transitions from one phoneme to the next may be above a child's current

Table 11.1 Common patterns of phonological development

Phonological pattern	Examples	Age (y) when no longer present in 90%
Reduplication of first syllable	'bobo' for 'bottle'	2½
Consonant harmony – articulated in the same place but different consonant	'guk' for 'duck'	3
Final consonant deletion	'caa' for 'car' 'moo' for 'moon	3½
Initial consonant deletion	'at' for 'cat'	3½
Devoicing	'ret' for 'red'	3½
Fronting – place of articulation brought forward	'tar' for 'car'	4½
Backing – place of articulation moved backwards	'goor' for 'door'	4
Stopping – fricative replaced by plosive	'tock' for 'sock' 'ban' for 'van' 'door' for 'four'	3 to 4½ depending on the fricative
Cluster reduction	'poon' for 'spoon' 'geen' for green	3½ for most clusters (5 for complex clusters)
Weak syllable deletion	'puter' for 'computer' 'nana' for 'banana'	4
Gliding	'wailway' for 'railway' 'wed' for 'red'	5½

articulatory prowess. In typically developing children neuromotor control of the speech apparatus matures and refines throughout the early childhood in response to phonological demand, in the same way as other systemic motor systems (e.g. the refinement in control of a pencil tip from 18 months until 7 or 8 years). Thus during the pre- and primary school years typical speech patterns reflect continuing neuromotor as well as phonological development.

With advances in expressive language the demands on the phonological and articulatory systems rise exponentially, because children need to select, summon up, organise and

Table 11.2   Development of articulation

Speech sound	Achieved by 50% emerging (y)	Achieved by 90% mastered (y)
'p' 'm' 'h' 'n' 'w' 'b'	1½	3
'k' 'g' 'd' 't'	2	3½
'ng' 'f'' 'y' 'r' 'l' 's'	3	4
'ch', 'sh', 'z', 'j' and 'v'	4	5
'th' (thin); 'th' (the); 'zh'	4½; 5[a]; 6[b]	6, 6½[a]; 7½[b]
'l'-blends	4	6
's'-blends	4	7
'r'-blends	5	8

[a]'th' as in 'the' achieved at this age; [b]'zh' as in 'measure' achieved at this age.

dispatch an increasing number of phonemes in the fulfilment of ever-longer and more complicated meaningful utterances in split seconds. The major role of the cerebellum and olivary nuclei in this process is currently becoming clearer (Koziol et al. 2014).

Age guidelines – What is normal?

Precise age norms are not available for phonological or phonetic development so the information that follows and in Tables 11.1 (Typical phonological patterns/simplifications) and 11.2 (Articulation) should be taken and used only as guidelines. The phonological processes are resourced from (Williamson G sltinfo.com) The articulatory guidelines are derived from studies and experience of specialists in the field including Sander (1972), Smit et al. (1990), Goldman–Fristoe Test of Articulation – GFTA-2 (2000) and Williamson G (2010) and http://www.speech-therapy-information-and-resources.com/articulatory-processus html.

Normal patterns of phonological development

There are several problems in constructing norms from available data. A large number of phonological patterns/simplifications have been described and the distribution of these within the population is very varied although some are much more common than others and virtually predictable. Time frame and intensity are also variable. Unlike other developmental sequences, phonological progress is indicated by the disappearance of patterns/simplifications that are typical of younger children rather than the appearance of the mature one. The data available therefore do not allow us to calculate when 50% achieve the mature pattern; however data are available for when the behaviour has disappeared in 90%. Some of the most common developmental patterns/simplifications are described in Table 11.1, together with the age in years at which they still persist in up to 10%.

Normal patterns of phonetic/articulatory development

In the normal course of development a sound may be achieved in one position in a word months or several years before it is achieved in others. Specialist professionals (speech therapists and speech and language pathologists) combine two criteria to describe articulatory achievement (1) age when 50% or 90% achieve and (2) achievement in at least *one* or *all* position(s) in words.

• Emerging – when 50% make the sound correctly in at least one position

• Mastered – when 90% make the sound correctly in all positions.

Vowels
Some vowel sounds are *mastered* in first words, i.e. by 18 months. The most complex vowel sounds are *mastered* by 3 years.

Consonants
In general the earliest sounds to *emerge* and be *mastered* in the shortest time interval tend to be the protophones that previously were 'practised' as babbling. Sounds made at the front of the mouth tend to *emerge* before those made at the back. The majority of single consonants *emerge* before consonant clusters/blends. The articulation of girls tends to be more advanced than that of their male peers; the difference is greatest between 4 and 8 years in mastery of consonant clusters

All but 3 (of 24) single consonants *emerge* by 4 years of age. The three are 'th' as in 'thin', 'th' as in 'that' and 'zh' as in 'measure'. Only a small proportion of children articulate more than a few consonant clusters/blends clearly before their fourth birthday. Some 'l' and 's' blends are achieved by 50% of 4-year-olds and 'r' blends by 50% of 5-year-olds.

A chart devised by *www.mommyspeechtherapy.com* derived from Goldman and Fristoe's (2000) standardisation sample gives age for mastery of single and clustered consonants by 85% of children.

Intelligibility
Intelligibility is a subjective estimate of the proportion of a child's speech that is under-

standable to a *non-professional* adult. Coplan and Gleason (1988) offered a method for remembering typical age-related proportions: create a fraction in which the nominator is the child's chronological age and the denominator is 4. Thus the fraction for a 1-year-old is 1/4 or a quarter; for a 2-year-old is 2/4 or *half*; for a 3-year-old 3/4 or *three-quarters* and for a 4-year-old 4/4 or *totally intelligible*. There are several factors that interplay to overestimate intelligibility when assessed by parents or professionals; the former are completely attuned to their own child's speech while the latter are so familiar with the phonological patterns of preschool children that they rapidly tune in. Moreover conversations with preschool children are usually related to events or objects in which both the adult and the child are currently engaged, thus providing an abundance of non-spoken contextual clues.

Assessment

The assessment of problems in speech production are the province of specialists in speech therapy/speech pathology, so the clinical pointers in this section are designed to help the reader decide whether or not development is within normal limits. Patterns of abnormality will be described in a later section.

History

Primary history

The primary history explores the medical and environmental risks for problems in speech production. Particularly relevant pointers for neuromotor disorder (e.g. dysarthria) are preterm periventricular leukomalacia and hypoxic ischemic episodes. A diagnosis or signs of craniofacial dysmorphia or a history of persistent feeding difficulties are 'alerts' for speech production difficulties. Deafness constrains phonemic development so primary questions should embrace intrauterine/postnatal infections and familial deafness in childhood. As the phonemic repertoire of languages varies, the first language of the family should be confirmed and also whether the parent or main caregiver has a speech impediment.

Secondary history

Parents do not always appreciate that their child has a problem with speech production, either because they have become 'attuned' to his speech or are unsure what to expect from a child of his age. On the other hand many parents worry unnecessarily about simplifications/patterns that are in fact part of typical development. Probably the most useful direct question to ask parents is 'how much/what proportion of Susan's speech do you understand – all of it, three-quarters, a half or a quarter?'

Examination

Procedure

Attention is switched to SSP once verbal comprehension, expressive language and symbolic play have been tested with the miniature toys or common objects. The assessor continues to engender conversation with the child (enlisting the parent's help as necessary) through interactive play with the toys or pictures, listening carefully to the child's SSP.

The assessor notes the following:

• The consonants and consonant blends used by the child.

• Several examples of the child's sentences in her 'personal' phonetic script; 'deh baba in deh baaf'; 'me wann aah boo won'; 'go de paa mummy? – 'bed fer guks in bag' for 'the baby is in the bath'; 'me want a blue one'; 'go the park mummy? – bread for ducks in bag'.

Age guidelines

Intelligibility: ¼ for a 1-year-old; ½ for a 2-year-old; ¾ for a 3-year-old; ⁴⁄₄ for a 4-year-old. The assessor should note the parental and his or her own estimates (Coplan and Gleason 1988).

Phonology: The assessor considers the *phonological* patterns in the context of chronological age using Table 11.1 and whether the simplifications/patterns are typical or deviant.

Articulation: The assessor checks whether or not the consonants heard represent a good range of those expected for chronological age using Table 11.2.
When levels are below those expected for chronological age she considers them in the context of expressive language age and the rest of the intellectual profile. If articulation is deviant she checks control of non-spoken movements and neuromotor status.

Examples

Susan's speech

• 'Dada gon ca' for 'Daddy gone car'

• 'Goggy dink wawa' for 'Doggy drink water'

Both samples are between 50% and 75% intelligible despite containing several phonological simplifications – age appropriate for a 2- to 3-year-old. The first syllable of the first sample is reduplicated in the word Daddy – fine up to 2½ years. The final consonant of the third word is deleted – fine up to 3½ years. In the second sample 'g' is substituted for the 'd' of doggy (backing) – acceptable until 4 years. A cluster reduction is heard in the word 'drink' – acceptable up to 5½ years. The first syllable of the third word is reduplicated – acceptable until 2½ years. Both utterances contain one pattern that should disappear by 2½ years. The phonetic content (d, g, n, c and g, d, k, w) is appropriate for a 2- to 3-year-old. Thus, if Susan is 2½ or less, her intelligibility is acceptable, her phonology and articulation are not of concern and her expressive language is reassuringly at a three-component level (slightly above average) with noun–verb–noun framework. However, if Susan is 4 years 3 months old, intelligibility and articulation are delayed, as are both phonology and expressive language. Phonological patterns/simplifications are all typical so phonology is likely to be delayed rather than disordered. However, as phonological patterns are in line with expressive language level, her phonological delay might be part and parcel of a language delay/disorder or of global developmental delay. Therefore, her non-symbolic cognition should be explored and taken into consideration when formulating a 'plan of action'.

John's speech – 3 years 6 months

- 'My doo in da bo' for 'my shoe's in that box'
Standing alone this utterance has low intelligibility (less than half), i.e. at a 1- to 2-year level, it can be understood only in the context of the question he had been asked, 'Where are your shoes?' and by his look towards a box whilst speaking. John's utterance contains phonological simplifications (e.g. stopping, backing and last syllable deletions) – all still used by up to 10%. All the consonants John articulated are from the youngest two groups that emerge by between 1½ and 2 years. Expressive language is a bit below average for age but not in the lowest 10%. Both articulation and intelligibility are delayed. Obviously, additional samples of his speech need to be considered before jumping to conclusions but if the findings were similar the advice of a speech therapist would be sensible.

Simon's speech – 6 years

- 'Cars and wailway trains don't go as fast as aeroplanes' for 'Cars and railway trains
  don't go as fast as aeroplanes'
Intelligibility is almost 100%, and the listener has no need of contextual clues. 'R' becomes 'w' in railway (gliding) – phonologically acceptable until 5½ years when it will have disappeared in 90% of children. In 10% of children it persists up to the age of 7 or 8 years. Articulation-wise there is a wide range of consonants and consonant blends and he produces a typical 'r' sound at the end of the word *car* and in the middle of the word *aeroplane*. Expressive language is above average. As long as other utterances are similarly clear, the assessor need have no concerns about Simon's phonological development.

Q If Simon was describing the colour of a tea-shirt he wanted for Christmas, which colour might contain a phonological simplification?
'Red' might be articulated as 'wed'.

Practice point If after listening to a child's speech production and considering intelligibility, phonological patterns and articulation in an otherwise typically developing child, the examiner is concerned about speech production the advice of a speech therapist should be sought.

Disorders of speech and sound production

Early behavioural pointers that 'all may not be well' with SSP include the following:

- High and/or variably pitched cry[1]

- Feeding difficulties

- Drooling

- Delay in canonical babbling

- Delay in first words

Differentiating between articulatory (phonetic/neuromotor) and phonological (phonemic) disorders in preschool children

In SSP the phonological system has a cognitive–linguistic role – abstraction, cognition and storage of the phonological rules governing language and on the speech production side retrieval and organisation of a phonological output plan. The role of the articulatory system is to execute the plan as a neuromotor event; thus it relies upon the integrity of the neuromotor and neuromuscular systems and the structural integrity of the vocal and respiratory tracts. In adults both the phonological and the articulatory systems are fully developed and open to evaluation as separate entities but in the preschool era while both are actively developing, distinctions are less 'clear cut' and precise diagnosis is more difficult. The main clinical characteristics of some common disorders of speech production are outlined here.

---

1   During crying air is expired through closed vocal cords so the muscles of respiration and of the vocal cords contribute most to the production of sound. During crying the cords of normal neonates vibrate at 496 ± 95 c/s.

Phonological disorders
Developmental phonological disorders are suspected in children aged 4 or more years in whom intelligibility is very poor and phonological patterns/simplifications for consonants are atypical or idiosyncratic, while those of vowel sounds are usually typical. These findings would be in the context of age-appropriate levels of language and cognition and age-appropriate findings on a Stimulability Test.[2] Phonological disorders are sometimes associated with literacy difficulties.

Developmental verbal dyspraxia[3]
Children with developmental verbal dyspraxia (DVD) have difficulty in controlling movements of the vocal tract and respiration in speech production in the absence of signs of upper or lower motor neuron lesions or muscle disorder. Speech is unintelligible and errors inconsistent, containing only a limited number of distorted vowel and consonant sounds. Breakdown in sequencing occurs as sentence length increases and idiosyncratic substitutions, omissions and glottal stops are common. Voice, intonation, resonance and prosody are affected in varying degree. Frequently, there is a history of speech, language (with the emphasis on expressive) and/or literacy difficulties in the family, and of early feeding difficulties and/or delayed babbling in the child. DVD is often associated with developmental oral dyspraxia (difficulty in coordinating isolated or sequenced *silent* movements of the oral musculature) and/or a mild to moderate degree of generalized developmental dyspraxia of the systemic musculature with or without difficulties with reading, writing and spelling. DVD, as other forms of dyspraxia, responds only slowly to treatment and does not tend to improve without therapy. The Nuffield Dyspraxia Programme is widely used (http://www.ndp3.org). *Developmental verbal dyspraxia* is another useful document that can be found at http://www.dyspraxia-foundation.org.uk/downloads/Developmental_Verbal_Dyspraxia.pdf.

Dysarthria
Dysarthria is a neuromotor disorder of speech production, due to functional disturbance of the musculature involved in speech, as a result of damage to the central and/or peripheral nervous system. The most common causes in children are cerebral palsy and traumatic brain injury. Dysarthria therefore usually presents as part of a more widespread neuromotor, neurocognitive and neurobehavioural disorder; severity of all components is very variable. The nature, sites and severities of the neurological lesions determine whether the speech musculature is predominately weak, spastic, dyskinetic

---

2   A disorder in SSP is considered to be phonetic when a child cannot pronounce age appropriate consonants correctly in isolation i.e. *outside* the context of words. Speech therapists use a Stimulability Test to explore articulation; the child is asked to listen and then imitate each of the 24 consonant sounds in isolation. Inability to pronounce age appropriate consonants correctly is considered to be indicative of a phonetic (articulatory) problem, whereas correct production in isolation but not in some positions in words or connected speech implies that the difficulty is phonological.

3   In the UK also referred to as articulatory dyspraxia and in the US as developmental or childhood apraxia of speech.

or mixed, which in turn determines the characteristics of speech. Speech may be erratic in terms of loudness or speed and slurred with imprecise articulation. Poor co-ordination also creates difficulties with pitch, intonation, prosody and voice quality (e.g. harshness or hypernasality).

Worster-Drought Syndrome (WDS) – suprabulbar palsy
WDS is a neuromotor disorder characterized by profound oromotor (feeding and dribbling) and speech production difficulties. The condition is often associated with tetraplegia, varying degrees of cognitive and behavioural problems and seizures. Bilateral dysgenesis (polymicrogyria) or damage to the perisylvian cortex at around 14 weeks gestation is now thought to be responsible. This syndrome is flagged up because the oromotor and speech production difficulties in this form of cerebral palsy are not responsive to conventional therapies, the former difficulty requiring specialized management from the early months.

Practice Point WDS is not a sequel of term 'hypoxic ischaemic encephalopathy' or preterm 'periventricular leukomalacia' (see Neville and Clark 2011).

Other
Abnormalities of speech production are also common in syndromic and non-syndromic craniofacial malformations and neuromuscular diseases (motor unit).

When oromotor or SSP disorders are suspected, a neurological or neurodisability opinion as well as a speech therapy opinion is advisable.

Key Points

- Phonological and articulatory templates are being primed from birth.

- SSP is a complex and highly refined domain.

- SSP in preschool children results from current levels in both domains.

- Most useful question: 'What proportion of X's speech do you understand?'

- Enhance gestalt of typical SSP by taking every opportunity to listen to preschool children talking (in the knowledge of their ages).

- Assessment – listen – record in your own phonetic script – consider intelligibility, simplifications and articulation in samples for age.

- Interpret SSP findings in context of age, rest of developmental and physical picture as appropriate.

- Phonological disorders do *not* have a neuromotor basis.

- Articulatory disorders have a neuromotor, neuromuscular or structural basis.

References

Coplan J, Gleason JR (1988) Unclear speech: Recognition and significance of unintelligible speech in preschool children. *Pediatrics* 82: 447–452.

The Dyspraxia Foundation (http://www.dyspraxiafoundation.org.uk/downloads/Developmental_Verbal_Dyspraxia.pdf).

Goldman R, Fristoe M (2000). *The Goldman-Fristoe Test of Articulation*. Circle Pines, MN: American Guidance Service.

Koziol LF, Budding D, Andreasen N et al. (2014) Consensus paper: The cerebellum's role in movement and cognition. *Cerebellum* 13: 151–177.

Neville B, Clark M (2011) Oromotor dysfunction due to cerebral hemispheric lesions. In: *Oromotor Disorders in Childhood*. Eds Roig-Quilis M, Pennington L Viguera, 9: 137–146.

The Nuffield Dyspraxia Programme NDP3 (2011) (http://www.ndp3.org).

Sander E (1972) When are speech sounds learned? *J Speech Hear Disord* 37: 55–63.

Smit A, Hand L, Freilinger J, Bernthal J, Bird A (1990) The Iowa articulation norms project and its Nebraska replication. *J Speech Hear Disord* 55: 779–798.

Watkins KE (2011) Developmental disorders of speech and language: From genes to brain structure and function. *Prog Brain Res* 189: 225–238.

Williamson G (2010) English speech sounds: Phonemes, allophones, and variations in connected speech. [eBook] http://www.kalgoo.com.

Chapter 12

Gathering domain assessments into a comprehensive whole

Perhaps this is the moment to reiterate that the primary purpose of this book is to give the reader the developmental know-how and confidence to explore the developmental status of the baby or young child before them; to dispel their reliance on manuals, forms and boxes to tick and rather to focus upon and engage with the child in a structured and informed interaction that is assimilated and modulated as it progresses. To do so requires a sound developmental knowledge base and a penchant for 'thinking developmentally ' about the tests one employs and the informal behaviours one observes. Once achieved for typically developing children and those with mild impairments or developmental disorders, the challenge of exploring the developmental status of those with more serious or multiple impairments no longer feels like climbing Everest.

To date, the quantitative and qualitative aspects of typical development and its assessment have been discussed within individual domains. The reader has been encouraged to complement the latter with developmentally thoughtful observation of babies and preschool children in everyday work and leisure settings. Both aspects are equally important to interpretation. When information from individual domains is gathered together everything clicks into place in children who are developing normally. Conversely, there are gaps or reduced levels in the profiles of those children with problems; the pattern of the profile often provides clues to the nature of the problem and signposts the next steps in the diagnostic process – see 'thinking in profiles' – Chapter 1, p. 16.

The gathering process discussed here utilises test protocols (materials, procedure, end-point criteria, age references/guidelines) drawn from the domain chapters. However, its purpose is to illustrate how to think through the developmental content of tests familiar to, or practiced in, the reader's area and to organise/scaffold them into a comprehensive scheme suited to a child's age or developmental level. Once digested, the assessor is free to focus on observation, assimilation and control, and upon developing an informed flexibility within this structured framework to accommodate children with neurodevelopmental disorders and disabilities. The rationale behind the order of testing, choice of materials and starting levels was introduced in Chapter 2 and is elaborated here.

Domain order

The suggested order of testing for 5-month-olds and over is different from the chapter order, i.e. it is sensible to start with a domain that is relatively undemanding, like manipulation,[1] in order to enhance relaxation, foster rapport and give the assessor space to assimilate the level of attention control. If the order at every age is similar, domains will not be overlooked. The suggested order for children from 5 to 30 months and over 30 months differ in only one minor respect – the test of visual 'acuity'. In babies and 1-year-olds the test of acuity and eye movements fits well after non-symbolic cognition. Tests for strabismus are minimally intrusive and therefore in order not to lose rapport are best left until later; similarly, letter matching is demanding for 2-year-olds so acuity testing is also better postponed. The domain listed is the primary one targeted by the test; however, there will be bonuses in the two supporting domains of varying relevance, i.e. when presenting an activity picture saying 'what's happening in this picture?' the primary domain is intellectual (expressive language); the bonuses are information about sensory (hearing[2]) and motor (articulation). Incidentally, tests of expressive language also provide bonus information about an additional domain of central processing.

Q Which domain?
Phonological processing.

The domain most difficult to place in terms of order is social communication because the best indications of a child's level will be observed during natural episodes of engagement with the parent or assessor rather than during a contrived procedure at a set time. Social Communication is therefore placed after language and speech production to remind assessors to review their observations to date and actively explore as required.

---

1 Gross motor, at most ages, is too exciting!!

2 Merely that hearing is adequate for the level of voicing used by the questioner if the response is appropriate.

Materials

Most test materials mentioned in the domain chapters cover a wide age range and often provide information about several domains – *core* materials and others that are *domain* or *skill specific*. They all fit into a briefcase, which implies that careful consideration was given to their selection. The selection in my 'developmental bag' is listed in Figure 12.1. The message to assessors is to consider carefully the versatility of the core materials when choosing a scheme. An example of a very versatile *core* material is a set of 16 (2.2cm) bricks in four colours because they are used to explore several domains and a very wide age range – at 4 months to test visual behaviour, from 5 months to 4½ years to test manipulation and multiple aspects of non-symbolic cognition such as permanence, relationships and the motor constructive series – from building a two-brick tower to six-brick steps (14 to 54 months), between 12 and 27 months to test verbal comprehension and expressive language and in some schemes hearing. In contrast the Sonksen logMAR Test pack is relatively domain specific but covers a wide age range, i.e. testing visual acuity from 33 months onwards and non-symbolic cognition at a 33-month level.

- Tissues and sticky labels
- Box of 16 x 1″ cubes (4 blue, 4 red, 4 yellow, 4 green)
- Stick rattle with bells
- Soft squeaker
- 12.5cm yellow and black woolly pom-pom ball on string
- 6.25cm plastic ball on string
- Pot with 1.2cm brick inside and lid (tight fit)
- Form boards (3 and/or 6)[a]
- Pencil, coloured pencils and crayon (fat)
- A4 sheets with and without geometric designs for R & L handers
- Peg board, wooden, 25 holes and pot of small plastic pegs (variety of colours)
- Pen torch with 'ooglie'
- Pot of hundreds and thousands, saccharins and Smarties (M&Ms)

- Tape measure or length of string knotted at 3m
- Sonksen LogMAR Test
- 15-18″ doll
- Real life objects – teacup (china), spoon, brush, comb, sock, shoe
- Miniature toys[b] – table, 2 chairs (different colours), china tea set, 2 spoons (different sizes), 3 dolls (1 without clothes, 2 that sit easily/automatically), bath (with taps), dog, car, aeroplane etc
- Action pictures (1 plural, 1 active, 3 every-day scenes)
- Egan Bus Puzzle Test
- High frequency rattle
- Picture Test of hearing
- Recording form

[a]If Bus Puzzle not included; [b]or Bus Puzzle

Figure 12.1 Contents of developmental bag.

In this scheme of preliminary assessment, test materials are generally introduced in the order in which they target the main aim of the domain under scrutiny. As some test materials subserve more than one domain, test material 1 is used to test domain A and then domain B; test material 2 is then introduced for domain A For example with a 9-month-old a 12.5cm woolly ball is first used to test permanence of objects (non-symbolic cognition) – by rolling it off the table so that it drops out of sight and then to examine eye movements before moving on to the next material for non-symbolic cognition. In other words *each test material is fully used before moving on to the next*, which gives the assessment a more natural feel (i.e. play with something fully and then put it away). Consequently the assessment flows more smoothly than in psychological scales where test materials may be produced and put away several times; repeat productions tend to be greeted with an expression that says 'Oh no, not those bricks again'. None of these suggestions are absolute and exceptions are the prerogative of experienced assessors. At 9 months, 'an index finger approach', is an important aspect, in fact a main target of assessment of manipulative development; it is also an *essential* aspect, though not the critical level, of the near detection vision (NDV) test. The Smartie fits more comfortably within the visual section than amongst the preceding manipulative or cognitive sections; therefore it is best to wait until the visual domain to present a Smartie as the introduction of the NDV test. At this moment the primary focus of attention must be the visual endpoint – fixation, so complete the NDV test with a hundred and thousand before placing a Smartie first to the child's right and then to her left to observe her approach, grasp, manipulation and release with each hand. Similarly, if planning to use the Bus Puzzle to test language it is not necessary to use a three or six-hole form board during the non-symbolic cognition section, nor introduce the Bus Puzzle early but wait until the language domain and flag up recognition of shape and orientation under non-symbolic cognition and the motor aspects under manipulation.

Choice of starting level

In some series, differentiation between ages depends on the endpoint becoming progressively more complicated (e.g. 'train, bridge, house, three steps, four steps' of the construction series). In others the task remains the same and differentiation between ages depends upon the level of achievement such as defined stages in levels of skill (e.g. level of fine finger control in peg and pegboard task; level of movement in catching, throwing and kicking); indeed, the manner in which ages are differentiated in a series is sometimes a mixture of the two, for example the motor constructive series with bricks – the number of bricks achieved for the tower – differentiates ages under 33 months and specific constructions of increasing complexity over that age.

When age differentiation depends upon increasing complexity of the endpoint, choose the one *below* that which at least 50% of the child's age group achieve, i.e. age-appropriate −1 as this

- saves time and risk of boredom when tasks are well below age level,
- gives the assessor maximal flexibility to move up or down subtly

  - Children who fail several age-appropriate −1 tests are likely to be below average and after the first few age- appropriate −1 introductions the assessor may decide to introduce tests in other areas at a younger age level (to avoid the parent and child sensing failure).

  - Conversely, children whose performance of several age-appropriate −1 tests is brisk and competent are likely to be above average. Continue to introduce new series at an age-appropriate level and follow through to the child's 'ceiling'. If ceiling levels are not explored there is a risk that significant discrepancies between domains (specific developmental delays/disorders) may be missed in bright children.

When age differentiation depends upon the level of achievement on the same task (e.g. a logMAR test of acuity), the assessor explains the task at age-appropriate level: if the child appears not to understand the instructions, he takes time to explain using simpler language, gesture and mime.

Constructing schedules for different ages

In the domain chapters tests are listed in the tables in order in which they appear in typically developing children, so that age-appropriate ones can quickly be identified and assembled into a test schedule that *draws together and interlocks the domains into a profile* .

Construction for a schedule for a 33 month old is depicted in Table 12.1, 33 months.

The columns from left to right indicate the following:

1. Main domain and subdomains within it

2. Materials

3. Tasks or procedures

4. Levels in typically developing children

5. Supporting domains.

Main domain (column 1) and supporting domains (column 5): Test tasks all involve 3 categories of domain sensory, intellectual and motor. The target category is listed as the main domain in column 1; the two that most support it in column 5. Mostly, the developmental levels of the supporting domains are much lower than those of the main. However if a supporting domain contributes positively to assessment of its home domain it is enclosed in square brackets and referred to as a bonus. Bonuses are flagged up in this way in order to remind the assessor to transfer them to the record sheet of their home domain when assembling findings into a profile of the child. Most bonuses are in the cognitive or motor domains rather than the supporting senses, because the levels of vision required to adequately see the material/demonstration and of hearing to hear a conversationally voiced instruction are already adequate before or by 12 weeks of age. The importance of identifying and transferring bonuses is clarified by looking at the non-verbal cognition section of Table 12.1 33months. Vision and Manipulation are noted as the supporting domains for all 4 sub-domains tested; Manipulation is flagged up as a bonus for the two tasks that actively contribute to the assessment of its home domain in a 33 month-old child – the nature of the contribution is signposted within the square brackets.[3]

Materials (column 2): Test materials are indicated; note that each material is introduced only once.

Tasks/procedures (column 3): Age-appropriate or age-appropriate-1 tasks are listed.

Levels (column 4): The level expected of typically developing children is briefly described. The age when all but 10% have achieved the level or moved to a higher stage/level can be sourced in the respective domain chapters. The list of tasks and levels is not exhaustive.

The thinking behind the adaptation of Table 12.1 33 months for children of 48, 24, 9 months, 19 and 9 weeks is discussed and illustrated in Tables 12.2, 9 weeks, 12.3, 19 weeks, 12.4, 9 months, 12.5, 24 months and 12.6, 48 months at the end of the chapter. Before consulting the tables think through the relative amount of alteration needed to each column. Readers who use different test regimes may also find it useful to construct schedules for these ages after thinking through the developmental content of the component tests, allocating them to their target domain and highlighting bonuses in the supporting domains column. Considering whether or not a test is currently allocated to the most appropriate domain is also a valuable exercise.

---

3   With the possible exception of the smaller optotypes in the logMAR Test.

Table 12.1 Assessment schedule: 33 months

Main domain and sub-sections	Material	Task or procedure	Level in typically developing child	Supporting domains [bonus findings for home domain]
Manipulation				
	Pegs/pegboard	Manipulation of pegs	Stage 1	Vision [Non-symbolic cognition: Colour—identifies 1 or 2]
Non-Symbolic Cognition				
Recognition of shape	Six-piece form board[a]	Select correct recess	6 selected correctly	Vision, Manipulation
Construction	Bricks	Build a tower	Tower of 8 or >	Vision [Manipulation: Cubes Stage 2]
Concept of shape	Pencil and paper	Draw after demonstration	Draws vertical line, horizontal line ± circle	Vision [Manipulation: Pencil Stage 2]
		Naming shapes on request	Names circle	Vision, Articulation
Symbolic cognition				
Expressive Language	Miniature Toy Test	Engendered and spontaneous utterances	3 key words including verbs, plurals, size	Hearing, [Phonology, Articulation]
Non-spoken Symbolic Cognition	Miniature Toy Test	Spontaneous arrangement of toys	Tea set, cutlery, dolls on mini furniture; transport on nursery table; ± PSPP	Vision, Manipulation
Verbal Comprehension	Miniature Toy Test	'n' component commands	Three component big/little, under plurals	Hearing, Manipulation

Table 12.1 continued

Expressive Language	Action pictures[b]	Replies to 'What's happening'	Three key words verb/plurals/prep	Hearing, [Phonology, Articulation]
Speech production				
Phonology	During language testing and general conversation	Assessor listens to range of immature patterns	Reduplication no longer present	Hearing, Articulation
Articulation	During language testing and general conversation	Listen to a range of consonants	'p' 'm' 'h' 'n' 'w' 'b' ± 'k' 'g' 'd' 't' present in at least one position	Hearing, Expressive Language
Intelligibility		Listen to speech	Half	Hearing, Expressive Language
Social Communication				
	Toys and happenings	Throughout assessment observe communicative interaction in spontaneous and adult-initiated situations	Shares interest and jointly attends to events/toys through body language, facial expression, gesture and age-appropriate comments	Vision, Hearing, Eye/facial/generalised movements
Hearing				
	Picture test five cards or large doll	Minimal voicing from right and left sides	Pictures or body parts correctly heard	Manipulation [Verbal Comprehension: 24/12]

Table 12.1 continued

Vision				
Acuity	Sonksen LogMar test pack	Acuity measures	BEO >10th centile (0.325 or better)	Manipulation, [Non-symbolic cognition:- Six letters matched 28/12]
Eye movements	'Oogly', glove puppet	Observation of the range and quality of eye movements	Full-range, normal quality	Vision, Non-symbolic cognition
Gross motor				
	Demonstration	Walk on toes	Heels tend to sink	Vision, Comprehension of spoken instruction or demonstration
		Stand on 1 foot	Succeeds 1–2 sec	
		Hop	Jumps with 2ft	
		Stairs up	1/step holding rail	
		Stairs down	2/step holding rail	
	Soft 12.5cm ball	Catch	Stage 2	
		Throw	Stage 3	
		Kick	Stage 2 girls/boys	

aA form board is not necessary if planning to use the Bus Puzzle to assess language. Wait until the Symbolic section to introduce the Bus Puzzle.

bAction pictures needed only if samples of expressive language, articulation and phonology to date are insufficient.

± on border of being typical

PSPP prompted sequence pretend play

BEO both eyes open.

48 months (Table 12.6): The domain and the material columns would remain the same, except replacement of a 6-hole form board with a 10-hole board and an increase in the number of pictures for the Picture Test to seven. There will be some task upgrades needed in column 3 and a few reminders about potential bonuses or their significance in column 5. Most of the task changes in column 3 are in the non-symbolic cognition section, e.g. 'tower' changes to 'bridge and train', 'draw from demonstration' changes to 'draw from model' and 'shape' is added to remind the assessor to test the language aspects of concepts of shape. In the manipulation section of column 5, the assessor is reminded to test comprehension and usage of words for concepts of number as well as of colour; also note that the non-symbolic cognition component of the SonkLT, and the expressive language component of the Picture Test are not highlighted because they are no longer close to being age appropriate at 48 months. The only column that requires a total upgrade is column 4 – typical levels. *Make a list from memory of the upgraded levels for column 4 and then crosscheck with Table 12.6 48 months at the end of this chapter.*

24 months (Table 12.5): Consider changes in the same way before reading further. The acuity aspects of the vision domain would shift up to below non-symbolic cognition for the reasons given earlier. Materials will change to a three-hole form board, a crayon rather than a pencil and the near detection vision scale (NDV) rather than the SonkLT. In the NSC section, two pots with easily pulled off tops of different sizes and another with a screw cap are added. The task and the supporting domain columns will reflect these changes, and the levels column will completely change. *Make a list from the memory of the upgraded levels column 4 and then crosscheck with Table 12.4 24 months..*

9 months (Table 12.4): The domain order will be the same as that for the 24-month-old, though now there will be major changes to materials in most domains except vision, as well as in the level column. The sheer number of items in the non-symbolic cognition domain emphasizes how important it is to recognise the cognitive achievements that these skills reflect. In contrast the language domain has shrunk; although very active at neuronal level, symbolic and phonological aspects are not observable until the second year.

Babies under 5 months

Traditionally, developmental assessment of newborn babies and babies of 5 months or less is heavily dependent on neuromotor and paediatric examination, with the emphasis on exclusion of neurological abnormality and dysmorphology rather than *a celebration of development.* This is not to say that the former are not essential aspects of examination at this age; but more time should be given to observation of dawning cognition in response to sensory input and the emergence of concepts that drive the different aspects of motor development. The most integrated cognitive networks at and shortly after birth are social communication and cognitive interest in looking. Interestingly, the two motor systems that develop most rapidly in the first 3 months are facial expression and control of the eyes, including accommodation and convergence. In contrast, the prerequisite concepts that drive gross motor and manipulative development, such as the potential of arms for prehension, the floor as a base, etc are not evident until 3½ to 4½ months and progress in these areas during the early months consists of preparatory adjustments of tone and weight distribution in prone and supine rather than active control of posture or movement. So in the context of this book, the focus is developmental celebration and the reader is referred to paediatric neurology and general paediatric texts for the traditional aspects.

The visible progress in social communication and non-symbolic cognition is largely in response to the visual component of sensory input, so start by establishing the integrity of visual system in terms of 'acuity' and movement control using age-appropriate visual targets from the NDV scale. As the smallest size of NDV target fixated also has age-related non-symbolic cognition implications, there is considerable overlap between the two domains and it makes sense to assess them in parallel. Babies in this age bracket are not shy and love a communicative situation, so there is no reason not to explore social communication through observation of both baby–parent interaction and then baby–assessor interaction; doing so also creates an opportunity to observe any difference in the immediacy and quality of baby's response to parent's and assessor's faces. Babies should be awake, content and alert – though if asleep on arrival remember not to 'waste a sleeping baby!' in the context of assessment of hearing (see Chapter 4). The developmental aspects of manipulation and locomotion are then targeted, followed by the rest of the neuromotor and the paediatric examination. From 12 weeks the emergence of concepts underpinning manipulative, gross motor, social communication, sound location and substantiality of sound sources add 'the meat' to each baby's profile. The schedules in Tables 12.2 and 12.3 illustrate progress between 9 weeks and 19 weeks.

Recording

A very simple form is recommended comprising well-spaced domain sections listed in 'standard order', for age, with an additional section at the top headed 'Attention Control'. The level of attention control needs to be established as soon as possible because it structures the assessor's delivery. Obviously, there are spaces at the top of the page for name, date of birth, age, etc. With preschool children, withdrawing from the interchange either to make notes after each test item or to read the instructions for the next item, courts disaster in the shape of loss of rapport, flow and control. Often the latter have been hard won; to put them at risk is neither sensible nor time efficient. Once an assessor has procedure and control increasingly on automatic, he can give more and more of his attention to analysing and storing the child's responses (short term) so that breaks to record become less frequent. Bonuses are recorded in their home domain. Brief qualitative comments, such as '++ trial and error' or '? clumsy' in addition to a tick or a cross beside each test item, are helpful in visualising the totality of the child's performance when writing the report. Samples of expressive language written in the assessor's personal phonetic code similarly heighten recall of expressive language, phonology and articulation, all in one. For example 'went kool in Daddy's buu tar' is more helpful than just ticking five keyword phrases and obviates the need to analyse phonology and articulation until later. There are too many aspects to social communicative behaviours to note them all down during an assessment; writing down what the child said is enough to conjure up all aspects of the event. For example, if you write 'What dat dere?' you immediately see Simon's eager face looking up with questioning expression and intonation as he points to an apple in a picture of two children making a cake. Three words bring to life the tick beside 'Initiates social communication' and 'shares interest in object' when writing the report.

Interpretation

Construct an intellectual profile and consider it in the context of findings in the sensory and motor domains. View these in the context of the developmental and medical history to date. Explore further through questions and paediatric/neurological examination if indicated. Construct a plan of action and discuss with parents – see Chapters 1 and 2.

Reporting

Most units have an agreed reporting format that includes an introduction, paediatric background, developmental background, developmental assessment findings, paediatric findings, summary/conclusions and finally medical followed by developmental recommendations. Obviously, format and content differ in complexity depending on whether the preliminary examination is at primary, secondary or tertiary level. The following comments reflect a personal viewpoint, born of personal experience and are in no way intended to be prescriptive, rather to engender discussion in the setting of the reader's practice.

Introduction

The introduction summarises the reason(s) for examination including the referrer's questions and the concerns of referrer and/or parents, plus details of the local professionals when a local team is already involved.

Paediatric background

The paediatric background will be increasingly long and complicated the more multi-ply impaired the child. To reiterate it at length is not time efficient and is not helpful to the referrer[4] or the parents, though a concise summary of developmentally relevant points will be.

Developmental background

Whatever the level of the assessment and complexity of the child, it is preferable to present the developmental background and the developmental assessment under separate headings; in each section the findings are reported under domain subheadings in the order indicated in Tables 12.1, 33 months, 12.2, 9 weeks, 12.3 19 weeks; 12.4 9 months, 12.5 24 months and 12.6 48 months.

Developmental assessment

Readers of developmental reports are much more likely to accept an assessor's opinion and recommendations when given sufficient information to see that these are soundly derived. Parents have a head start in this regard as usually they have been present throughout the assessment. Most professional recipients will not have had that privilege. Therefore, description brings the assessment of each domain to life and provides the relevant information rather than listing successes and failures. Reading the reports of others with a critical eye is a good learning exercise as it highlights faults in one's own technique; however, perhaps more importantly it draws the reader's attention to common and widespread inadequacies that reduce the validity of the report.

Often measurements and findings are given without providing the name of the test used and/or other information relevant to interpretation. Paediatric Ophthalmology Clinics are frequently guilty of this one, recording visual acuity as 6/12 without naming the test or indicating whether the optotypes were presented singly or in linear array or whether the measure was monocular (R or L) or binocular, or whether the child was wearing glasses or contact lenses. Without these details the result is meaningless and potentially misleading. Similarly, descriptions of progress are frequently so vague as to be positively unhelpful. 'Jenny has made progress with her language since I last saw her'. The reader thinks 'When did you last see her?' 'What was her level then and what is it now?!' 'Six months ago Jenny was understanding two-component commands and currently is managing three-component commands; this represents steady progress' would be more informative.

---

4   Indeed it may irritate the referrer to plough through all that he already knows and risk him jumping straight to the summary – an opportunity for the writer to spread interest in developmental medicine lost!

Last but not least, the tone of the language used in many reports can have a negative psychological impact. The effect of qualifying every developmental attribute with words like *can't* or *is unable* or doesn't can have a negative impact on parents. Use of the more positive *can* or *is able* or *does* is little better, as both constantly remind parents of the negative counterpart and create a growing impression that the assessor was trying to find things wrong with their child, rather than confirming and enjoying his normality or helping them to plan how to help him reach his potential. *A parent would much rather read 'Johnny crawls upstairs'* than *'Johnny is able to crawl up stairs.' 'Johnny is unable to walk upstairs even with both hands held'* (the *even* rubs it in further). Using a simple present or past tense has the least judgemental impact, and at the end of the assessment section, leaves the reader with a clear-cut picture of what Johnny *is* doing rather than a confusing hotchpotch of positive and negative attributes.

Paediatric findings

It is helpful to detail findings of the paediatric examination that shed new light on diagnosis or are relevant to medical management.

Summary and conclusions

Reiteration of the assessment findings in the summary/conclusions is common practice, but to my mind is neither needed nor helpful. If everything has been normal simply say so ('Michael' below). If suspicious of a developmental disorder at the end of a preliminary assessment ('Jeremy' below) set the domain profile in the context of the paediatric, social and developmental background and any new paediatric findings of diagnostic import, emphasizing aspects that are naturally transformed into medical and developmental/educational recommendations. After a more in-depth assessment of a multiply disabled child ('Mary' below), referred for advice on communication strategies, it is even more important not to reiterate the assessment findings, but to summarise the nature and degree of severity of the sensory, cognitive and physical impairments. Subsequently, to discuss the developmental profile, commenting on how the various deficiencies impact on function. Care is needed to ensure that these comments will underpin the developmental recommendations.

Michael
'Michael is a delightful 2½-year-old who is developing well in every way.'

Jeremy
'Jeremy's intellectual profile is uneven with understanding of speech and expressive language significantly below non-verbal, imaginative play and social communicative skills. Hearing responses to the distraction test (used as verbal comprehension inadequate)

are prompt to – high, medium and low frequencies at minimal levels and his vision and manipulative skills are age appropriate. Attention control at level 2b is responsible for some of his parent's behavioural concerns. Gross motor development and strength are within the normal range though visuomotor skills (catching throwing and kicking) are slightly below age level. These findings suggest that Jeremy may have specific developmental language delay.

Mary
Mary is a charming 5-year-old with multiple impairments following a series of complications associated with extreme preterm birth. As a consequence she has severe physical disability with moderate learning disability and severe visual impairment (of mainly cortical origin). Poor acuity, very variable visual attention and difficulties sustaining gaze combine to make use of visual materials for learning and communication problematic. Mary's manipulative problems and eye movement disorder further constrain her ability to communicate through hand or eye pointing. Happily Mary's hearing is acute and although dysarthria impairs the intelligibility of her speech she spontaneously chooses to communicate using single or two keyword utterances, etc.

Recommendations

It is useful to divide recommendations into two sections: medical and developmental/educational. Medical recommendations may be of diagnostic, investigative or therapeutic portent, and care should be taken to support and not to undermine the local team.

Michael
Michael does not require any medical recommendations.

Jeremy
With the profile outlined earlier and the assessor confident that Jeremy's hearing responses are satisfactory and that Jeremy has not been subject to repeated attacks of OME, the priority referral is to the Community Developmental Team (CDT). The composition of the team will vary by area but will probably include a Community Paediatrician and Speech Therapist and a Psychologist, who work closely with the Community Paediatric Audiology Service.

Mary
A referral to ophthalmology is pertinent, as Mary has not seen an ophthalmologist since the age of 18 months to review her gaze problem and strabismus and to check whether she has developed a significant refractive error that could be corrected. Liaise with local speech therapist regarding communication strategies.

Table 12.2 Assessment schedule: 9 weeks

Main domain and sub-sections	Material	Task or procedure	Level in typically developing child	Supporting domains [bonus findings for home domain]
Vision				
Acuity	Face and 12.5cm ball	Fixation	Fixates face and 12.5cm ball	[Non-symbolic cognition: Interest in Looking] Eye movement
Eye movements	Face	Following, convergence	Briefly follows and some convergence	
Non-Symbolic Cognition				
	Face	Faces are communicative	Facial expression, responsive smile	Vision, Facial movements
Pre-Symbolic				
Vocalisations	Assessor/parent	Cradle, smile and coo/talk to baby	Coos, gurgles or moist sounds	Hearing, Articulation
		If crying	Quality of cry	
Social Communication				
	Assessor/parent	Cradle, smilingly talk to baby and/or observe the parent doing so	Returns gaze, listening expression; ± coos and moist sounds; ± finger and mouth movements	Vision, Hearing, Eye/facial movements
		Cradle, smilingly engage baby	Smiles, intense sparkling eye contact	Vision, Hearing, Eye/facial movements

Table 12.2 continued

Hearing			Gross motor
Noisy rattle/bell	Sudden, loud 3 to 6 sec from right and left sides	Startle or reflex eye and head turning or stilling	
Gross motor including upper limb			
Assessor	Observation of tone, symmetry, weight distribution, posture and movement in: Prone	See Tables 9.1, 9.2 and 9.8	
	Supine		
	Pull to sit		
	Supported stand		
	Ventral suspension		
	Primitive reflexes		
	Neurological and Paediatric examination		

± on border of being typical.

Table 12.3 Assessment schedule: 19 weeks

Main domain and sub-sections	Material	Task or procedure	Level in typically developing child	Supporting domains [bonus findings for home domain]
Manipulation				
Grasp	Jingle bell rattle	Stroke under surface of fingers with rattle	Grasps rattle but doesn't visually inspect it	
Release			Passive drop	
Vision				
Acuity	6.25cm stationary ball	Fixation on ball at 30cm	Fixates ball	[Non-symbolic cognition: interest in looking] Eye movements
Eye movements + other AA visual behaviours see Chapter 3	12.5cm spinning ball	Following, convergence	Follows ⇔ and ⇑⇓ Converges symmetrically	Vision, [Non-symbolic cognition: Interest in looking]
Non-Symbolic Cognition				
Understands potential to reach	Supine baby Dangling toy 12.5cm or >	Active swipe at toy	Visually directed swipe	Vision, [Manipulation; Reach]
Substantiality of sound/ permanence of people	Parent	Parent calls in greeting when out of sight	Alerts, excited movements and visual search	Vision, Gross motor: eye movement and visual search
Pre-Symbolic				
Vocalisations	Assessor/parent	Listen to spontaneous or engendered vocalisations	Spontaneous tuneful cadences of vowel sounds	Hearing, Articulation

Table 12..3 continued

	Assessor/parent			
Receptive		Adult vocalises back to baby	Pauses in own vocalisations to listen to adults	Hearing, [Non-symbolic cognition: Voices are communicative]
Social Communication				
Communicative interaction	Assessor	Observe for the baby's attempts to attract adult attention	Baby vocalises and tries to catch adult's eye, ± excited movements	Vision, Hearing, Eye/facial/generalised movements
Hearing				
	Bell rattle, baby well supported in sitting	Moderate intensity, duration 3 sec from right and left sides at ear level	Slow turn to correct side	[Non-symbolic cognition: Substantiality of sound-making objects and location relative to self] Gross motor
	Distraction test Items	Minimal intensity, from right and left sides at ear level	Stills or slowly turns to correct side	[Non-symbolic cognition: Substantiality of sound-making objects and location relative to self] Gross motor
Gross motor including upper limb				
	Assessor	Observation of tone, symmetry, weight distribution, posture and movement in: Prone / Supine / Pull to sit / Supported stand	See Tables 9.1, 9.2 and 9.8	Vision [Non-symbolic cognition: Early stages of concept of floor as a base]

Table 12.3 continued

	Ventral suspension	Primitive reflexes	Neurological and Paediatric examination

AA   age appropriate
±   on border of being typical
⇔   to either side
⇑⇓   up and down.

Table 12.4 Assessment schedule: 9 months

Main domain and sub-sections	Material	Task or procedure	Level in typically developing child	Supporting domains [bonus findings for home domain]
Manipulation				
Reach	Bricks	Manipulation of bricks	Smooth, direct	Vision, Non-symbolic cognition
Grasp			Scissors or IP	
Transfer			Some act relax	
Placement & release			No act relax	
Non-Symbolic Cognition				
Cause and Effect	Rattle	To produce effect	Shakes	Vision, Manipulation
	Bricks		Bangs on table	
Permanence	Bricks	Number held	2	
	Woolly ball	Roll out of sight	Actively searches	
		Rotate around head	Anticipates side of reappearance.	
	Car and cloth	Find under cloth	±Finds car	
Relationships	Car and cup	To separate	Shakes as one	
Problem solving	Ball on string	How to retrieve	Retrieves by string	
Vision				
Acuity	Near Detection Vision Scale	Fixation	100/1000 1.2mm	[Manipulation: Smartie IP, Non-symbolic cognition: interest in looking HT] Eye movements

Table 12.4 continued

Eye movements	'Oogly', glove puppet	Range and quality of spontaneous, following etc	Full range normal quality	Vision, Non-symbolic cognition
Pre-Symbolic				
Vocalisations	Assessor/Parent	Engender and listen to spontaneous vocalisations	Repetitive double syllable babble	Hearing [Articulation]
Verbal Comprehension	Assessor/Parent	Recognition of name	Recognizes and responds to name. Alerts to FPhP non-specifically	Hearing, Gross motor
Speech Production				
Articulation	Assessor/Parent	Listen to the range of consonant and vowel sounds	2 or more of each	Hearing, Vocalisations
Social Communication				
Communicative interaction	Assessor/Parent	Engender and observe social communication episodes	Visually engages adult and/or vocalises for attention, two-way dialogue peek-a-boo, laughs, ±imp pointing	Vision, Hearing, Eye/facial/generalised movements
			Looks at and is responsive to communicator's facial expression/simple gestures	Vision, Hearing, Eye/facial/generalised movements

Table 12.4 continued

Hearing	High frequency rattle, Voice, Warble tones , Jingle bell rattle	Distraction Test Minimal levels from right and left sides at ear level	Turns and looks	[Non-symbolic cognition: sound localisation 2-stage]
			Locates (2-stage)	Gross motor
Gross motor	Assessor/ parent Motivating toys	Facilitate in: Prone	Up on hands and knees, early crawl ⇔sitting, ±pulls to stand	Vision, Non-symbolic cognition
		Supine	Roll⇔	
		Sitting	Straight back	
		Standing	With support,	
		Saving	Present, right, left, forward in sitting, FP	
		Postural	Emerging in sitting	

IP inferior pincer
±   on border of being typical
FPhP familiar phrase pattern
⇔   to and from
HT hundred and thousand.

307

Table **12.5** Assessment schedule: 24 months

Main domain and sub-sections	Material	Task or procedure	Level in typically developing child	Supporting domains [bonus findings for home domain]
Manipulation				
	Pegs/pegboards	Manipulation of pegs	Stage 1	Vision, Non-symbolic cognition
Non-Symbolic Cognition				
Recognition of shape	Three-piece form board[a]	Select correct recess	3 selected correctly	Vision, Manipulation
Construction	Bricks	Build a tower	Tower of 5–7	Vision, [Manipulation: Stage 1 or 2]
Concept of shape	Crayon and paper	Draw after demonstration	Circular scribble ± vertical and horizontal line	Vision, [Manipulation: Stage 2]
Concept of size	Pots/lids two sizes	Put lids on pots	Lids on correctly	Vision, Manipulation
Concept of screwing	Pot + screw cap	Takes off lid	Unscrews	Vision, [Manipulation: planning]
Vision				
Acuity	Near Detection Vision Scale	Fixation	100/1000	Non-symbolic cognition, Eye movements
Eye movements	'Oogly', glove puppet	Range and quality of spontaneous, following etc	Full range, normal quality	Vision, Non-symbolic cognition

Table 12.5 continued

Symbolic cognition				
Expressive Language	Miniature Toy Test	Engendered and spontaneous utterances	One and two-word phrases, present participle	Hearing, [Phonology, Articulation]
Non-spoken Symbolic Cognition	Miniature Toys	Spontaneous arrangement of toys	Tea set, cutlery, dolls on nursery table; transport separated, SRP	Vision, Manipulation
Verbal Comprehension	Miniature Toy Test	'n' component commands	Two component	Hearing, Manipulation
Expressive Language	Action pictures[b]	Spoken answers	Two key words enumeration	Hearing, [Phonology, Articulation]
Speech production				
Phonology	Miniature toys or conversation, spontaneous utterances	Listen	Any combinations of the patterns in Table 11.1 may be present	Hearing, Articulation
Articulation	Miniature toys or conversation, spontaneous utterances	Listen to the range of consonants	'p' 'm' 'h' 'n' 'w' 'b' Present in at least one position	Hearing, Expressive Language
Intelligibility		Listen to utterances	A quarter to a half	Hearing, Expressive Language

Table 12.5 continued

Section	Equipment	Task	Observation	Notes
Social Communication	Toys and happenings	Throughout assessment observe communicative interaction in spontaneous and adult-initiated situations	Shares interest and jointly attends to events/toys through body language, facial expression, gesture and age appropriate comments	Vision, Hearing, Eye/facial/generalised movements
Hearing	Large doll or Picture Test five cards	Minimal voicing from right and left sides	All identified correctly	Manipulation, [Verbal comprehension: 24/12]
Gross motor	Demonstration	Walk on toes	Momentary	Hearing, Vision, Comprehension of spoken instruction or demonstration
		Stand on 1 foot	Tries but unable	
		Hop	Unable	
		Stairs up	2/step holding rail	
		Stairs down	2/step hands held	
	Soft 12.5cm ball	Catch	Stage 1	
		Throw	Stage 1 or 2	
		Kick	Stage 1 or 2	

aA form board is not necessary if planning to use the Bus Puzzle to assess language. Wait until the Symbolic section to introduce the Bus Puzzle.

bAction pictures only needed if samples of expressive language, articulation and phonology to date are insufficient.

SRP   self-related play
VC   verbal comprehension.

Table 12.6 Assessment schedule: 48 months

Main domain and sub-sections	Material	Task or procedure	Level in typically developing child	Supporting domains [bonus findings for home domain]
Manipulation				
	Pegs/pegboard	Manipulation of pegs	Stage 2 or 3	Vision, [Non-symbolic cognition: Colour – names 6 or >, Number – counts 8 to10]
Non-Symbolic Cognition				
Recognition of shape	10 piece form board	Select correct recess	10 selected correctly	Vision, Manipulation
Construction	Bricks	Bridge and Train	Bridge and Train	Vision, [Manipulation: Cubes Stage 3]
Concept of shape	Pencil and paper	Draw from model	Draws circle, cross, ±square	Vision, [Manipulation: Pencil Stage 3]
		Naming shapes on request	Names circle, cross, square; may name triangle	Hearing, Vision, [Expressive Language, Articulation]
Symbolic cognition				
Expressive Language	Miniature Toy Test	Engendered and spontaneous utterances	Four key words, past and future tense, pronouns, concepts	Hearing, [Phonology, Articulation]
Non-spoken Symbolic Cognition	Miniature Toy Test	Spontaneous arrangement and play with toys	Arrangement precise, PSPP ±USPP	Vision, Manipulation
Verbal Comprehension	Miniature Toy Test	'N' component commands	Four components, colour, shape, etc	Hearing, Manipulation

Table 12.6 continued

Expressive Language	Action pictures[a]	Replies to "What's happening?"	Four key words, past tense, pronouns, concepts, questions	Hearing, [Phonology, Articulation]
Speech production				
Phonology	During language testing and general conversation	Assessor listens to the range of immature patterns	Redup, initial and final consonant deletion or harmony, devoicing, most stopping & fricative reduction no longer present	Hearing, Articulation
Articulation	During language testing and general conversation	Listen to the range of consonants	All except 'th' 'th' 'zh' and complex blends present in at least one position	Hearing, Expressive Language
Intelligibility		Listen to speech	Almost complete	Hearing, Expressive Language
Social Communication	Toys and happenings	Throughout assessment observe communicative interaction in spontaneous and adult-initiated situations	Shares interest and jointly attends to events/toys[b] through body language, facial expression, gesture and age appropriate comments	Vision, Hearing, Eye/facial/generalised movements
Hearing	Picture test (7) or large doll	Minimal voicing from right and left sides	Picture test or body parts all heard correctly	Manipulation, Verbal comprehension

Table 12.6 continued

Vision				
Acuity	Sonksen logMAR Test pack	Acuity measures	BEO/EES >10th (0.125/0.200 or better)	Manipulation, Non-symbolic cognition
Eye movements	'Oogly', glove puppet	Observation of the range and quality of eye movements	Full-range normal quality	Vision, Non-symbolic cognition
Gross motor				
	Demonstration	Walk on toes	Runs on toes	Vision, Comprehension of spoken instruction or demonstration
		Stand on 1 foot	3 to 6 sec	
		Hop	1 to 6 hops (ots)	
		Stairs up	1/step no hands	
		Stairs down	1/step holding on	
	Soft 12.5cm ball	Catch	Stage 3	
		Throw	Stage 3	
		Kick	Stage 2 (girls) 3 (boys)	

aAction pictures only needed if samples of expressive language, articulation and phonology to date are insufficient.
bWith peers as well as adults.

±, on border of being typical; PSPP, prompted sequence pretend play; USPP, unprompted sequence pretend play; Redup, reduplication; Stop, stopping BEO both eyes open; EES, each eye separately; ots, on the spot.

Chapter 14 is devoted to developmental guidance so guidance for Jeremy and Mary is not covered in detail here.

Jeremy

When, as in Jeremy's case, a developmental disorder is suspected, developmental guidance is an important interim measure as it will help his parents to realise that there are positive things that they and professionals can do to improve his language. A valuable account of the principles underlying the generation of guidance for children with developmental language delays and disorders is given in Cooper et al. (1978).

Q Which areas are going to be the primary focus of your interim guidance for Jeremy?

Attention Control, Verbal Comprehension and Expressive Language. Attention control is paramount – Jeremy will only benefit significantly from the language aspects of his intervention programme once he moves from Attention Control Level 2b to Level 3.

Mary

Mary was referred to a specialised team for advice on communication systems. The summary makes it clear that Mary has better and more attentiveness and more consistent access to auditory than visual information; also that control of motor output is more functional for speech than for eye or finger pointing. Thus, for learning and communication auditory input, processing and speech should take priority. The specialised team would liaise with their local counterparts and offer to review their recommendations if Mary's acuity is, for example, significantly improved by glasses.

The benefit of this style of preliminary assessment is that it gives the knowledgeable assessor freedom to be flexible, to make use of events outside the test protocol and is economical of time and space and adaptable to children with developmental disorders and neurodisabilities.

Key Points

- Carefully consider domain order and materials.

- Plan to use materials only once.

- Know the content, procedure and age-appropriate levels of the tests you use.

- Go in at age-appropriate or age-appropriate –1 level.

- Go up to ceiling (to avoid missing discrepancies in bright children).

- Channel bonuses to their correct domain.

- Appearing to see test material and to hear instructions does not obviate the need to definitively test both senses.

- Be alert to discrepancy in attention given to different sensory inputs.

  - Suspect the integrity of the sense less well attended to.

  - Significant discrepancy has implications for guidance.

- Celebrate concepts in the first 5 months!

- Recording: develop personal 'shorthand'.

- Reporting: consider the reader.

Reference

Cooper J, Moodley M, Reynell J (1978) *Helping Language Development: A Developmental Programme for Children with Early Language Handicaps*. London: Edward Arnold Ltd.

Chapter 13

Preliminary assessment of children with developmental delays and disorders and with severe single or multiple impairments

In this chapter the focus shifts to the preliminary comprehensive assessment of children with developmental delays and disorders or with single or multiple impairments. Hopefully, the reader will become convinced that the preceding chapters with their emphasis on neurodevelopmental process, typical progress and the developmental content of tests were essential stepping stones to looking with confidence into the development of babies with severe or multiple impairment and preschool children.

Many of the tests described in the preceding chapters will, with thoughtful selection and/or minor alteration, be appropriate for a preliminary examination of children with developmental delays and disorders and with single impairments of mild to moderate degree. As the severity and number of impairments increases, so does the pressure on the assessor's developmental 'know-how', to select and modify interaction while preserving the integrity of the target measurement. Assessor skill in preliminary assessment of children with severe and multiple disabilities will be better founded if training and experience is gained first with children with a wide range of mild to moderate problems.

Children with developmental delays and disorders or single impairments of mild to moderate degree

Children with even mild impairments or developmental disorders need to put more effort than typically developing children into completing test procedures; this is greatest when the impaired domain is the target of the test, e.g. a test of manipulation in a motor impaired child. They are most likely to persevere if they see encouragement and interest in the assessor's eyes. Thus the assessor needs to work harder to ensure the child's interest is sustained and the flow of the test procedure uninterrupted, i.e. without pauses to make notes, or find the next test item.

As soon as impairment/s are suspected the assessor needs to consider adjustments to the schedule plan and adaptations to individual tests. From the outset a wise assessor assimilates findings and modifies the rest of the schedule in the light of them. For example, as soon as cognitive impairment is suspected the assessor adjusts both the cognitive content/level of further tests and the profile of the child that is formulating in her head and flags up pertinent aspects requiring further questioning, and/or paediatric and developmental examination. The following case vignette illustrates these points.

Colin

Colin, age 4 years 3 months comes for a routine check. Findings so far are Level 2 attention control, Stage 2 manipulation of pegs, names one colour, doesn't count, doesn't build a bridge or a train, doesn't draw a circle from the model, replaces six pieces in the 10-hole board, arranges cutlery and crockery on the miniature table, gives the assessor three of four requested items, puts only the dog under the table, when asked to 'put the dog and cat under the table'. Colin's spontaneous utterances include 'dolly dinkin tea', 'in de bot', 'daddy gone werr' and 'op owes de easel'

Q What are you thinking?
   *Colin presents with skills between 30 and 36 months. He may be **globally developmentally delayed**.*

Q At what point would you have expected the assessor to introduce a modification?
   Certainly after he failed to construct the bridge or train (four age appropriate, NSC failures in a row + a red alert with attention control level 2 at 4 years).

Q What would you have done at that point?
   Drop back to building a tower. When he achieved 7, re-introduce drawing by demonstrating a vertical and horizontal line and when his maximum achievement was an imperfect circle, launch into testing verbal comprehension with a two- rather than a four-component command.

Q What developmental stage of expressive language does 'pop goes the weasel' represent?
Situational phrase rather than four-component phrase

Q Are phonology and articulation acceptable?
Yes, for his cognitive and language ages.

Q What materials would you pick up to test vision?
The Sonksen logMAR Test, because it is suitable for children NSC level of 2½ years and over.

Q Would you plan to modify the vision test? If so in what way(s)?
Introduce the test and training procedure as detailed in the SonkLT manual for 2½-year-olds rather than for 4-year-olds – see Chapter 3, p. 57

Q What materials would you pick up to test hearing?
The Picture Test because it is suitable for children with verbal comprehension of 24 months and over.

Q Would you plan to modify the hearing test? If so in what way(s)?
Use five pictures rather than seven (seven is too intellectually demanding at 2½ years old); explain the procedure as you would to a child under 27 months rather than to a 4-year-old – see Chapter 4 p. 106.

Q Would you modify the gross motor examination in any way?
Use more demonstration to ensure understanding of what is required and start at the baseline of each sequence.

Q Levels in which domain, not yet mentioned, would you include when constructing Colin's developmental profile for planning action?
Social communication.

Q With the profile to date what aspects of history would you flag up to ask about?
Family history of learning and developmental delays; antenatal, perinatal and postnatal history.

Q With the profile to date what aspects of paediatric examination would you flag up to prioritise?

Dysmorphology, cutaneous stigmata, head circumference, signs suggestive of fragile X syndrome, etc.

Q If Colin's cognitive level had been below 24 months how would you plan to test (a) his vision (b) his hearing?
(a) Use the Near Detection Scale (NDV) (b) If language adequate the Doll and Body Parts Test, otherwise the Distraction Test.

Assimilation of Colin's emerging profile ensured that relevant aspects of the history and paediatric and developmental examination were not missed. The assessor chose to stay with the Sonksen logMAR test (SonkLT) because modifications are aimed at ensuring understanding of the response task and do not degrade the measure.

Q Would it have been equally acceptable if the assessor decided to use single optotypes or the Sheridan Gardner Test?
No, because both tests compromise the optometric content and hence the acuity measure.

Likewise, the modification to the Picture Test of hearing is a cognitive adaption and does not affect the sound levels or the phonetic discriminations.

Test construct and the nature and degree of a child's impairment(s) are taken into account when planning adaptations of individual tests. As emphasized in Chapter 1, the construct of every test embodies three categories of domain: sensory, intellectual and motor. The main target of the test lies in one of those categories and is **not open** to modification, whereas the two supporting categories **are open** to modification. The first question the assessor should ask himself when a child fails a test is *'Why did he fail?'* i.e. which domain is responsible for the failure? If it isn't the target domain he can consider adapting either or both the supporting ones, and/or the medium or level of giving instructions. Finally, the assessor checks that none of these will corrupt findings in the target domain. Modifications for the three brick bridge, the distraction test and the peg board test for children with different impairments are used to illustrate this process.

Three-brick bridge test (Vivian and Monty)

The target domain in the three-brick bridge test is NSC (intellectual category) so the child must demonstrate this three-dimensional concept. The two supporting domains are sensory and motor – primarily vision (sufficient vision to see the model) and manipulation (sufficient motor control to grasp, place and release the bricks). Vivian has moderate visual impairment; acceptable modifications for her might be the use of larger bricks in three colours that contrast strongly with each other. Monty has mild–moderate motor impairment (developmental coordination disorder); acceptable modifications for him might be to use slightly larger bricks that are easier to grasp and release. Vivian places the first two bricks a suitable distance apart and then the third on top of the left hand brick. Monty positioned the third brick across the gap; he over-pushed and exerted asymmetrical pressure during release scattering all three bricks.

Q Would you credit either or both children with the concept and why?
Vivian's positioning of the third brick was not across the gap, so she should not be credited with this concept. Monty's positioning of the third brick was correct so he should be credited with the concept; his failure was clearly because of motor disorder not cognitive status.

Q If the assessor wanted to check Monty's performance do you think it would be acceptable for her to steady the two base bricks once he had placed them?
Yes, because she would have been facilitating the manipulative rather than the cognitive aspect of the task.

Distraction test (Monica)

The target domain in the distraction test is *hearing* (sensory category) so the sound sources (nature, quality, loudness) are sacrosanct. The two supporting categories are intellectual and motor – NSC (substantiality of sound sources and their position relative to self), and sufficient neuromotor control to turn head and eyes in supported sitting. In this example the NSC element is requisite; so if a baby or toddler is cognitively below this level, the assessor would have to consider using a hearing test procedure for babies under 4-month-old. However, Monica is 10 months and 'floppy' (hypotonic cerebral palsy) so the assessor needs to reduce the attention she is giving to postural control by laying her supine on a narrow table and making the test sounds to either side just below the table edge, i.e. outside Monica's field of vision.

Peg and pegboard test (Veronica)

The target domain in the peg and pegboard test is *manipulation* (motor category) – grasp, intradigital manipulation, placement and release of small objects, so the size of both pegs and recesses are not open to modification. The supporting domains are sensory and intellectual – visual acuity for pegs and recesses and NSC for two-component relationships respectively. For Veronica aged 25 months with moderate visual impairment, the assessor could heighten colour contrasts between pegs, board and holes without jeopardising the evaluation of manipulation. Understanding of the two-component relationship is requisite and, as it should be in a test of motor function, emerges at a younger age than the motor skill. The assessor would need to choose a test with lower cognitive requirement if Veronica did not have the concept.

The above-mentioned examples are starkly stated to stress that before adapting any test the assessor should have the target and two domains that most support it clear in his mind. In real life the situation is not so 'cut and dried', with other domains contributing to instructions, delivery, rapport and creation of a natural and encouraging atmosphere. In some ways an assessor conducting a preliminary assessment has privileges denied to one administrating a fully standardised psychological scale, for example, the licence to adapt materials or give a degree of physical support in order to demonstrate presence or absence of an intellectual concept. The following cases provide further examples of adaptations for children with different disorders.

Hilary, Henrietta and Langley

Hilary, Henrietta and Langley are all 3 years 3 months old. Hilary has a mild to moderate degree of hearing impairment (MHI), Henrietta is severely/profoundly deaf (PHI) and Langley has significant developmental language delay (DLD). Hilary and Henrietta cannot hear the assessor's instructions, whereas Langley doesn't understand them. The assessor might raise his voice[1] when giving instructions or testing Hilary's language. Raising his voice when communicating with either Henrietta or Langley is likely to be counterproductive; it might be better for the assessor to simplify his speech and complement it with gesture, mime and facial expression when giving instructions for non-language tests to Langley.

Q How else might the assessor convey instructions to Henrietta for non-verbal tests?
Through gesture, facial expression and/or signing if Henrietta is a British Sign System (BSS) or Makaton user.

Q and for visual acuity testing?
The letter matching instructions can be conveyed through demonstration using the parent, through mime or through sign language.

Q If Hilary or Langley hesitates to place the fourth brick of a four-brick train, should the assessor point to or tap the top of the front brick of the three already lined up?
No, because that degrades the main objective of the test – NSC motor constructive.

Q How could the assessor approach the question of Henrietta's language levels?

---

1   It goes against the grain to raise one's voice to children but if a child is hearing impaired, a raised voice is helpful rather than alarming. It is a good idea for tester to forewarn parents.

Henrietta's level of comprehension of spoken language could be assessed through lip reading, and of expression through her utterances. Similarly, for the sign system through her comprehension and expressive use of signs. N.B. If the assessor is non-conversant in the sign system, the parent or visiting therapist can be carefully instructed to translate exactly what the assessor says into signs and what the child signs into words. Careful observation will provide the assessor with ample evidence of the signer's providing additional clues to tests of verbal comprehension and of elaboration of child's expressive language, e.g. 'He said "the dolly is washing herself" ' when the child signed a single word!

Andrew

Andrew is 3 years 6 months old. The staff at Andrew's nursery have expressed concern about his speech and relationship with other children. Preliminary observations and history suggest that he may be autistic. He throws a tantrum when the assessor tries to separate him from his toy car and the more she tries to engage with him or get his interest in other toys the more distressed he becomes. What is she to do? An 'ignoring' technique sometimes works. The assessor makes a model of a bridge on a small table on the other side of the room, knocks it down, leaves the three bricks on the table and returns to her chair. She and the parent continue their conversation ignoring Andrew. After a few minutes he may go across the room and make a bridge when he thinks no one is looking! Another variation of the ignoring technique can be used to test hearing; minimally voice 'it, it, it,' or words from the doll or picture hearing test while pretending to be focused on your notes. Andrew may imitate them a few moments later while he continues to play with his car. Similarly, if the assessor suspects that one of a multiply impaired baby's difficulties is autism it may be best, when doing for example, a grating acuity test, if she doesn't try to attract the baby's attention forwards or try to reposition herself where the baby's gaze happens to be, but to wait patiently until he spontaneously directs it forward and instantly present the test card.

The above-mentioned cases also illustrate how demands upon the assessor to multi-task escalate even when assessing children with moderate problems. In particular, the importance of the assessor having, test content, procedure and typical responses 'on automatic' in order to allocate sufficient attention to assimilation, analysis and adaptation while keeping rapport and flow smooth and constant. They also highlight how every aspect of the consultation is likely to take longer, as soon as developmental disorder or impairment is suspected (e.g. developmental examination, history taking, paediatric exam, discussion, counselling, guidance and reporting/letter time). In practice, the time requirement to complete a comprehensive preliminary examination increases with the complexity and severity of the disorders/impairments. Clinic managers need to base time allocation on the findings of the clinical audit.

Severe single and multiple impairments

Age levels in terms of typically developing children become less and less relevant in the assessment of children as the developmental disorders, single or multiple impairments become more severe. Identification of functional levels and constraints within each domain, become the neurodevelopmental priority as they provide the information required to design individualised developmental guidance. A severe single impairment may constrain development in domains other than its own, because a specific level in its own domain underpins the developmental sequence within the others. Constraints become more numerous, complex and cumulative when impairments are multiple. The first job of an assessor is to think through the possible constraints and try to ascertain which are operant. Observation and a few targeted questions, rather than chronological age, inform starting levels. If these involve cognitive aspects of a supporting domain the assessor may need to select tests suited to a cognitively younger child. If they involve the motor aspects in a supporting domain he may need to adapt response tasks to suit the child's motor capabilities. If they involve the sensory aspects in a supporting domain he may need to convey the instructions via a different sense or through the standard sense at greater intensity. The objective is to preserve the scientific integrity of the target domain. The next sections provide examples of adaptations for children with severe single and/or multiple impairments.

Adaptations for children with severe and profound visual impairment (SVI, PVI)

Tests of hearing

Distraction test
The distraction test is underpinned by two cognitive concepts (1) substantiality/permanence of sound sources and (2) location (position of the source relative to self). PVI constrains both. The standard response task is eye and head turning to the side of the sound source. PVI also constrains motor development. In sighted babies responses to sounds of unfamiliar quality are less definite and often at lower level than to familiar sounds; this is even more pronounced in babies with PVI. Babies with PVI also tend to still with passive facial expression rather than become more animated in response to sounds. A wise assessor therefore checks out several things before embarking on the test. He and the distracter should observe and familiarise themselves with the baby's responses to moderately loud familiar sounds when made to either side (e.g. own rattle, splash of juice in his bottle, the parent's voice etc). If the baby tends to still in response to sounds the sound maker may decide to wait until the child's face is actively expressive before making a test sound. On the other hand, if the baby becomes animated when he hears sounds, the sound maker may wait until the baby's expression is relatively still.

Q What might the distracter use to distract?
The baby is visually impaired so visual lures are not appropriate. Sounds lures may well confuse the baby especially if the test sound comes from a different location. Often it is best simply to put the baby in listening mode by asking for quietness.

Q How would you interpret the baby leaning and reaching forwards when sounds are made to the side at ear level?
The baby has concepts of the substantiality of sound sources and of the potential of his hands for reaching but not for the position of the source relative to self. His response indicates that he hears the sound and can therefore be credited.

The assessor also notes the level of motor development. If inadequate for supported sitting on a lap he can place the baby as indicted for Monica (earlier). The stage is now set for test sounds at minimal levels to be introduced to each side; as for sighted babies, the decibel level should gradually be raised until a response is noted.

If *unfamiliarity* is suspected for lack of response (e.g. to the high frequency rattle), the assessor may attempt to familiarise and motivate the baby to a sound of similar quality (e.g. shake an open pot of hundreds and thousands in front of the baby and hand her a raisin). Repeat several times at increasingly low decibel levels, observing her response. Once she regularly alerts, substitute the *high-frequency rattle* shaking it minimally out of her visual range.[2] If she responds positively reward her and repeat on the other side; if she doesn't respond raise the dB level until she does and check dB level with a sound level meter. Three quarters of the assessor's time has been spent familiarising and motivating, but worth the effort if the baby bounces up and down excitedly when the high frequency rattle is shaken minimally! The integrity of the test sound has been preserved and the baby may have been spared (depending on responses to other frequencies) an anaesthetic and brainstem evoked response.

Language based tests
The visual contribution to the Picture and Doll tests is considerable. Verbal comprehension for the test items is requisite but significantly delayed by PVI, as experience of objects is limited to tactile exploration and pictures are totally meaningless. The standard response task is pointing. The characteristics and location of test items are assimilated 'at a glance' by sighted children, but truly laborious for those with PVI. Thus these tests are inherently unsuitable. Repetition of words is an alternative

The child repeats words after the assessor. A period of training with the assessor speaking at moderate conversational levels is required before the assessor gradually drops

---

2   If the baby has PVI the optimal position within the semicircle will be directly in front of her, because this is where most things are proffered. If she has sufficient form vision to see the tester or rattle the sounds need to be outside her field of vision at ear level.

the decibel level to minimal voicing. Phonetically the words used for testing should be discriminatory and taken from a recognised hearing test for young children. The child's diction needs to be clear so this adaptation is not appropriate for children with many phonological immaturities or articulation difficulties. The alternatives are to abandon language and use-:

Free Field Pure Tone Audiometry (FFPTA): This test requires a NSC level of 2 years 6 months or over in sighted children, i.e. to understand that they should listen for a tone and make a specific response each time they hear one. Children with PVI are later in achieving understanding of this concept. Standard response tasks such as placing a plastic cup on top of another cup, or putting rings on sticks are very taxing for a child with visual impairment because visual monitoring is not available to them and tactile monitoring is laborious and diverts their attention from task. A simple soft squeaker makes a good response task as no visual monitoring is required and the idea of squeaking a squeaker each time a sound is heard is easily imparted.

Tests of intelligence – non-symbolic cognition (e.g. concepts of permanence)

In the first 4 months babies quietly absorb visuo-perceptual information about the animate and inanimate world that surrounds them. Babies with PVI are denied the opportunity to construct these perceptual templates upon which to base non-symbolic concept formation. As PVI also *directly* constrains visual and manipulative development, opportunities for conceptual learning through visually directed manipulation of everyday objects and toys is further delayed. In addition vision is the modality normally responsible for arousing and sustaining a baby's interest to explore and experiment with a toy/object. Altogether a PVI baby faces a cumulative circle of constraints that impact on NSC development and on standard methods of testing. For example, both the method of introduction and that used to judge the presence or absence of concepts of permanence in tests for sighted babies utilise the visual system – in the ball dropping out of sight test the procedure involves the baby watching a woolly pom-pom ball roll back and forth across the table then off the end and out of view. A baby with permanence of objects bends and visually searches for the ball on the floor; one lacking the concept looks back at the table or assessor. This test is totally unsuited to adaptation for a baby with visual impairment. The case of Vincent, aged 10 months, described here, illustrates how permanence might be tested in babies with visual impairment. Some guidance is included to show how every finding/observation in an assessment can be assimilated into generating ideas that will consolidate and take forward a child's current level.

Vincent: Profound visual impairment
As mentioned in Chapter 6 permanence of people (P of P) develops before permanence of objects (P of O). Babies become animated and visually search for Mummy when she says 'mummy's home' from out of sight. When Vincent is quietly lying on the assessment mat the assessor asks his parent not to speak for a few minutes and then to say

'Mummy's here'. Vincent stills and listens.

> Q How would you interpret this response in the context of P of P?
> *Stilling and listening only indicates that Vincent has heard. Without animation one can't be confident that he recognises her voice, so not P of P.*

> Q How might you advise the parent to help promote P of P.
> *Suggest that as soon as he alerts, she lightly touches his side or cheek and repeats 'mummy's here' and bends forward to kiss him.*

After two weeks of building this into his daily routine he smiles and wriggles excitedly, when she first says 'mummy's here'.

> Q In terms of P of P how do you interpret the post guidance response?
> *His animation and anticipatory movements confirm that he knows she is there, i.e. P of P.*

> Q Which other base line concept would you now credit Vincent with?
> *The substantiality of sound sources.*

> Q How might you check that he also has this for sound making objects?
> *Give him a rattle and let him shake it. Take it away and shake it in front of him.*

If Vincent just stills and listens, he hasn't demonstrated permanence for sound making objects.

> Q How might you advise the parent to help promote permanence for sound making objects?
> *Suggest that when removing a rattle she shakes it in front of him and immediately guides his hand to it.*

> Q What else does this guidance activity promote?
> *Location of sound.*

However, if Vincent reaches in any direction he could be credited with permanence for sound emitting objects.

Now the assessor needs to explore whether Vincent has permanence of silent objects. She gives him a woolly ball to play with, then takes it back and places it on the table/tray surface in front of him, or if Vincent is sitting or lying on the floor, beside him.

Q What response would earn Vincent credit?
Exploratory searching of either the table, floor or near space with his hands.

Q What is the assessor's first consideration when setting out to test verbal comprehension in a 3-year-old child with visual impairment?
Is standard material suitable, i.e. (a) miniature toys and (b) Bus Puzzle.

Q Are miniature toys and/or The Bus Puzzle suitable?
No; representation in miniature is very delayed in SVI children and they could not see the pictures on the inserts.

Q What could the assessor use instead?
Four to six real objects, some of which sensibly relate to each other.

Q What adaptations to introduction might the assessor make?
As the child cannot see, the assessor will need initially to guide her hand to each object in turn, let her feel it, ask her to name it (expressive language) and if she doesn't name it for her. Subsequently ask her to find each object on request (verbal comprehension for single words), then to carry out two-component (put the spoon in the cup), then three-component commands (give me the car and the brush), etc.

Q Has she made the task easier?
No, if anything it is still more difficult than for a sighted child, because a child with visual impairment has to remember the position of each object and tactilely verify it, while holding on to the instruction in her mind – a very laborious task.

Consider adaptations for testing other domains.

Adaptations for children with severe neuromotor disorders with or without additional impairments

The characteristics and distribution of the motor disorder are very variable in children with severe degrees of cerebral palsy and most have additional impairments of varying severity. Adaptations for one child are not necessarily suited to another and the following examples are for illustration, not for blanket application. When contemplating the intellectual and sensory examination of a child with severe cerebral palsy time is saved, if a little is taken early on, to identify, through observation and discussion with parents, the motor systems and movements available to her and the ways in which she uses them and if speech is not an option to establish how she indicates 'yes'/'no'. Even though speech is often impaired, language, particularly verbal comprehension, is frequently easier to test than NSC. Time is also well spent ensuring that positioning and seating are optimal for the child to give attention and to enact her response; in all children who have sufficient use of their hands or can eye-point, the wheelchair tray should be set up before assessment starts. Assessment strategies for Molly and Matthew are discussed below.

Molly
Molly is a 3-year-old with Worster-Drought Syndrome. She has a generalised motor disorder but can walk and control hand movements sufficiently to achieve a 30 to 33 month level of verbal comprehension and a 27 to 30 month level of NSC. Molly's oro-motor difficulties are profound and her speech incomprehensible.

Matthew
Matthew is 4 years 3 months. Matthew understands three-component commands; his hand movements are too limited to point reliably but his eye movements are concomitant and he can direct and maintain gaze for a few moments. Speech is dysarthric.

Tests of vision

Molly is unable to letter match – a cognitive requisite for the SonkLT. Alternatives might be the Sonksen Picture Test (SPT) which is a more discerning alternative than the NDV at Molly's developmental age, but the standard response task is for the child to *name* the picture – see Chapter 3, p. 52. Impossible for Molly, so adaptations could be (1) to give her a second set of pictures for her to point to when the test card is present or (2) to utilise her Yes/No response (nodding/shaking head) by offering her four verbal alternatives with the item depicted on the test card randomly positioned amongst the others. 'Is it a ….?'

Q Which alternative maintains the integrity of the test target (visual acuity) best?
   Adaptation 2.

Q Why does Adaptation 2 maintain the integrity of the test task better than Adaptation 1?
   Adaptation 2 requires Molly to discern fine detail in the test picture; adaptation 1 only requires her to see and match gross visual clues such as distribution of blobs of colour.

The possible pitfalls with adaption 2 are that the range of possibilities is reduced from infinite to four and that either the assessor or others in the room could give clues through voice inflection, facial expression or body language.

Matthew's language level suggests that he may be able to match letters and be tested with the SonkLT. Letters on the key card are too close together for the assessor to interpret eye pointing, though she could space 3 × 3cm black wooden letters widely on the tray of Matthew's wheel chair. After training Matthew to use eye pointing to match letters in the training booklet to the ones on his tray, the assessor takes the test booklet to 3m and tests acuity.

> Q What practical tips might you give the assessor?
> *To be careful not to direct her own gaze to the correct letter on the child's tray and to check that the black wooden letters contrast well with the background, i.e. are placed on a white rather than a black background.*

The response task has been adapted leaving the test of acuity intact.

Suppose during training Matthew had only reliably matched four of the six letters; the assessor could remove the other two and subsequently 'skip' them when presenting the test booklet. This adaptation will impact on the accuracy of the measurement, but in a child with multiple disabilities it may be of more value to know that he can see 2 out of 4 logMAR 0.1 letters and 3 out of 4 logMAR 0.2 letters from a linear array, than that he can see a hundred and thousand! (i.e. the assessor is much better placed to give advice to therapy teams about vision for symbol systems based on this slightly corrupted log-MAR finding). Of course the adaptation and the reason for it should be detailed in the report. On the other hand, suppose during training the assessor suspects that matching failure is visual, two sets of cards each displaying single size 60 letters can be substituted for the training booklet and the key card; subsequently the assessor uses the log MAR 1.0 to 0.8 test booklet from 3m or nearer as appropriate.

> Q Is the acuity measure corrupted?
> *No.*

Although laborious, the SonkLT can be administered to older children with very severe neuromotor problems, affecting eye and arm movements and speech production using the 'Is it a …?' and the child's 'yes/no' response.

Tests of hearing

Both Molly and Matthew have adequate verbal comprehension and vision to use the Picture test or the Distraction test. The test pictures can be arranged normally for Molly as she points clearly; however Matthew's manipulative impairment will require the cards to be widely spaced so that he can eye-point. Matthew could probably manage free field audiometry, asking him to vocalise/grunt or to look up when he hears a tone, i.e. altering the response task to suit his motor skills without interfering with the audiometric content.

Tests of intelligence

Molly

Q How might the assessor modify tests for Molly?
Motor constructive
Larger bricks, steady the base brick(s).

Pencil and paper
Use a crayon instead of a pencil; steady the paper for her.

Size, colour and number concepts
Use well-spaced items. Possibly real rather than miniature items e.g. tablespoon and teaspoon; set of coloured bricks rather than little pegs.

Verbal comprehension
Be accommodating of a degree of clumsiness as long as she is carrying out the command; e.g. the chair falls over when she tries to sit dolly on it; if size rather than co-ordination is the problem use Wendy house sized or real objects.

Expressive language
Expressive gestures or signs if she uses Makaton.

Non-spoken symbolic cognition (NSpSC)
Be accommodating of a degree of clumsiness – after her intention is clear assist the final parts of the placement or if the item falls put it back where she intended. It is important not to let physically impaired children become too frustrated with themselves or to assist too quickly!

Q Do any of the modifications corrupt the target measures?
No.

Matthew

Q How might the assessor modify tests for Matthew?
Motor constructive
Motor constructive tests are not modifiable for Matthew.

Pencil and paper
Pencil and paper tests are not modifiable for Matthew.

Size, colour and number concepts
Space items widely and use eye-pointing or "Is it ..?" as the response task.

Verbal comprehension
Space items widely and give n-component commands without action words e.g. "Where is ..." or "look at the doll, the bath and the spoon". "Where are the red chair and the aeroplane"

Expressive Language
Use questions about visually suitable objects/pictures.

NSpSC|
NSpSC tests are not modifiable for Matthew.

Q Do the modifications corrupt the target measures?
No.

Children with severe physical disability associated with severe learning difficulties and some sensory impairments.

Molly and Matthew both had serious, though different, motor impairments. Although their learning potentials were limited, standard tests (thoughtfully modified) could be used to test the special senses and some areas of the intellectual profile. However, when severe physical impairments are combined with severe learning difficulties and/or sensory impairments the assessor steps back from standardised tests and applies his developmental knowledge base and powers of observation to actively explore the child's developmental status with his parents and to develop an individualised programme of developmental and medical management.[3]

When standard tests cannot be applied valuable information, especially about the special senses, can sometimes be gathered from a mixture of formal and informal observations. For hearing the following procedure proves helpful in Jonathan The assessor keeps her eyes and ears open throughout the face-to-face period for signs of auditory responsiveness. She notes and lists the nature and loudness of parentally reported, incidental and assessor contrived sounds, together with the child's response to them For example (1) *'pasta', moderate/conversational, alerted and turned with mouth open, 2) door shutting,*

---

3   Although diagnostic and medical management questions are often included in neurodevelopmental referrals they are too wide ranging to be covered in this book.

very loud, startled etc. Other examples can be *added* to the list by asking the mother or father about responsiveness to vocalisations (raspberries), situational phrases ('row, row, row the boat.'), or words (pasta', 'crisps') that make the child laugh, smile or react in a specific way and subsequently observe his response to them spoken quietly.[4] When reporting on hearing the assessor can state 'Standard testing was unsuccessful. However, informally Jonathan was noted to respond to quiet environmental noises and to hear and respond appropriately to the following words/phrases when quietly spoken'. This information is helpful to the assessor in formulating a profile of Jonathan's difficulties, in evaluating whether or not there are serious hearing constraints impacting on intellectual functioning and in prioritising referrals and formulating guidance. However the above examples of 'stretching the rules' are *not a licence* to credit children in the absence of definitive evidence or sufficient experience.

It is hardly surprising that children sometimes tire and give up mid test; this is particularly common with tests of the special senses, especially when that sense is itself impaired or the child has multiple problems. Suppose half way through a letter or a grating test of visual acuity Millicent appears to give up; the problem could be visual or behavioural. One way of checking is to return to larger grating or letter and if, Millicent is immediately co-operative and subsequently loses interest again at the same point, the failure is likely to be visual. If she doesn't respond to the larger stimulus it is more likely behavioural. If the assessor is left uncertain of the reason for failure it may still be of practical value to explain in the report that 'Millicent's logMAR near acuity is at least 0.275 and that this may not be the limit', i.e. it could be better. Millicent's teachers may then be able to stop worrying whether or not the materials they are currently using are too small.

Before starting a developmental examination a wise assessor takes time to explore the following questions and observations during the preliminary discussion with parents:

1. To what extent and how the child spontaneously explores, reacts and interacts with events and people at home and in a new environment; the motor systems and movements and the visual, auditory, social and motor behaviours available to him. To observe his current positioning – in wheelchair or on the parent's lap – and to note degree of trunk and neck control and amount of support currently given. To discuss with the parents alternative positions in which he has to give less effort to control of head and trunk, and hence can give more to the developmental task. Indeed arm and hand movements may be freer when a child is optimally supported.

2. To observe the pattern of unprovoked involuntary movements. Subsequently to explore triggers that provoke startling and 'spasms – the child attempting to move, presentation of tactile, visual or auditory stimuli and whether the pattern of provoked

---

4   Voicing level is likely to be consistent when delivered by the assessor but if there are problems with familiarity use mothers or father's voice. Peak levels of voicing and environmental sounds can be checked using a sound level meter.

and unprovoked movements are the same. The pattern of unprovoked movements is important when *timing* the presentation of test stimuli during tests of hearing and vision; responses to stimuli presented just before the next 'spasm' is due, are more open to misinterpretation than those presented shortly after one.

3. To observe for evidence of seizure activity, especially myoclonic episodes, focal jerks or periods of reduced awareness or confusion. Tests need to be paused during such episodes. If awareness does not fully return or persists for a long period, testing should be abandoned and seizure control reviewed, because developmental findings will not be truly representative of the child's abilities or useful as a basis for designing guidance.

4. To observe for evidence of significant impairment of either hearing or vision, i.e. in addition to severe learning and severe neuromotor difficulties. The assessor's suspicion should be raised by any discrepancy between the amount of attention paid to visual and to hearing stimuli and/or in the developmental levels of hearing and of visual behaviours.

With these preliminary observations the assessor starts his interaction with the child at appropriate levels, in the most suitable position and with his own eyes open to pitfalls such as seizure activity and involuntary spasms. Maurice illustrates some of these points.

Maurice

First visit to a Developmental Vision Clinic – age 3 years 3 months.

Maurice suffered hypoxic ischemic encephalopathy at birth and had neonatal seizures. Initially he was hypotonic; gradually signs of spastic quadriplegia emerged worse on the right than the left. Nocturnal episodes of grand mal seizures ceased by 24 months and anticonvulsants were tailed off. Six weeks earlier the local paediatrician became concerned about Maurice's vision and the advent of dystonic movements and referred him to a Developmental Vision Clinic.

Preliminary observations

Mother carries Maurice into the clinic and sits him on her lap with his head supported on her right arm. Granny follows with all their belongings on the back of a pushchair – Maurice has no special seating. Maurice's large blue eyes are open and spontaneously move concomitantly in all directions. Nothing in the surroundings appears to arouse his visual interest. When a person, he appears to be gazing at, moves his gaze does not follow them. In this position he has frequent spasms – his eyes widen, his body extends, his head and eyes turn to the right and his right arm partially extends; these occur if mother shifts his position but are mostly unprovoked. He startles when a door bangs down the corridor. When asked about development mother replies that in the last year

Maurice has become less interactive with them and less interested in his surroundings; he used to smile responsively, two-way vocalise, laugh when his father blew 'raspberries', and hold a rattle for a few moments in his left hand. His right hand has always been fisted. When asked if she thinks Maurice can hear she immediately answers 'yes', but to a similar question about vision she hesitates then says "a year ago I would have said 'yes', he definitely looked at me but now I'm no longer sure". She is enthusiastic to demonstrate that he smiles and squeals when she bounces him about in her arms or up and down on her lap; he does not gaze at her during these games. On one occasion his eyes jerk a few times rhythmically to one side, then lock in extreme gaze, accompanied by a change in the rhythm of his breathing. On another, the index finger of his right hand twitches and the twitching spreads to his arm before settling. Mother said these episodes had been happening more in recent weeks and she thought it was part of his muscle problems. Mother feels he is most relaxed in cradled sitting on her lap.

These provisional observations tell us that currently Maurice

- Has severe spastic quadraplegia affecting the right more than left.

- He is experiencing two types of focal seizure intermittently.

- He has frequent involuntary spasms

- He hears loud sounds and moderately loud conversational voicing

- His visual behaviour is more concerning than his hearing behaviour

- He has very limited movement available to him

- He appears to be functioning at < a 3½ month level.

- The history suggests loss of skills from a 5- to 6-month level.

Medically we are alerted to the possibility of an undercurrent of seizure activity that could account for loss of skills. Developmentally, we are alerted to pause the assessment whenever seizure activity is clinically apparent and to time presentation of stimuli when testing hearing, vision and intellectual status optimally between spasms.

Developmental aspects of assessment

Details of motor development, neurological and general paediatric examination are not given.

We start our interaction with Maurice, cradled half lying on his mother's lap. First we check that the spasms are not visually or auditorily provoked by using novel stimuli of moderate intensity (e.g. the NDV tinsel ball spun on the spot about 20cm in front of his eyes and a music box opened after a period of relative quiet.) By varying the timing of presentation we find that his spasms are neither auditorily nor visually induced. He stills when the assessor quietly coos, 'you are a lovely boy', blows raspberries as quietly as possible and when the music box plays (peaks at 65dB) though there is no other behavioural reaction. There is no eye or head turning directly linked to more formal distraction test sounds made to his right side – (note that his left ear is cradled against his mother's chest). He does not fixate or follow any of the large light reflecting NDV targets nor does his expression change.

We lay him supine on a gym mat and note a decrease in his spasms. We repeat the hearing and vision tests with better access to the left side. The findings are similar except that he now alerts and briefly follows the 'Oogly' on a pen torch in a darkened room. When the assessor strokes the palmar surface of the fingers of his left hand with hers or with his own toy he doesn't grip or withdraw; his right hand is less tightly fisted than when sitting on mother's lap. When a tissue is gently placed over his face in a peep-boo game he stills and briefly holds his breath. When his own toy is jiggled on his chest he alerts but doesn't move his left hand towards it. Several times during the developmental and paediatric aspects of the examination seizures similar to those described earlier are noted and twitching can be felt after it is no longer visible.

Today Maurice is functioning as profoundly visually, intellectually and motor impaired although this may not reflect his true status or his potential. The priority is to liaise with the local paediatricians and to offer to review Maurice as soon as his epilepsy is under control. This is explained to his mother.

Second visit to The Developmental Vision Clinic – age 3 years 5 months.

Preliminary observations

Mother reports that Maurice responded quickly to reintroduction of anticonvulsant therapy becoming more alert and more visually responsive and interactive. She feels that he is now doing all the things he had done (and maybe more) before his epilepsy returned. Note that the skills she reported at their first visit had been at a 4- to 6½-month level of sighted development. She picks Maurice out of his pushchair and sits him upright on her lap. He lifts his head and looks up at her and smiles briefly before his head drops forward; she tips him back a little so that his head is supported on her arm and he continues to gaze at her for a few moments. The assessor speaks to him from about one metre; he listens but doesn't smile back until she leans forward smiling to about a third of a metre. No epileptic episodes are observed and spasms are both less forceful and less frequent. In response to the question, 'Do you think he understands anything you say', she replies, 'I think he knows his name because he alerts when I call "Morri"'. 'How about his vision?' Mother replies 'He looks at the television and gets excited during The X Factor, but I don't know how much he sees or how much of his response is to the cheering and music; he looks at me when I'm close to him – I'm not sure about further away'. 'Overall is that worse, the same or better than before he first stopped anticonvulsants?' 'I'd say the same.'

Q What could you suggest she does to clarify whether his excitement during The X Factor was to the visual or auditory aspects?
Turn the volume down.

Developmental aspects of assessment

In order to illustrate how to use developmental findings in the construction of a programme to promote ongoing development in each area, the report format described in Chapter 12 is not used; the level achieved by Maurice is often followed by one not achieved in order to highlight the target of intervention/guidance.

The assessment starts with exploration of positions in the context of their suitability for administration of tests e.g. supported sitting on a lap, supine and side lying. Head and trunk control in supported sitting is currently inadequate; head and trunk are supported in supine and side lying so for testing these positions will mainly be used. Currently Maurice has no special seating. Seating has been assessed locally since his first appointment and is expected to be available in the near future.

Vision

- NDV-VI: visually alerted to 12.5cm black and yellow woolly ball spun on spot at 30cm – not to 6.25cm yellow plastic ball

- Follows woolly ball slowly to each side but not up down – convergence minimal but both eyes to similar degree.

- Loses interest in woolly ball at between a third and half a metre

- Watches adult to a distance of ¾m

- Alerts to approach of a 'silent' adult at about 1m

- Seems to recognise his mother visually, two of his favourite toys [teddy and music box] from about a ¼m, i.e. shows greater excitement to them than to other faces or unfamiliar toys.

- Grating acuity (Keeler Acuity Cards) – does not preferentially look at largest grating at 39cm – Card 18, xx c/d 39cm.

Practice Point Examination to establish field defects, differences in acuity of the two eyes, eye movement disorders, etc. are essential parts of the visual examination and highly relevant to prescription of developmental guidance and referral onwards; they are omitted here in the cause of clarity.

Manipulation

Maurice accepts guidance of his left arm by the assessor in supported sitting, in supine and in side lying. A more limited range is found on the right.

- Left arm less tense and left hand more open than the right; lifts arm slightly when sees a familiar proffered toy – no directed reach.

- Left hand: grasps when pads of fingertips are stroked with a finger or a rattle – not when dorsum of fingers stroked – grasp not yet adaptive.

- Right hand: fisted – no active grasp. Arm moves mainly at shoulder and elbow when excited.

- No attempt to transfer.

- No attempt to reach towards a near toy or face he is looking at.

- Release – passive relaxation of grasp – no active release.

Cognition

- Visual interest in faces and large toys within 30cm, bell rattle – red with shiny jingle bells, 12.5cm woolly and tinsel balls, music box – pink and white, 15 × 10 × 10cm, yellow squeaker 12.5 × 10cm.

- Cause and effect: Looks surprised when hits self with rattle – does not actively shake. Feels soft squeaker briefly –does not squeak it.

- Smiles and squirms when toy jiggled on chest –does not reach for toy.

- Stills and smiles to familiar sounds –no orientation of eyes or head towards the sound source, e.g. his own music box.

- Object permanence. Maurice sometimes makes a distressed noise when a toy is removed from grasp –does not attempt to search for it visually or manually.

- Peep boo – shakes head in attempt to remove tissue from face –does not attempt to use hands to pull it off.

Prelanguage

- Takes part in two-way proto-conversation – unformed vowel sounds and raspberries. N.B. His speech apparatus affected by neuromotor disorder – drooling and dysarthria.

- Gets excited and vocalises when mother sings a rhyme game –e.g. round and round the garden – doesn't show anticipation of the 'tickle you under there'.

- Alerts preferentially to the assessor calling his name in a conversational voice. The assessor asks 'Does he understand any every day phrases like "up you come" or "clap hands"?' The moment the assessor says 'clap hands' Maurice makes uncoordinated clapping movements with a big grin. Mother is thrilled because she has been playing 'clap hands' with him and this is the first time he has spontaneously clapped to the words alone!

Social communication

- Maurice becomes most animated when people engage him in two way interaction – smiling and vocalisations – not seen to initiate interaction.

Hearing

- Maurice stills and listens to minimally voiced 'it, it, it' and 'is is, is', 'ooooh' and 'Morri'. He claps his hands and smiles to minimally voiced, 'clap hands'. He smiles and his face 'lights up' to a 'raspberry' blown as quietly as possible. His body tenses and he looks excited when he hears our music box (peaks at 65 dB).

Gross motor

- Mobility in supine

  - Pushes self 'up the mat' with heels – not goal directed.

  - No attempt to sit up or to roll over.

- No forward parachute reaction; no downward parachute reaction – scissors.

- No righting responses of head on neck or of trunk.

Adaptations

Position: Although most tests are routinely carried out with the child in sitting, most can be carried out in supine if the examiner moves his own position.

Order: The priority for Maurice was to establish whether or not he is visually impaired, because this will affect the visual characteristics of the materials used to test other areas; vision was therefore explored first.

Functional aspects: Functional aspects have been added to the assessments of the special senses that are not necessary in the assessment of typical children. These explore additional parameters of vision and hearing to illustrate how a child with a sensory impairment sees and hears in different every day and educational circumstances. For example for Maurice (1) the distance at which he is visually aware of a person's approach and the distance at which he can identify them, (2) the size, luminance, colours and distance at which he can see objects/toys sufficiently clearly to learn about if novel, or recognise if familiar (his teddy and music box) and (3) the level of voicing required for him to hear words within his vocabulary like 'clap hands'.

Test materials: Ensuring that objects/toys and voicing levels used for testing intellectual domains comply with the findings of the functional visual and hearing assessments.

Developmental profile

Maurice's developmental profile shows severe delay in all areas. However his prelanguage and social communication are clearly ahead of non-verbal cognition, and both hearing behaviour and the attention he gives to auditory events in the room are strikingly greater than their visual counterparts. He is using audition to make sense and to interact with the world. The NDV-VI and the grating acuity tests suggest that he has very severe visual impairment in addition to severe learning and severe neuromotor problems. Obviously Maurice's neuromotor disorder impacts considerably on his speech, gross motor and manipulative development; also on his intellectual progress by restricting his access and ability to use learning opportunities. Similarly, his primary cognitive impairment constrains development in its own and other areas.

For a fully informed programme of developmental guidance, therapy and treatment the assessor will need to embrace the developmental and neurological aspects of Maurice's condition and liaise closely with multidisciplinary specialists in Maurice's local team. Such depth is beyond the scope of this book but hints at the high levels of specialisation and time commitment of multidisciplinary professionals required to optimally care for children with multiple impairments. Guidance is therefore confined to aspects of Maurice's assessment described above and is followed by the findings on review at age 4 years 5 months (see Chapter 14 p. 352 -358).

Marcus

Marcus age 2 years 11 months is referred for a functional assessment of vision. He presents an even greater challenge in terms of technique and test adaptation than Maurice. Severe hypoxic ischaemic encephalopathy at birth resulted in severe dystonic motor disorder – Gross Motor Function Classification System level V. Local attempts at assessment have been frustrated by the frequency of dystonic movements and extensor jerks of his neck, which cause him great distress. His parents report the expression in his eyes is pained and they often glisten with tears during these spasms and that he is most content when 'left quietly' cradled on his father's lap or laying on the sofa. Experimenting with positions the assessor finds him most relaxed on a beanbag. Even then he startles, grimaces and cries out whenever the assessor touches, attempts to move him or introduces a toy (silent or sound making), however gently, into his near space. When left alone he lies still and free from spasms apparently quietly listening and watching background events. One's instinct is to remove a stimulus that causes someone to startle violently. While presenting grating acuity cards the assessor notices that if the card is left in place through the spasm, Marcus then looks from one to other grating and selects a test grating. By keeping the stimulus in place through the spasm the assessor achieves a reliable measure of grating acuity (2.9 c/d at 38cm), an assessment of eye movements for a 12.5cm spinning ball in near and middle distance and tracking of an adult walking to a distance of 3m. She extends her remit to demonstrating hearing for a quiet music box (peaking at 50dB) and quiet conversational voice to either side.

We have journeyed from very small changes to supporting domain aspects of tests to a complete change in approach, hopefully without ever losing track of the target domain of our test or observation. The integrity of the target domain must always be assured by the assessor and be apparent to the readers of her report.

Key Points

Schedule modification: From outset

- Assimilate findings and modify accordingly.

- Construct profile to highlight priorities of paediatric and neurological history, examination and to inform plan of action.

Good test design:

- Level of target domain should be higher than those of supporting domains.

Test adaptation:

- Protect integrity of target domain.

- Only adapt supporting domains.

Multiple or severe impairment

- Aim to construct personal developmental and impairment profiles that inform individual programmes of guidance rather than compare with typical development.

- Demands on the assessor to multitask increase with the severity and multiplicity of impairments in the child.

- Carefully chronicled responses to incidental happenings provide valuable information for developmental/educational management.

Message from Marcus' case study

- Informed observations, logical thinking and common sense are the keys to finding a way.

Chapter 14

Developmental guidance

The findings of developmental assessment often contribute significantly to diagnosis when viewed in the context of neurological, paediatric and social findings. However, the generation of intervention strategies that promote development is an equally important outcome.

Constructing developmental guidance tests builds a paediatrician's developmental knowledge base, as it requires comprehensive insight into typical development and into the constraints on progress imposed by different impairments. Thus, inexperienced assessors should not jump into the deep end of severe and/or multiple impairments, but practice generation of ideas for cases with minor developmental delays and disorders and discuss these with more experienced multidisciplinary colleagues. Similarly, before recommending a particular programme it is advisable to look into its developmental foundation and the strength of any evaluation studies. The remit of clinics at every level of service varies; guidance is usually reserved to those with a secondary or tertiary developmental remit and when suitable developmental provision is not already in place.

The discussion post-assessment is a stressful event for parents of a child with a significant problem and demanding for the assessor. Parents are naturally distressed to hear about their baby's impairments and the implications in terms of medical investigations and/or interventions, long term development and education. Generation of ideas with the team that will help the baby achieve his developmental potential restores their confidence in themselves as parents and arms them with positive things to do while they wait for appointments and local services to come online. Thus, developmental guidance is an additional arrow in a paediatrician's therapeutic bow and one with a more positive flavour than medical and surgical interventions.

In this chapter the approach to design of guidance strategies for children with developmental disorders, single and multiple impairments is founded on principles pioneered by Joan Reynell for children with specific developmental language delays and disorders (Cooper et al. 1978). The objective of developmental management is achievement of the child's developmental potential. Potential varies innately, with the nature and severity of the impairment, associated medical conditions, additional impairments and quality of the emotional and developmental climate. Thus, blanket prescription of developmental intervention according to a child's age is unlikely to be sufficiently finely tuned to be optimally effective. Ideas to remedy, circumvent or counter the factors constraining progress are based on each individual's assessment findings and generated both to consolidate current levels and to foster progress towards the next. The case vignettes below are of children with a variety of disorders and impairments and illustrate how assessment findings can be used to design individualised intervention strategies to promote multiple aspects of development.

Harley

Attention control is frequently delayed in children with mild to moderate hearing impairment or specific language delay. Harley aged 35 months comes for a developmental check. His mother is stressed by his negative behaviour and frequent tantrums but is otherwise happy with his development. The assessor finds that she has to work hard to switch Harley's interest from one task to another: he sweeps all the bricks off the table and screams when she tries to take them away. He says 'No' and turns away when she asks 'would you like to do some drawing'? Manipulation and NSC are age appropriate and when she gets his full attention he carries out three-component commands. He names the pictures in the Picture Test of hearing but then tries to 'escape' and reaches out demanding 'car' when she uses minimal voicing. As she raises her voice to moderately loud he begins to co-operate and hands her all five pictures. On questioning the parent says he has had constant colds and always has a stuffy nose and that she finds herself getting angry and shouting at him more recently. Otoscopic examination suggests chronic OME.

Q What developmental advice could the assessor give the mother while she waits for the audiology appointment?
Explain that Harley's attention control has got stuck in the toddler stage as a consequence of not being able to hear conversational voice levels. Suggest that she doesn't shout at him from across the room, but goes up to him, calls 'Harley' in a moderately loud but not angry voice and as he looks up smilingly say, 'Come, it's

dinner time' or 'get your boots we're going to the park' at the same moderately loud voicing level. To counter his negative behaviour she drops all invitations to say 'no' by removing all the 'would you like', 'shall we', etc. from her communications so that they are framed as directives in a pleasant voice (as the two above). Alternatively, she can give him a choice 'Where shall we go today – to the park or the wood?' as this format asks for a positive response.

Visual impairment will be used to illustrate that the first stage in programme development is clarification of the impact of the impairment and hence the constraints acting on other aspects of development (Sonksen 1983 , Sonksen et al. 1984); ideally a population of babies with severe uncomplicated impairments need to be studied longitudinally. Our team studied those with congenital disorders of the peripheral visual system e.g. microphthalmia, cataract, glaucoma, retinal dysplasia, retinal coloboma etc.

Vision is a 'magic carpet' to the formation of basic concepts that underpin development across several domains. Thus every ounce of vision is developmental gold dust, and it is vital, that the potential for vision of a baby with severe visual impairment (SVI), is achieved at all times, and that available/residual vision is utilised optimally in all learning situations. Thus for babies with visual impairment a programme to promote general aspects of development (PGD) needs to be complemented with one to promote visual development (PVD) and one to make optimal use of available vision (OUAV). The findings of standard tests of visual acuity (see Chapter 3) are not suitable building blocks upon which to design intervention for babies, so alternative more functional measures were needed. As more than half the babies attending our Developmental Vision Clinic were unable to see the largest grating of the preferential looking cards, there was an urgent need for a way of grading very low levels of vision. More levels were added to the near detection vision scale to create the NDV-VI, to monitor visual progress and to inform guidance (Sonksen 1983 , Sonksen and Dale 2002). For example, NDV-VI findings inform the visual characteristics (size, colour, luminance) of toys used for activities in the general programme and the baseline of PVD. The NDV-VI was the 'first born' of a group of functional measures of binocular vision[1] collectively known as a Functional Assessment of Vision (FVA). Scales were designed to inform a PVD; others to demonstrate 'vision for' the everyday scene from which young children learn. The everyday scene (people, objects, pictures, photographs) is composed of subtle shades and hues that merge into one another and require relatively higher acuity to resolve than the high-contrast black on white of standard vision tests. It is easy for parents, caregivers, teachers and other professionals to overestimate the amount of detail seen by a visually impaired child when he obligingly names or finds a picture on request, because he may be using gross visual clues such as colour to do so; for example, once familiar with a picture of a Teddy he only needs to see a brown blob on a blue background to name or find it.

---

1   Functional measures are (binocular) because we naturally function with both eyes open.

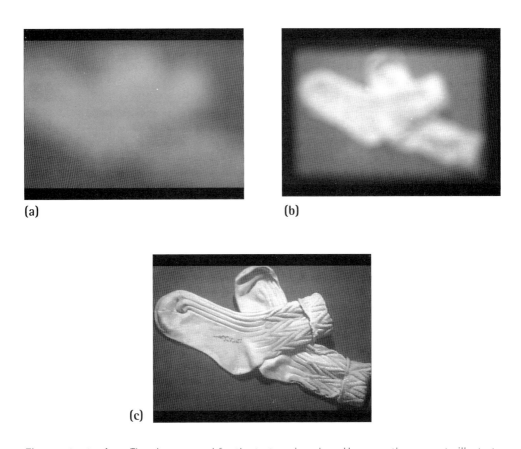

(a)   (b)

(c)

Figures 14.1a, b, c The pictures used for the test are in colour. However, they serve to illustrate three levels of vision for a picture of a pair of socks: Figure 14.1a is too nebulous to arouse cognitive interest in looking. Children seeing the socks as depicted in Figure 14.1b for the first time often say 'aeroplane', 'bird' or 'butterfly'; once told that it is a pair of socks they identify subsequent viewings correctly. Figure 14.1c - Picture as seen by a fully sighted person.

Therefore, pictures used for functional testing (e.g. those in the Sonksen Picture Guide to Visual Function [SPGVF]) should not already be familiar to the testee (Sonksen and Macrae 1987). SPGVF pictures are grouped into three grades of visual complexity and presented one at a time from a distance of 3 meters. The assessor progressively moves closer from 3 to 2 to 1 to ½ to < ½ meter(s) until the child identifies the picture. The identification distance indicates the distance at which the child can see sufficient detail to learn about new items of similar visual complexity. When the pictures are shown a second time the identification distance is likely to be greater and now reflects that at which the child can recognise familiar items from their gross visual parameters. Figures 14.1a–c show how a picture of a pair of socks is seen at three levels of vision.

Examples of the process – assessment → guidance – for each of the three programmes are given in the following section. The drawn illustrations in this chapter are from the Developmental Vision team's developmental guide for parents and professionals of visually impaired babies entitled 'Show me what my friends can see' (Sonksen and Stiff 1991).

Programme of general development (PGD)

Vina

Vina is 15 months old and has no vision (anophthalmia) so will serve well to illustrate the design of a PGD – for brevity only two domains are discussed.

Assessment findings

Motor: Vina sits well on her parent's lap and bangs the table surface in front of her. On the floor she sits securely with straight back feeling the toy in her hands, but never disturbs her centre of gravity or searches the floor space beside or in front of her for a dropped toy.

Postural control: Complete head control. Truncal righting is emerging side to side and forwards, though she becomes anxious if tilt is more than minimal. Backwards righting is absent.

Saving responses: Downward parachute is absent. Forward parachute is absent. Saving in sitting is absent.
There are no signs of neuromotor disorder.

Non-symbolic cognition: Vina sits on her mother's lap up to the table (except where specified).

Touch location: When supine Vina reaches for a toy jiggled on her chest and tummy but not on her knee or thigh.

Sound location: Vina reaches forward for familiar sounds made to her right or left at ear level.

Cause and effect: Vina shakes a rattle with enthusiasm and tentatively squeaks a soft squeaker (assisted demonstration). She does not manually explore a music box but stills and clearly listens in delight.

Permanence of objects: Sound making – present; silent – absent.

Relationships: Vina promptly pulls her vest off her face, but not socks while being undressed. Projecting rattle in a cup – Vina does not attempt to separate the rattle from the cup when one hand is placed on each item.

Programme of general development

The following activities will enhance Vina's motor development – equilibrium responses..

1. Sit Vina across your knee facing forwards; hold her well supported around the trunk and bounce her straight up and down to a 'bouncy' nursery song. Once she relaxes slide your hands down so they are around her hips and introduce small sideways tilts. If she shows any sign of alarm it means she feels insecure, so back track and rebuild her confidence and increase the size of the tilts very gradually – Figure 14.2a Do the same with her sitting sideways and tilting her forwards and backwards.

2. Vina is ready to learn that she can use her hands and feet to save herself when she feels unstable in sitting.

   Playfully bounce Vina up and down on the bed; make each rise about 30 cm. Once she spreads her feet to land, vary the height of the rise.

   Sometimes tip her forward with a 'wheee' while a second adult guides her hands to the surface (Fig 14.2b).

   Sit on the floor behind Vina and to a 'See-saw' song gently swing her arms to each side and diagonally so her hands alternately touch the floor.

Vina is ready to learn the following:

   To locate touch more extensively. Jiggle a favoured toy on her thigh and guide her hand to it. Once she actively reaches, add other sites (thigh/knees).

   To locate sound more accurately. When proffering something (beaker, rattle, biscuit tin, crisp packet, etc.) shake it in a position along an arc in front of her at her ear level. As she reaches forward nudge or guide her arm to the source (Fig 14.2c). Avoid moving the source into her hand as this may confuse her as to its original position. Once accurate at ear level, make sounds slightly above or below her ear level.

   Cause and effect. Try to find a musical toy with a simple switch e.g. a roller or soft push button that starts up a nursery tune: alternatively, a music box. Help Vina move the switch or open the lid until she realises the relationship between the sound and her action and starts to do it herself.

   Permanence of silent objects: Vina reaches out for noisy toys but needs help to understand that silent ones are still there. Play a 'give and take' game in several ways. Give Vina a toy, after a moment or two say 'thank you' or 'my turn' as you take it away and then quickly say 'here it is' as you guide her hand back to it. Sometimes hold the toy in front of her and sometimes place it on her highchair tray.

   Relationships: The aim is to extend Vina's understanding of the relationship of her clothes to herself. During undressing loosen Vina's sock and then guide her

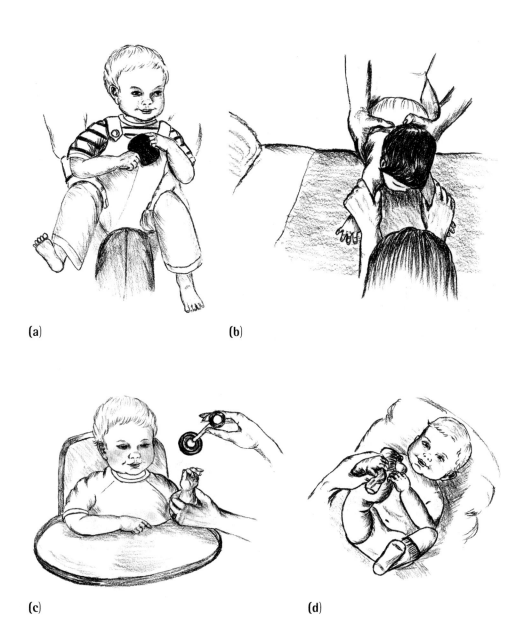

(a)

(b)

(c)

(d)

Figure 14.2(a) Encouraging the development of truncal postural reactions in a child with profound visual impairment. (b) Guidance to encourage the development of saving reactions in a child with profound visual impairment. (c) Guidance to develop sound location in a child with profound visual impairment. (d) Guidance to encourage concepts of two-component relationships in a child with profound visual impairment.

hand to the loosened tip and help her pull it off with an 'off it comes' (Fig 14.2d).

Put a favourite item in a small biscuit tin; rattle the tin as you place it on Vina's tray. Guide one hand to the item and one to the tin and help her remove the item and then replace it while saying 'out it comes' and 'in it goes'.

Programme to make optimal use of available/residual vision

The following is an extract from Violet's developmental assessment.

Violet

Violet is 10 months old. Violet stills and listens to sounds made to either side at ear level. She sits unstably with a rounded back. When lifted aloft and tipped to one side playfully no righting response is seen. When bounced her feet spread in anticipation after several bounces but when tipped forwards she clasps her arms to her chest. Similarly, she clutches herself rather than reaches for the floor when gently destabilised from sitting.

The assessor expands the Functional Visual Assessment to reveal the attributes of Violet's vision with reference to each target skill.

For sound localisation the assessor would check the following:

• Vision for silent rattle-sized objects

• Within arms' reach

• To each side and in an arc in front of her at ear level

The assessor found a difference in Violet's vision in the left and right fields. In the right temporal field, Violet was visually aware of a 12.5cm woolly ball at 30cm. In the left temporal field she was not aware of the woolly ball but was aware of the tinsel ball.

For postural and saving reactions the assessor would check Violet's awareness of the following:

• A large mirror with a dark frame at 1m

• A large brightly coloured patterned scarf at ½ a metre

Violet was visually aware of both.

Programme to make optimal use of available vision

For sound localisation: Carry out the sound localisation programme using any brightly coloured rattle of at least 12.5cm in length in the right side of the arc; use a bell rattle with three or four shiny bells or sew bells onto a glowing toy when presenting in the left side of the arc.

For saving reactions: Carry out the saving programme with a multicoloured duvet on the bed and a bright piece of carpet on the floor.

For righting responses: Carry out the righting programme with Violet facing a wall mirror or well-contrasted room upright (Brown door/cream wall) at a distance of about 1m.

Programme to promote visual development

Connectivity at neurological level proceeds particularly rapidly during the first 4 months in response to visual input. In the 1970s, it was assumed that the rate in visually impaired babies reflected the degree of visual impairment. Our teams' observations suggested that visual development 'took off' in babies with minimal vision when their hands were taken to a toy or their mother's face of which they were only dimly aware. Moreover, the phenomenon was not confined to babies in the first year but was seen up to at least 27 months. Thus, connectivity within the visual nervous system is not a passive response to visual input, but is dependent on that input being of sufficient quality to convey reality/substantiality to the target and to arouse cognitive interest in looking. Thus there is a difference between *looking* and *seeing*: the former requires cognizance and the latter does not; for example when lying on one's back, gazing at the stars, one will be *looking* if actively searching for the Great Bear and *seeing* if just relaxing.

Feedback from the hands confers reality to vague visual impressions, and hence interest in looking is aroused. Once achieved, currently suitably sized visual targets are used to encourage improvement of detection vision and acuity (first in near distance and then further away) and eye movement control (following and tracking), in near and subsequently at gradually increasing distance and speed (Sonksen et al. 1991). The assessor bases the initial distances and size of visual targets on the findings of the FVA – usually starting slightly closer and with the size of the object the child sees easily. Parents and advisory teachers of the visually impaired are given ways to take each section of the programme forward, between formal assessments, as the child's performance improves. The PVD was evaluated and found to be effective when introduced before or after the age of 6 months. However, the importance of earlier introduction is to ensure that a higher quality of vision is available earlier for all aspects of development and to maximise the opportunity for neuronal connectivity and achievement of full visual potential (Sonksen et al. 1991). Our later research revealed another powerful reason to introduce a PVD as early as possible; the achievement of form vision (SVI status) by 10 to 16 months reduces the risk of developmental setback (Dale and Sonksen 2002, Sonksen and Dale 2002).

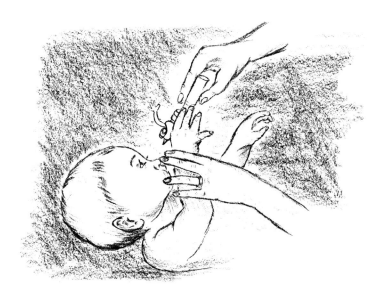

Figure 14.3 Guidance to impart 'substance' to vague visual impressions and thus develop cognitive interest in looking in a child with minimal perception of light.

Valerie, age 8 months

Parental observations: Screws up eyes in bright sunlight.

Findings of Functional Visual Assessment
Valerie visually alerts to an 'Oogly' on a pen torch in a darkened room, but does not attempt to reach for it. She does not follow it to either side nor vertically, and does not alert to 12.5 cm tinsel ball in a well-lit room. Her eyes widen when overhead lights are switched on in a darkened room.

Programme of visual development

Parents often find an explanation of the purpose of the PVD helpful.
The images perceived by her brain have probably been too hazy to arouse her visual interest in looking, and this may have slowed his visual development. The purpose of the visual programme is to

- consolidate Valerie's dawning *interest in looking*, i.e. realisation that that the hazy visual impressions that she currently sees are real, information carrying and reachable;

- improve her acuity;

- improve her eye movement control;

- expand her visual horizons, i.e. sphere of visual attention and interest'.

Take Valerie's hands to a glowing light source in a darkened room (Fig 14.3). This will help her realise that hazy visual impressions are real, reachable and of interest. Once she shows interest sometimes move the Oogly slowly from side to side or up and down, as this will encourage the development of following.

Verity, age 13 months

Findings of Functional Visual Assessment

Grating acuity: No response to the largest grating.

NDV-VI: Both eyes open; alerts to a face, to a 12.5 cm yellow and black spinning woolly ball and to a 6.25 cm yellow spinning ball at 30 cm. (She saw and reached for a stationary 12.5 cm woolly ball on the tabletop but was not visually aware of a stationary 6.25 cm ball.)

Following: She follows slowly moving ball horizontally but not vertically; no convergence.

Sphere of visual attention: To a distance of 40 cm for 12.5 cm woolly ball and to 1.25 m for a person.

Tracking: She watches a 20 cm multicoloured plastic ball roll across the floor at a distance of 0.75 m.

Programme of visual development

1. To encourage acuity place a toy (at least 12.5cm) on the tray of Veronica's highchair and encourage her to look for it verbally and by tapping the under surface of the tray. Gradually reduce the size of the toy in tune with her performance. Once she is locating crisp-sized objects, foods like tangerine segments, cheerios, etc. offer a safe in-built reward! (Fig 14.4).

2. To encourage development of eye movements: when Verity is looking at your face slowly move your head horizontally and vertically. As her following improves, gradually increase the speed of movement; sometimes move your face closer to encourage convergence and focusing. Substitute an attractive spinning toy (at least 12.5cm) for your face and gradually smaller ones.

3. Sometimes, call Verity and do a little jig about 1 m away. As she looks at you, zig-zag across the room and further away, singing as you go, until she stops watching; move closer and repeat. This activity helps her learn to track and increases her sphere of visual interest.

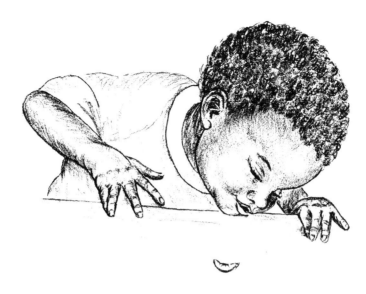

Figure 14.4 Guidance to develop cognitive interest and improve visual acuity for increasingly small items in a child with severe visual impairment.

4. When three adults (A, B and C) are available sit on the floor with Verity supported between A's legs. Initially place B and C about ¾m away, as the base of a triangle of which you and Verity are the apex. Help Verity to roll the ball *slowly* to C who pats it on to B and back to Verity. As before, gradually increase the speed of the roll and distance of B and C from Verity and finally reduce the size of the ball. This game will help Verity learn to track moving objects 'across' her visual field and 'to and fro', to alert to movement in her peripheral fields and improve distance acuity.

Guidance for children with multiple impairments

The basic principles of a developmental approach still apply. However, as with assessment, it is essential to ensure that the child can give maximal attention to the guidance activity and that other demands on his attention are kept to a minimum, i.e. that he is well supported when the aim of guidance is not motor control. Consultation with a therapist regarding optimal positioning, seating, head support, etc is advised and should be among the guidance and educational recommendations.

Maurice

Maurice was introduced in the last chapter. He is 3 years 5 months and has cerebral palsy with severe physical, intellectual and visual impairments. Maurice has a local physiotherapist, occupational therapist and Portage teacher who have to date been treating him as ' sighted', so the following advice is confined to counteracting the impact of SVI on some aspects of intellectual, motor, hearing and visual development and how to use his residual vision optimally in his general programme. Maurice's mother already knows and has accepted that he has severe learning and physical difficulties and epilepsy, requiring ongoing medication. She will be upset to hear that he also has severe visual impairment, but may feel more positive once she realises that visual impairment may account for some of his intellectual and physical delays and may be open to developmental remediation together with his visual development.

Developmental guidance

The reader should refer to the assessment findings (Chapter 13, p. 336—339) while reading the guidance and Practice Points.

Positioning: Until Maurice's special seating arrives, most activities can be enjoyed with him supine. Once seating arrives the activities can be further consolidated and extended in sitting. A tray fitted to his wheelchair will provide him with better access to toys for visual and manual inspection and help to prevent them dropping 'out' his visual space.

Programme for Visual Development

Maurice's PVD is not included but would be based on the findings of his visual assessment in the same way as for Verity and Valerie above.

Optimising Use of Available Vision

Toys and objects: Toys need to be at least 12.5 cm in one parameter, brightly coloured or shiny with good contrast between component parts, and presented within 30 cm of his eyes – his current visual space.

People: He will be aware of people moving within 1 m but not see them clearly enough to recognise from gross visual clues until within a third of a metre.

Programme for General Aspects of Development

Manipulation: Maurice's visual impairment makes it difficult for him to learn about the potential of 'his arms for reaching' and grasping.

Adaptive grasp: It will help Maurice to learn to adapt the shape and position of his hand for grasping if you stroke the dorsum of the fingers of his left hand and over the tips with your finger or a toy. As his vision improves, this learning will be visually reinforced if you hold the toy close to his hand.

Guiding: Maurice was happy to allow his left arm to be guided. The best way to do this is to lightly grasp his forearm[2] and guide his hand so that his fingertips are first to touch the object. This gives him the opportunity to choose whether or not to grasp, thus reducing the risk of tactile defensiveness that can occur if objects are pushed into the palm. Therapy for the right arm needs discussion with his physiotherapist.

Reach: When Maurice is supine, lean over him and attract his attention to your face, to a toy in your hand or to a dangling toy on a baby gym within 30 cm. Once he is looking, guide his left arm to it.

Sensory feedback from the motor system and vision although limited gives him the feel of a normal pattern of movement and consequently helps build templates for arm movements at neurological level.

Non-symbolic cognition

Interest in smaller objects – as per PVD

Cause and effect: Encourage Maurice to watch you shake a bunch of keys (distance about 20cm) so he learns that it makes a noise when shaken. Then help him shake it, making sure that the action is within his visual space. Similarly, demonstrate squeaking a soft squeaker and then help him to do so.

Touch and sound location: Maurice is clearly aware and interested in both touch and sound and now needs to learn to locate where he is touched and where sounds are coming from.

- *Touch* – Sighted babies learn to locate touch first on their chest. Jiggle a toy on his chest and guide his left hand to it. Sometimes shift the position of the toy on his chest and tummy.

- *Sound* – Take his hand to your face as you lean over and talk to him gently moving your head from side to side. Shake a rattle or squeak a squeaker within his visual space (centrally and just to R and L of midline) and guide his hand to touch it. Sometimes talk close to one ear (out of sight) and take his hand to your cheek. Always guide his hand to the sound source; moving the sound source into his hand could confuse him about its original location.

Object permanence: Sighted babies learn that silent people and objects still exist when

---

2   The movement is more natural for you if you are behind rather than in front of him.

not in physical contact through their vision. Side lying will be the best position for this activity. Give Maurice a sound-making toy, take it gently away, tap the floor space in front of him saying, 'where's it gone?' and immediately guide his hand to it with a 'here it is'. Once he is familiar with the game, substitute a favoured silent toy. Subsequently, whenever he drops a toy immediately say 'where is it?' and guide his hand back to it.

Relationships: When you take off Maurice's vest, leave it on his face and with a 'where's Maurice?' guide his left hand to it and help him pull it off 'there he is'. Similarly, play peep-bo with him.

Language

Understanding: Maurice is ready to extend his understanding of situational phrases like 'clap hands'.

• Play 'wave bye bye' using his left hand.

• Introduce a pause in 'round and round the garden' for Maurice to tighten in anticipation of the 'tickle you under there'.

• With Maurice comfortably cradled sing 'row, row, row the boat' rocking him gently. After a few weeks put in a pause and see if he starts to rock himself; if he doesn't, sing and rock him again.

• Use consistent phrases for daily routines, e.g. 'open up', 'arms up', 'up you come', 'this foot', 'night-night', 'where's Maurice?' 'there he is'.

• Maurice only sees well enough to learn the names of large objects and people when they are very close and his capacity to feel is reduced. Help him hold a much-loved toy in his visual space and say 'here's Teddy' or 'here's music box'. Ask family members to say, 'here's Grannie' as she bends over him and to take his left hand to her face.

Expressive language: Maurice's motor difficulties make speech difficult for him. We will liaise with his speech therapist regarding expressive strategies and development of a yes/no response.

Hearing

The assessor is not concerned about hearing impairment; Maurice needs help with the cognitive aspects of learning to locate sounds (see non-symbolic cognition above).

Gross motor

Maurice's physiotherapist may be glad to receive information on the constraints imposed by poor vision on this area of development, e.g. that in sighted development vision helps integrate the feedback from balance apparatus, muscles and joints to effect right-ing responses. Similarly on the role of vision in the development of saving reactions. An assessment carried out a year later is summarised here so readers can reflect on Maurice's progress and, if they wish, devise a follow-on programme.

Assessment at 4 years 5 months

Maurice came smiling into the clinic in his wheelchair looking at each of us in turn (2 m). He responded to 'Hallo' with a smiling and dribbly but correctly intonated 'ahh-ohh'. He appeared to listen to mother's report and raised both arms and vocalised 'ang' loudly and laughed when she spoke of a firework display they had seen.

Main points from the developmental examination:

Vision

NDV-VI: Visually aware of 2.25 cm yellow cube at 30 cm (but not a yellow Smartie 1.25 cm)

Grating acuity: Card size 15. 0.36 c/d at 38 cm (Snellen equivalent 6/500; 20/1700)

Tracking: (1) Tracks the assessor walk across the room at 3 m. (2). Watches 16 cm colourful plastic ball roll at slow speed at 1.5 m across the room and to and fro.

Vision for people: Recognises mother from physiotherapist (both wearing blue jeans and white shirt) at 2 m.

Alerting to novel visual stimuli in distance: Face from behind screen at 1.25m (not at 2m).

Manipulation

Left – Reaches for toy on tray or held in front of him. Orientates hand for grasp. Grasp raking (no radial specialisation). Release passive relaxation.

Right – Hand more open than before; grasps when pads of fingers touch object. No reach. Arm partially mirrors movement of left arm when excited.

Non-symbolic cognition

Cause and effect: Shakes bell rattle. Bangs table enthusiastically with brick in imitation. Tries, but is physically unable to squeeze squeaker.

Tactile location: Locates toy and reaches for it on chest and tummy.

Sound location: Locates sound to right and left at ear level (but not above or below ear level)

Permanence of objects: (Doesn't look for woolly ball when rolled off tray). When side lying on the right Maurice searches the floor with his left hand for object lost from grasp.

Permanence of people: Actively looks around to see where face will appear next (see vision test).

Relationships: Reaches and pulls tissue and vest off his face.

Language

Verbal comprehension: Situational phrases: anticipates. 'tickle you under there' and 'screams' when pause at the end of 'Row, row, row the boat' after 'don't forget to scream'. Tries to lift head, shoulders and arms in response to 'up you come'.

Noun labels: Eye points and attempts to reach with left hand to 'car', 'beaker', 'ball' and 'teddy' from choice of three. Looks at Mummy and Grannie when asked 'Where's …?'

Expressive language: A few appropriately intonated vowel sounds convey meaning in context of given situation (see above).

Social communication

Responds to a greeting from a stranger sociably. Loves attention and vocalises to attract it when not included in adult discourse. Vocalises and eye-points to something he wants. Loves socially interactive games like peep-bo and rhyme games. Uses general body movement, facial expression and vocalisation to request a repeat. No clear 'yes/ no' responses but smiles broadly when something he likes is mentioned.

Hearing

Distraction test – Responded to high- and low-frequency speech sounds at minimal levels on both sides.

Gross motor: Not included.

Q Do you suspect that Maurice may have autism as well as learning disability?
No, his social communicative development is one of his strengths!

Maurice has made definite progress in all areas of intellectual development and aspects of visual development. Progress in motor development is less marked because of the severity of his neuromotor disorder; manipulative advances are greater than in gross motor and speech production areas. Think through some guidance from this assessment.

Marcus

Marcus was also introduced in Chapter 13, p. 340, with findings of a functional visual assessment (FVA). The FVA confirmed a moderate to severe degree of visual impairment, in addition to his known severe neuromotor and learning difficulties.

Developmental guidance

Frequent severe dystonic extensor spasms are triggered by movement and by tactile, visual and auditory stimuli introduced into Marcus's near space, which cause him pain and distress and render interaction and play an averse and unhappy experience. A calm, gentle, quiet and 'not too busy' environment will best promote Marcus's development.

Positioning: During assessment Marcus was most relaxed, observant and interactive when lying on a beanbag; he clearly felt more comfortable and secure than when lying on a gym mat and he experienced less frequent spasms. Lying on a bean bag is therefore recommended for learning as well as comfort.

Introduction of new stimuli: Any incursion into his near space triggers spasms. New stimuli beyond a metre are less likely to induce spasms unless strong or sudden. It may help to introduce things from just over a metre distance and *slowly* bring them closer while you talk to him about them (e.g. his Teddy). 'These are Teddy's eyes, nose….' etc. Whenever he does startle during introduction leave the toy in place through the spasm – if you withdraw the toy he may well have a repeat spasm when you try to introduce it again.

Daily routines like suctioning, changing nappies, moving him or therapy are likely to induce spasms. It may help to use a consistent verbal cue for each activity before entering his near space. Hopefully, as Marcus learns to associate the phrase with the activity the forewarning will serve to minimise his startle response and benefit his language development. If he startles the phrase should be repeated before the routine begins.

Marcus experiences spasms whenever he tries to move. However, he has a full range of voluntary eye movements that don't induce spasms. Currently he uses these to good advantage watching what is going on in, and learning from, the everyday scene. During testing he demonstrated that he could use eye pointing to communicate the position of the grating.[3] This ability could be further developed as a communication strategy (e.g. for him to communicate choices and a 'yes/no' response).

Visual development

Marcus has a full range of concomitant movements but no convergence. In order to lessen the risk of a startle, present the visual lure in the midline at eye level at about 1m and very slowly bring it closer to his nose. Your smiling face would be a good initial lure; talk quietly as you approach. In the distance position him in the room so he can watch what you are doing from about 1.5 m; this may mean placing his bean bag on a table or the sofa.

Marcus teaches us that the answer for some children, particularly those with a 'hypersen-

---

3   This appeared to be active selection, rather than preferential looking, because he looked carefully from one to other image before selecting the one with the grating.

sitive nervous system', is not masses of 'stimulation' but a little, carefully and logically thought through. The possibility for relief of spasms through medication also requires discussion with a paediatric neurologist.

A developmental approach to the generation of guidance has been illustrated. There are other sound approaches. The Portage System was an early programme established in Wisconsin in 1970 in which developmental stages are broken down into small steps. Parents of babies with learning difficulties and a trained Portage teacher work together at weekly home visits to monitor progress and discuss how to achieve the next small step (www.portage.org.uk). Over the years strategies to help children with autistic spectrum disorders, challenging behaviours and profound and multiple learning difficulties have been embraced. The system is widely used but the evidence base for its effectiveness is limited. From the late seventies numerous programmes, targeting different developmental disorders have been developed and implemented by individual clinicians and university research teams across the Western world. Among these is the Early Bird programme (National Autistic Society) for preschool children with autism (www.autism. org.uk/earlybird). In a recent review of collaborative intervention studies in Europe for the treatment of autism, the authors demonstrated a need for more rigour in controlled trials and recommend that measures of parent–child interaction style and adherence to treatment are included (McConachie and Fletcher-Watson, 2014). The last two decades have seen increased efforts to compare and evaluate programmes scientifically. For example attempts have been made to evaluate task-orientated and process-orientated programmes for developmental coordination disorder, and even though the evidence for effectiveness remains inconclusive the studies represent a move in the right direction (Gibbs et al. 2007). There have been government initiatives to formalise both procedure, content and parental access to early support. For example in England the government initiated an Early Years Programme to provide appropriate developmental experience for all children during the formative years (www.earlysupport.org.uk). Part of this initiative is the production of Developmental Journals to help parents, supported by their teachers and therapists, to provide optimal developmental experience. Currently, there are Journals for babies and preschool children with Down syndrome, with deafness, and with severe visual impairment. The Developmental Journal for Infants and Young Children with Visual Impairment is based on the work of the Developmental Vision Team, University College London (Salt et al. 2006). The knowledge base is growing and the impetus should be sustained.

Development of the human infant brain is wondrous to observe. There is so much more that thoughtful observation can tell us, particularly when combined with the insights that modern technology can reveal. How I wish I could start all over again!

Key Points

Guidance is an

- important outcome of assessment,

- additional arrow in the assessor's therapeutic bow,

- expands the assessor's developmental knowledge base.

Talking through and demonstrating guidance activities gives parents:

- a timely psychological boost;

- ways to forward their babies' development;

- back their joy, pride and confidence in parenthood.

Programmes based on individual findings aim to

- consolidate current levels and foster progress towards the next.

Profound visual impairment

- is a developmental emergency/networking disaster,

- requires urgent intervention to promote

  - visual development

  - general development

  - optimal use of available vision.

Children with physical impairment

- should be optimally supported when assessing or promoting intellectual and sensory domains.

Message from Marcus

- Knowledge needs to be applied with care.

References

Cooper J, Moodley M, Reynell J (1978) *Helping Language Development: A Developmental Programme for Children with Early Language Handicaps.* London: Edward Arnold Ltd.

Dale N, Sonksen PM (2002) Developmental outcome, including setback, in children with congenital disorders of the peripheral visual system. *Dev Med Child Neurol* 44: 613–622.

Gibbs J, Appleton J, Appelton R (2007) Dyspraxia or developmental coordination disorder? Unravelling the enigma. *Arch Dis Child* 92: 534–539. doi: 10.1136/adc.2005.088054

McConachie H, Fletcher-Watson S (2014) Building capacity for rigorous controlled trials in autism: The importance of measuring treatment adherence. *Child; Care Health Dev* 41: 169–177.

Salt AP, Dale N, Osborne J, Sonksen PM (2006) *Developmental journal for infants and young children with visual impairment*. London: Early Support Programmes, DfES Publications. www.earlysupport.org.uk.

Sonksen PM (1983a) Vision and early development. In: Wybar R, Taylor D, eds. *Paediatric Ophthalmology: Current Aspects*. New York: Marcel Dekker.

Sonksen PM (1983b) The assessment of 'Vision for Development' in severely visually handicapped babies. *Acta Opthalmologica* Supplement 157: 82–91.

Sonksen PM, Dale N (2002) Visual impairment in infancy: Impact on neurodevelopmental and neurobiological processes. *Dev Med Child Neurol* 44: 782–791.

Sonksen PM, Levitt SL, Kitzinger M (1984) Identification of constraints acting on motor development in young visually disabled children and principles of remediation *Child: Care, Health Dev* 10: 273–286.

Sonksen PM, Macrae AJ. 1987. Vision for coloured pictures at different acuities: The Sonksen picture guide to visual function *Dev Med Child Neurol* 29: 337–347.

Sonksen PM, Petrie A, Drew KJ (1991) Promotion of visual development in severely visually impaired babies: Evaluation of a developmentally based programme. *Dev Med Child Neurol* 33: 320–335.

Sonksen PM, Stiff B (1991) *Show Me What My Friends Can See: A Developmental Guide for Parents of Babies with Severely Impaired Sight and their Professional Advisors*. London: The Wolfson Centre, Institute of Child Health.

Index